Handbook of Sports Medicine and Science
Volleyball

Volleyball

IOC Medical Commission
Sub-Commission on Publications
in the Sport Sciences

Howard G. Knuttgen PhD (Co-ordinator)
Boston, Massachusetts, USA

Harm Kuipers MD, PhD
Maastricht, The Netherlands

Per A.F.H. Renström MD, PhD
Stockholm, Sweden

Handbook of Sports Medicine and Science
Volleyball

EDITED BY

Jonathan C. Reeser MD PhD

Department of Physical Medicine and Rehabilitation
Marshfield Clinic
1000 North Oak Avenue
Marshfield
Wisconsin 54449
USA

Roald Bahr MD PhD

Oslo Sports Trauma Research Centre
University of Sport and Physical Education
PO Box 4014 Ullevål Stadion
0806 Oslo
Norway

Blackwell
Science

© 2003 by Blackwell Science Ltd
a Blackwell Publishing company
Blackwell Science, Inc., 350 Main Street, Malden, Massachusetts 02148-5018, USA
Blackwell Science Ltd, Osney Mead, Oxford OX2 0EL, UK
Blackwell Science Asia Pty Ltd, 550 Swanston Street, Carlton, Victoria 3053, Australia
Blackwell Wissenschafts Verlag, Kurfürstendamm 57, 10707 Berlin, Germany

First published 2003

Library of Congress Cataloging-in-Publication Data

Volleyball / edited by Jonathan Reeser.
     p.   cm. — (Handbook of sports medicine and science)
  Includes index.
  ISBN 0-632-05913-3
  1. Volleyball players — Wounds and injuries.
  2. Volleyball — Training. I. Reeser, Jonathan. II. Series.
  RC1220. V65 2002
  617.1′027 — dc21

                      2002011083

ISBN 0-632-05913-3

A catalogue record for this title is available from the British Library

Set in 8.75/12 pt Stone Serif by SNP Best-set Typesetter Ltd., Hong Kong
Printed and bound in India by Replika Press Pvt. Ltd.

Commissioning Editor: Andrew Robinson
Production Editor: Alice Emmott
Production Controller: Chris Downs

For further information on Blackwell Publishing, visit our website:
www.blackwellpublishing.com

Contents

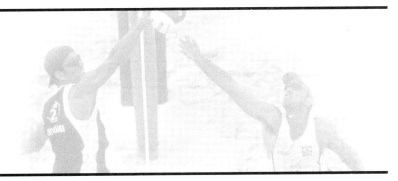

List of Contributors

Elizabeth Arendt MD
Medical Director, Varsity Athletics, Department of
Orthopaedic Surgery, University of Minnesota, 401 East
River Road, Minneapolis, Minnesota 55455, USA

Roald Bahr MD, PhD
Oslo Sports Trauma Research Group, Sports Medicine
Department, University of Sport and Physical Education,
P.O. Box 4014 Ullevål Stadion, 0806 Oslo, Norway

Tudor O. Bompa PhD
Tudor Bompa Training Systems, P.O. Box 95, Sharon,
Ontario L0G 1V0, Canda

Steef W. Bredeweg MD
Centre for Sports Medicine, University Hospital
Groningen, P.O. Box 30001, 9700 RB Groningen,
The Netherlands

William W. Briner, Jr. MD, FACSM
Lutheran General Hospital, 1775 Dempster Street,
Park Ridge, Illinois 60068, USA

Sven Bruhn, PhD
Institute for Sport Sciences, University of Freiburg,
Schwarzwaldstrasse 175, D-7800 Freiburg, Germany

Michael C. Carrera MSc
Tudor Bompa Training Systems, P.O. Box 95, Sharon,
Ontario L0G 1V0, Canada

Angelo De Carli MD
Sant'Andrea Hospital, Department of Orthopaedic
Surgery, University of Rome "La Sapienza", Via de
Grottarossa 1035/1039, 00189 Rome, Italy

Andrea Ferretti MD
Sant'Andrea Hospital, Department of Orthopaedic
Surgery, University of Rome "La Sapienza", Via de
Grottarossa 1035/1039, 00189 Rome, Italy

Michael Gasse PhD
Landesinstitut für Schule, Arbeitsbereich 2.4,
Lehren, Lernen, Begabungsforderung und
Unterrichtsentwicklung, Paradieser Weg 64,
59494 Soest, Germany

Albert Gollhofer PhD
Institute for Sport Sciences, University of Freiburg,
Schwarzwaldstrasse 175, D-7800 Freiburg, Germany

Karim Khan MD, PhD
School of Human Kinetics and Allan McGavin Sports
Medicine Centre, University of British Columbia, 6081
University Boulevard, Vancouver V6T 1Z1, Canada

Darlene A. Kluka PhD
Department of Human Performance and Leisure Studies,
Grambling State University of Louisiana, P.O. Box 1193,
Grambling, Louisiana 71245, USA

Heiner Langenkamp PhD
Fakultät fur Sportwissenschaft, Ruhr-Universität
Bochum, 44780 Bochum, Germany

D. Enette Larson-Meyer PhD, RD
Division of Health and Performance Enhancement,
Pennington Biomedical Research Center, Louisiana State
University, 6400 Perkins Road, Baton Rouge, Louisiana
70808, USA

Fernando A. Pena Gomez, MD
Orthopaedic Surgery, Clinica Santa Elena, Cl. La Granja,
8, 28003 Madrid, Spain

Jonathan C. Reeser MD, PhD
Department of Physical Medicine and Rehabilitation,
Marshfield Clinic, 1000 North Oak Avenue, Marshfield,
Wisconsin 54449, USA

Jaci L. VanHeest PhD
Department of Kinesiology, 2095 Hillside Road, U-1110,
University of Connecticut, Storrs, Connecticut 06268,
USA

David Wang MD, MS
University of Minnesota, Department of Family Practice,
Boynton Health Service, 410 Church Street SE,
Minneapolis, Minnesota 55455, USA

Forewords by the IOC

Volleyball has truly become one of the most popular events for the international sports world, especially as regards the number of competitors.

The sport of volleyball places great demands on the athlete in terms of both the biomechanics and the physiology involved in successful performance. As with any sport involving vigorous movements, there are a variety of injuries and other medical problems for which the professional personnel working with volleyball players and teams must work to prevent and to treat. The objective of this Handbook is to provide information on the scientific and medical aspects of volleyball that will be of great interest and aid to physicians, therapists, trainers, coaches and athletes.

The co-editors and the contributing authors have done an excellent job in presenting the information important to conditioning and preparation for competition, injury prevention, the treatment of injuries, and the special considerations for male and female athletes participating at all levels of competition.

We are deeply indebted to Dr Jonathan Reeser and Dr Roald Bahr for their leadership in organising this excellent publication and to all of the participating authors for the quality of their various contributions. This Handbook will constitute the basic source of information for the science and medicine of volleyball for many years to come.

Prince Alexandre de Merode
Chairman, IOC Medical Commission

Volleyball originated in 1895 and the sport spread rapidly throughout the world, both as a recreational activity as well as a sport involving high levels of competition at regional, national and international level. The Fédération Internationale de Volleyball (FIVB) was established in 1947 and currently includes the national federations of over 200 countries.

The volleyball competition has been an integral part of the Olympic programme since 1964 when the sport made its debut at the Games of the XVIII Olympiad in Tokyo. Interestingly, the competition was open for both men and women on that occasion and for all succeeding years.

It is, therefore, both fitting and appropriate that the sport be included in the IOC Medical Commission series, Handbooks of Sports Medicine and Science. The editors and authors have included the basic and applied science of the game, injuries and other medical aspects, performance enhancement, and special considerations for the young, women, the elite, and disabled volleyball athletes.

I wish to extend my congratulations to the co-editors, to the contributing authors, and to the IOC Medical Commission for producing this outstanding publication.

Dr Jacques Rogge
IOC President

Foreword by the FIVB

In today's world of professional sport, where athletes are driven to ever greater heights of athletic achievement, there can be nothing more important than preserving, as far as it is possible, the health of our players and to take the necessary preventative action to avoid injury.

Volleyball is currently enjoying a boom in popularity and is penetrating into increasing numbers of countries. It is played everywhere from refugee camps in East Timor, right through to the pinnacle of international competitions — the Olympic Games and World Championship tournaments and, for this reason alone, we have a great responsibility to carry out research and present the findings to the public.

This Handbook goes far beyond being a mere study of volleyball-related injuries and prevention; it is also a scientific study into the mechanics of the sport and its consequences, and a guide to the volleyball medical professional. It also deals with serious topics connected with the health of volleyball players at all levels, and in a variety of situations.

We therefore welcome this Handbook as a vital tool in dealing with our sport and we do so on behalf of the FIVB, its five Continental Confederations, its 217 affiliated National Federations and indeed, everyone who plays volleyball.

Dr Rubén Acosta
FIVB President

Preface

Preparing a work for publication, like volleyball itself, is a team endeavor. It is therefore appropriate that at the outset we acknowledge a select few of those individuals who contributed to bringing this project to fruition. The complete list is lengthy, and it is humbling to realize that without their myriad contributions, both large and small, this handbook would not have been possible. Our thanks, first and foremost, go to our families for their patience, support, and understanding of our passion for volleyball. Ms Julie Elliott and Ms Alice Emmott at Blackwell Publishing provided expert editorial assistance. Ms Catherine Chapuis and Ms Alexandra LeClef were most helpful in providing Olympic action photographs from the IOC Museum archives for inclusion in the text. Professor Howard G. Knuttgen, coordinator of the IOC Sub-Commission on Publications in the Sport Sciences, proved himself an invaluable friend and mentor in seeing us through from conceptualization to completion of this undertaking. We are grateful for the support of Dr Rubén Acosta, President of the

FIVB, and for that of our colleagues on the FIVB Medical Commission. Finally, we wish to thank the IOC Sports Medicine Commission and its chair, Prince Alexandre de Merode, for giving us the opportunity to share our insights into sports medicine and science applied to the sport of volleyball. On behalf of our fellow contributors to *Volleyball*, it is our pleasure to present this volume in the Handbook of Sports Science and Medicine series. We have attempted to create a work that is at once comprehensive in approach, practical in content, and accessible in delivery. We hope that we have succeeded in meeting our objective, and that this handbook will help to improve the medical care provided to volleyball athletes around the world. We invite your comments and suggestions, so that we may improve in the future.

Jonathan C. Reeser
Marshfield
Roald Bahr
Oslo

Chapter 1
Introduction: a brief history of the sport of volleyball

Jonathan C. Reeser

Volleyball was invented in 1895 by William G. Morgan in Holyoke, Massachusetts, USA (Fig. 1.1). Morgan, a physical education instructor at the local YMCA, intended volleyball to serve as a less strenuous sporting alternative to basketball for local businessmen. In slightly more than one century, volleyball has grown into one of the most popular participation sports in the world. The Fédération Internationale de Volleyball (FIVB), the international governing body for the sport, has conservatively estimated that over 500 million people worldwide play volleyball at one level or another. It is a "lifetime" sport that may be enjoyed by young and old, male and female, able bodied and disabled, and recreational and elite athletes, both indoors and outdoors. However, the game as it is presently enjoyed bears only passing resemblance to the sport that Morgan invented.

Morgan initially named his creation "mintonette," since (it is thought) he consciously borrowed some aspects of the new sport from badminton. In 1896 the name was changed to "volley ball," after Alfred T. Halstead of Springfield College remarked following an exhibition of the new sport that the participants appeared to be "volleying" the ball back and forth. In 1951 the compound word "volleyball" appeared in print in the United States for the first time.

Early in its history, the game suffered from a lack of consistent rules regarding court dimensions, net height, and the number of participants per side. The first "official" compilation of volleyball rules was published by the YMCA in 1897, but apparently had

little effect in bringing uniformity to the game. Only after an early rules revision in 1912 did the sport begin to grow. In 1916 the net height was established at 8 feet (2.43 m), and the rotation of service rule was adopted, in addition to the convention of limiting indoor teams to six players per side. These changes paved the way for the first United States men's national championship, which was contested in New York City in 1922. In 1928, the United States Volleyball Association was established, and it soon supplanted the YMCA as the major organizing force behind the game in the USA. It was in the same year that separate rules for women were adopted, some of which (such as eight players a side and two service attempts per rotation) persisted until the 1950s. The first women's national championship in the United States was held in 1949, and since then the popularity of volleyball among females has skyrocketed.

Once popularized, the style of play evolved quickly. Although invented in the United States, volleyball probably would be a very different sport today had it not spread overseas. Perhaps the most effective volleyball "missionaries" were the YMCA—which introduced the sport to Canada, Cuba, and Latin America—and the American military, whose servicemen enjoyed the sport while stationed in Europe during World War I and in both the European and Pacific theatres during World War II. The precursor of the spike was developed in the Philippines after World War I, and it was in that country that the three-contact rule gained acceptance as well. The forearm pass, or "bagger," was developed in Eastern

Europe in the 1940s. As the number of countries in which volleyball was played increased, it became evident that an international governing body was needed to oversee further development of the game. The Fédération International de Volleyball was incorporated in Paris in 1947, with 14 charter member countries. The first World Championship was held in 1949, but the first World Championship to draw participants from more than two continents took place in 1956. By then the sport was growing in worldwide popularity, and indoor volleyball subsequently joined the pantheon of Olympic sports when the first volleyball gold medal was contested among both men and women during the 1964 Tokyo summer Olympic Games.

Since its Olympic debut, volleyball strategy and tactics have changed at a rapid pace. With World Championship and Olympic medals to be won (Table 1.1), innovative volleyball minds have created new, evolving offensive and defensive systems

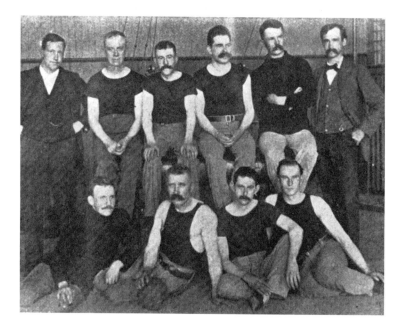

Fig. 1.1 History's first volleyball team, *c.* 1895. William G. Morgan is standing on the left in the second row. (Courtesy of the Volleyball Hall of Fame, Holyoke, Massachusetts, USA.)

Table 1.1 World champions and Olympic gold medalists in indoor volleyball.

World champions			Olympic gold medalists		
Date	Men	Women	Date	Men	Women
1949	USSR		1964	USSR	Japan
1952	USSR	USSR	1968	USSR	USSR
1956	Czechoslovakia	USSR	1972	Japan	USSR
1960	USSR	USSR	1976	Poland	Japan
1962	USSR	Japan	1980	USSR	USSR
1966	Czechoslovakia	Japan	1984	USA	China
1970	East Germany	USSR	1988	USA	USSR
1974	Poland	Japan	1992	Brazil	Cuba
1978	USSR	Cuba	1996	The Netherlands	Cuba
1982	USSR	China	2000	Yugoslavia	Cuba
1986	USA	China			
1990	Italy	USSR			
1994	Italy	Cuba			
1998	Italy	Cuba			
2002	Brazil	Italy			

that have dramatically changed the character of the sport over time. In its infancy, volleyball was not overly demanding and therefore quickly developed a reputation as a genteel sport for less athletically inclined individuals. At its highest level, volleyball is now a sport of explosive, powerful skills demanding athleticism and precise teamwork (Fig. 1.2). The history of indoor volleyball is peppered with the accomplishments of superb athletes, intense competitors, and coaches who have fashioned teams with indomitable spirit. In recognition of the rich history of the sport, the FIVB recently named its male and female athletes, coaches, and teams of the century (Table 1.2). These are but a few of the champions who have contributed to volleyball's tremendous growth over more than 100 years.

For the uninitiated, the objective of the game is to keep an inflated ball aloft, preventing it from contacting the ground or playing surface on your side of the net, while attempting to score points by putting the ball into play on your opponent's side of the net with such force or skill that it cannot be returned. The modern game requires true teamwork, and is an elegant blend of power and finesse, speed and quickness, jumping and leaping. Over the years, volleyball players have become quite specialized in their skills and duties on the court. Today, "setters" are relied upon to "set" the volleyball to an "attacking" teammate who typically attempts to powerfully "spike" the ball over the net. Opposing players in the

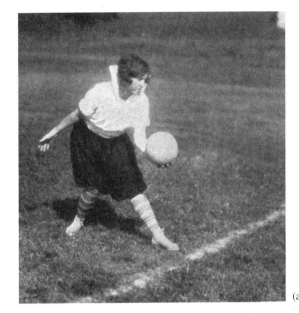
(a)

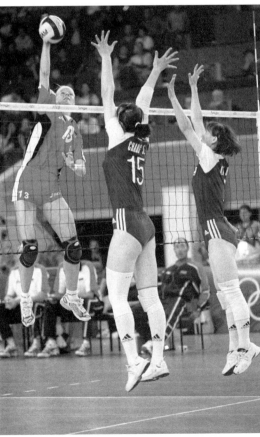
(b)

Table 1.2 The century's "best."

Men's team of the century:	Italy (1990–98)
Women's team of the century:	Japan (1960–65)
Male athlete of the century:	Karch Kiraly, USA (1984–96)
Female athlete of the century:	Regla Torres, Cuba (1992–2000)
Men's coach of the century:	Yasutaka Matsudaira, Japan (1964–74)
Women's coach of the century:	Eugenio George, Cuba (1990–2000)

Fig. 1.2 These photographs provide a striking contrast in juxtaposition, and demonstrate just how greatly the sport of volleyball has changed since its inception. (a) Female participant, c. 1915 (courtesy of the Volleyball Hall of Fame, Holyoke, Massachusetts, USA) and (b) female Olympians competing in the 2000 Sydney Games. (© Allsport/Clive Brunskill.)

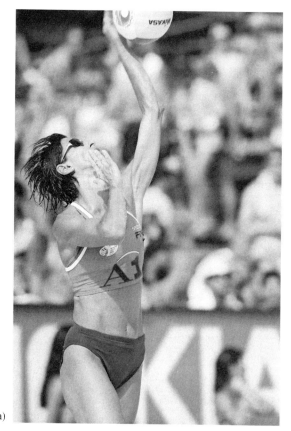

(a)

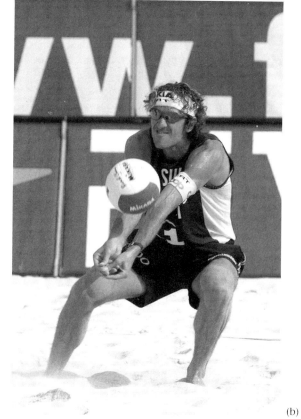

(b)

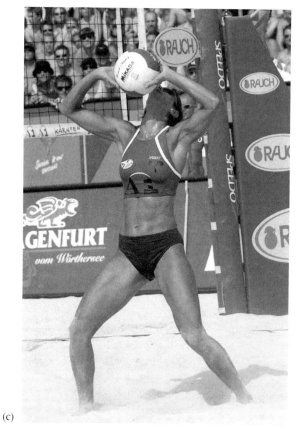

(c)

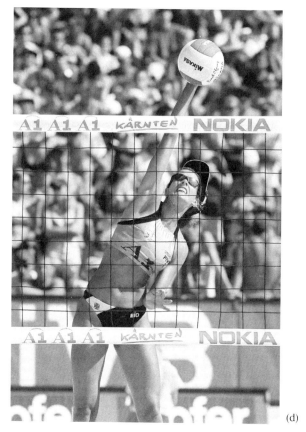

(d)

Fig. 1.3

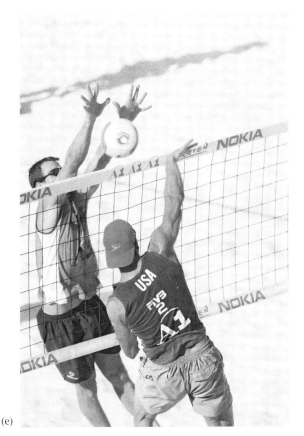

(e)

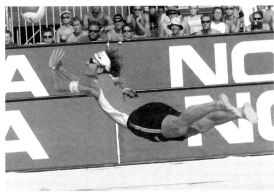

(f)

Fig. 1.3 The essential skills of volleyball are the same whether the sport is played indoors or on the beach, and consist of (a) serving, (b) passing, (c) setting, (d) spiking, (e) blocking, and (f) defending. (Courtesy of the FIVB.)

"front row" attempt to "block" the ball from coming over the net, while a second line of defense is supplied by the "back row" players who attempt to pass or "dig up" balls that penetrate the block (Fig. 1.3).

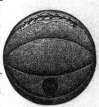

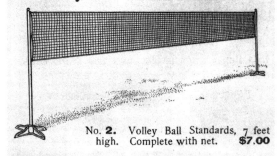

Volley Ball

Volley Ball is a new game which is pre-eminently fitted for the gymnasium or the exercise hall, but which may be played out of doors. Any number of persons may play the game. The play consists of keeping the ball in motion over a high net, from one side to the other, thus partaking of the character of two games—tennis and hand ball. Made of white leather. Constructed with capless ends and furnished with pure gum guaranteed bladder.

No. **V.** Regulation size; best quality. Each, **$4.00**
No. **W.** Regulation size; good quality. " **2.50**

Volley Ball Net and Standards

No. **2.** Volley Ball Standards, 7 feet high. Complete with net. **$7.00**

Fig. 1.4 The first volleyball, designed and produced by Spalding Sports Worldwide in collaboration with William G. Morgan, was quite different from those in use today. Note the net height, which had not been standardized at the time of this 1903–1904 Spalding catalogue. (Courtesy of Spalding Sports Worldwide, Inc.)

One of the appealing aspects of the sport is its simplicity. Little equipment is required, other than a ball and a net. The first volleyball was actually a basketball, but it proved too heavy and a soccer ball was substituted. Eventually, at Morgan's request A. G. Spalding & Bros (now Spalding Sports Worldwide, Chicopee, Massachusetts, USA) fashioned the first volleyball (Fig. 1.4). Over time, modifications of the ball's size and weight have been authorized to suit the age of the participants and the environment in which the game is being played. For example, volleyballs intended for use by young children just learning the game are lighter in weight than regulation volleyballs. The FIVB publishes a listing of the companies that manufacture volleyballs and other volleyball-related equipment (such as modern net systems and uniforms) that meet International Fédération specifications.

As implied above, volleyball is more than a six-person-a-side indoor contest. Indeed, perhaps the greatest area of the sport's growth in recent years has been "beach volleyball." Beach volleyball (Fig. 1.5), now considered a distinct discipline of the sport, began as a recreational pastime on the beaches of California, USA. Originally, beach volleyball was also played with six people per side, but it soon evolved into a demanding sport featuring two people per side. With its combination of sun, sand, surf, and skin, beach volleyball has become associated with the "southern California" lifestyle, and is burgeoning in popularity worldwide. The FIVB sponsors a World Tour of beach volleyball, as well as a biannual World Championship competition, and beach volleyball has been a medal sport for both

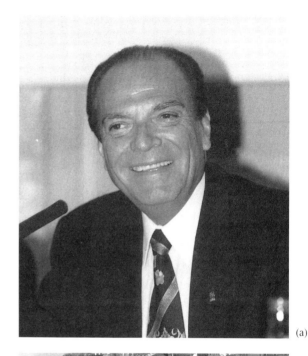

(a)

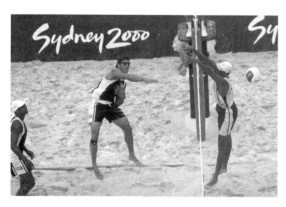

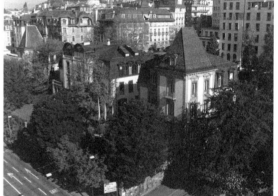

(b)

Fig. 1.5 Beach volleyball, an Olympic medal sport since 1996, is burgeoning in popularity worldwide. (© Allsport/Shaun Botterill.)

Fig. 1.6 The FIVB, under the direction of President Rubén Acosta (a) since 1984, is headquartered in Lausanne, Switzerland (b). (Courtesy of the FIVB.)

Table 1.3 World champions and Olympic gold medalists in beach volleyball.

World champions			Olympic gold medalists		
Date	Men	Women	Date	Men	Women
1997	Para-Guilherme (Brazil)	Jackie-Sandra (Brazil)	1996	Kiraly-Steffes (USA)	Jackie-Sandra (Brazil)
1999	Emanuel-Loiola (Brazil)	Behar-Shelda (Brazil)	2000	Blanton-Fonoimoana (USA)	Cook-Pottharst (Australia)
2001	Baracetti-Conde (Argentina)	Behar-Shelda (Brazil)			

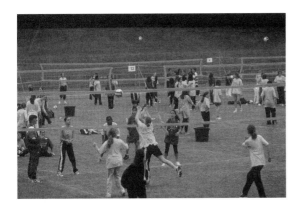

Fig. 1.7 Park volley is designed to appeal to recreational-level athletes of all ages. Further information on park volley is available from the FIVB.

men and women since the 1996 Atlanta Olympic Games (Table 1.3). Perhaps to an extent even greater than the indoor game, the history of beach volleyball is strewn with colorful personalities who contributed to its development and popularity—many of whom have been inducted into the International Volleyball Hall of Fame in Holyoke, Massachusetts, USA.

The future of the sport appears bright. The FIVB (Fig. 1.6) now counts 217 national federations among its membership, more than any other international sports federation. A new discipline has re-cently been introduced—park volley—designed to appeal to the outdoor recreational participant (Fig. 1.7). Professional leagues for men and women draw thousands of spectators in Europe, Asia, and South America, and the FIVB-sponsored World League (for men) and Grand Prix (for women) annually feature the world's best national teams in competition for substantial prize money and international prestige. Finally, in recent years the rules of volleyball have gradually evolved in order to enhance spectator interest and to grow the game. No doubt the next 100 years will witness ongoing evolution, but the status of volleyball as one of the most popular and exciting sports in the world would seem to be assured.

Recommended reading

Fédération Internationale de Volleyball (1996) *100 Years of Global Link*. FIVB, Lausanne, Switerland.

Shewman, B. (1995) *Volleyball Centennial*. Masters Press, Indianapolis, IN.

United States Volleyball Association (2001) *USA Volleyball 2001 Official Guidebook*. USA Volleyball, Colorado Springs, CO.

Additional information is available at the following internet addresses: www.aahperd.org/nagws; www.fivb.org; www.usavolleyball.org; www.volleyball.org; www.volleyhall.org.

PART 1
BASIC AND APPLIED SCIENCE

Chapter 2
Energy demands in the sport of volleyball

Jaci L. VanHeest

Introduction

From a physiological standpoint, volleyball traditionally has been described as a high power, predominantly anaerobic sport. Due to the rules of the game and the structure of matches, volleyball athletes experience repetitive bouts of intense exercise, but also have an opportunity to recover between bouts. The "work period," defined as the total time during the match in which the ball is in play, is typically slightly shorter than the "recovery (or rest) period," which may be defined as the total time during the match in which the ball is not in play. In practical terms, the work period represents the time spent contesting each point, while the recovery period represents the time between points. Volleyball athletes must therefore be capable of generating energy rapidly and also must be capable of recovering rapidly in anticipation of the next point. Consequently, both the aerobic and the anaerobic systems must be well developed to enable the volleyball athlete to perform maximally. This chapter describes the biochemical systems that provide energy to the volleyball athlete and discusses their relative importance in the sport of volleyball.

Energy-generating systems within the body

Adenosine triphosphate (ATP) is the principal energy currency of the human body. The nutrients consumed by an athlete are broken down by the gastrointestinal system into building blocks that are used at the cellular level to produce ATP through a series of interconnected biochemical pathways as depicted in Fig. 2.1 (Brooks *et al.* 1999). ATP, in turn, is used by the body in general and by the skeletal muscles in particular to generate the energy necessary to run, jump, and perform volleyball-specific skills. Energy demand dictates how ATP is utilized by the body, while training influences the regulation of the biochemical processes that cells use to produce, store, and distribute ATP. Therefore, an athlete's training methods should be designed to increase both energy availability and the efficiency of ATP utilization in a sport-specific manner.

In addition to the intracellular stores of such "high-energy phosphates" as ATP and creatine phosphate (CP), humans have several other potential sources of metabolic fuel available within the body. These include stored lipids (muscle triglycerides and adipose tissue), stored glucose (glycogen in the liver and muscle), and stored proteins (muscle tissue itself) (Brooks *et al.* 1999; Wilmore & Costill 1999). Each of these fuel sources may be used in the production of ATP during training or competition. The complexity of the biochemical composition of these different energy sources affects the ease and speed with which each is utilized. Some, like ATP itself, are immediately available sources of energy while others require additional chemical manipulation in order to provide ATP. Each, however, ultimately serves as the substrate for ATP production by one of

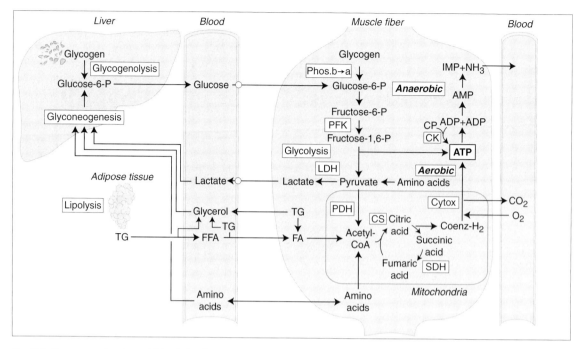

Fig. 2.1 Energy production within skeletal muscle. ADP, adenosine diphosphate; AMP, adenosine monophosphate; ATP, adenosine triphosphate; CK, creatine kinase; CP, creatine phosphate; CS, citrate synthase; Cytox, cytochrome oxidase; FA, fatty acids; FFA, free fatty acids; IMP, inosine monophosphate; LDH, lactate dehydrogenase; NH_3, ammonia; PDH, pyruvate dehydrogenase; PFK, phosphofructokinase; Phos., phosphorylase; SDH, succinate dehydrogenase; TG, triglycerides. (From Bangsbo 1994.)

three biochemical pathways: the ATP-CP system, anaerobic glycolysis, or oxidative metabolism.

Of these three metabolic pathways leading to ATP synthesis, two (the ATP-CP pathway and the anaerobic glycolytic system) produce limited quantities of ATP at high rates in the absence of oxygen. The third pathway, which requires oxygen and consequently is referred to as the oxidative or respiratory system, produces nearly 20 times as much ATP as the anaerobic pathways. However, more chemical reactions are necessary to produce this quantity of ATP and thus the rate of ATP production is relatively slower than for the anaerobic pathways (Stryer 1995; Nelson & Cox 2000).

ATP-CP system

The ATP-CP or high-energy phosphate system is often referred to as the "speed" or "power" system. Intracellular ATP is immediately available to fuel

muscular work, and when replenished by CP this system yields energy at a very high rate. The ATP-CP system is therefore used primarily at the beginning of exercise and in situations that require short bouts of powerful muscular work. However, the energy supply of the ATP-CP system is limited, since within each muscle cell there is only a finite quantity of ATP and CP. The total amount of ATP stored within the body is approximately 85 g—enough to perform maximal work for only a few seconds (Brooks *et al.* 1999; Wilmore & Costill 1999). Training this system allows adaptations that may increase intracellular ATP storage capacity and the efficiency of the ATP-CP system. The average intracellular concentration of CP is about three to five times that of ATP. Once the high-energy phosphate bond of ATP is broken and the potential energy liberated, adenosine diphosphate (ADP) is produced (i.e. ATP → ADP + Pi + energy). Like ATP, energy is released when the high-energy phosphate bond of CP is broken. The reaction generates a free phosphate molecule that is then available to combine with ADP to regenerate ATP (i.e. $ADP + CP \rightarrow ATP + C$) (Sharkey 1997). In the presence of adequate concentrations of CP, ATP can be regenerated at a high rate (equivalent to 35–40 kcal·min^{-1} or 145–170 kJ·min^{-1}) via this pathway (Brooks *et al.* 1999). The total capacity of the high-energy phosphate system is limited: sufficient substrate is available to fuel only 5–15 s of intense muscular work (Wilmore & Costill 1999). After this point, another source of energy must be available for muscular activity to continue.

Anaerobic glycolysis and oxidative (aerobic) metabolism

Anaerobic glycolysis and the oxidative system are the body's two primary energy-generating pathways. It is important to resist the temptation to think of muscular work as being either strictly aerobic or anaerobic, since even during light exercise both aerobic and anaerobic mechanisms are used in the process of energy production.

The preliminary sequence of reactions in carbohydrate metabolism (summarized in Fig. 2.1) involves the breakdown of carbohydrate sugars through a process called glycolysis. Simple sugars such as glucose are provided through the digestion of carbohydrate-containing foods. The body also stores glucose in the form of glycogen. Glycogen is stored both within the liver and skeletal muscle. Approximately 6,300 kJ worth of glycogen is stored by the body at any given moment—sufficient to fuel 1–2 h of intense exercise (Brooks *et al.* 1999; Wilmore & Costill 1999).

Replenishing glycogen stores between workouts is critical to performance and endurance, as training intensity can be compromised when glycogen stores are depleted.

If oxygen is available, pyruvate (the end product of glycolysis) enters into the mitochondria and aerobic metabolism proceeds via the citric acid cycle. The citric acid (or Kreb's) cycle consists of a series of biochemical reactions that lead to the production of ATP via oxidative phosphorylation (aerobic metabolism). The mitochondria found within skeletal muscle—particularly slow-twitch oxidative (type I) muscle—serve as the "energy powerhouses" where

the reactions of the citric acid cycle occur and ATP is produced (Stryer 1995; Nelson & Cox 2000). The details of the citric acid cycle are beyond the scope of this chapter, and the interested reader is referred to the excellent references by Stryer (1995) and *Lehninger's Principles of Biochemistry* (Nelson & Cox 2000) for further information. However, one point worth emphasizing, which is apparent from studying Fig. 2.1, is that the metabolites of carbohydrate, fats, and protein all can enter the citric acid cycle and thus each of these types of nutrients can serve as fuel for the production of ATP. However, without the breakdown products of carbohydrate metabolism the reactions of the citric acid cycle could not occur, and it may therefore be said that "fats burn in a carbohydrate flame."

Similar to a waterwheel that harnesses the energy of falling water, the products of the citric acid cycle are used in subsequent reactions to form ATP via the electron transport chain. Aerobic metabolism generates roughly 90% of all the ATP produced by the body, while anaerobic metabolism produces the remaining 10% (Stryer 1995; Brooks *et al.* 1999). By definition, oxygen is required in the final series of aerobic metabolic reactions, combining with hydrogen ions to produce water. Oxygen is extracted from inspired air by the lungs, where it is bound by hemoglobin and transported to the tissues by red cells within the bloodstream. One measure of an athlete's ability to utilize oxygen to efficiently produce ATP is the maximal oxygen update, or $\dot{V}_{O_{2max}}$. Although respiration is the principal source of oxygen utilized during aerobic metabolism, it is important to note that skeletal muscle does store a small amount of oxygen bound to myoglobin, a heme-carrying molecule that can provide an immediately available source of oxygen in the absence of adequate respiratory oxygen delivery.

If oxygen is in short supply, perhaps because the metabolic demand has exceeded the respiratory supply (the anaerobic threshold), pyruvate can be metabolized via an alternate anaerobic pathway to produce a small amount of ATP. This anaerobic glycolytic pathway, which can fuel up to 60–90 s of intense muscular work, is particularly important in "fast-twitch" muscle cells. The fast-twitch glycolytic muscle fibers (type IIb) contain fewer mitochondria than their slow-twitch counterparts, and are—as

Decrease	Increase
Resting and maximal heart rate	Maximal cardiac output
Resting blood pressure	Resting and maximal stroke volume
Resting ventilation	Heart volume
Resting ventilation rate	Blood volume
Muscle fiber area (type I, IIa, IIb)	Maximal blood pressure
Blood lactate concentrations	Maximal ventilation
	Maximal ventilation rate
	Arteriovenous oxygen difference
	Capillary density
	Enzyme activity (citrate synthetase, hexokinase, lactate dehydrogenase)
	Running economy

Table 2.1 Physiological adaptations to endurance training (Brooks *et al.* 1999; Fleck & Kraemer 1999).

their name implies—particularly important in developing muscle power (Wilmore & Costill 1999). The end product of this anaerobic pathway is lactic acid, or *lactate*. Under conditions of persistent oxygen deficiency, lactate can accumulate within the cell, creating a suboptimal working environment for the muscle. In the presence of high concentrations of lactic acid, skeletal muscles are less capable of generating force. Furthermore, muscle groups acting about a joint may become less coordinated in controlling joint motion in the presence of a high lactate concentration. Lactic acid also activates pain receptors, often resulting in a burning sensation in the muscle. Training above this "threshold" of lactate accumulation is both physically and mentally demanding. Athletes often cannot tolerate the intensity of this anaerobic work and must either reduce their intensity or discontinue the exercise (Fleck & Kraemer 1999).

Fortunately, lactic acid does not remain in the body indefinitely. In fact, once lactic acid is produced it is quickly transported out of the muscle cells into the bloodstream where it is delivered to other organs, including the liver and the heart. The lactic acid produced by intensely working muscles is itself subsequently metabolized in one or more ways, including: (i) incorporation into newly synthesized proteins, (ii) removal through sweat and in urine; (iii) synthesis into glucose or glycogen by the liver; and/or (iv) conversion back into pyruvate, which then can serve as a source of oxidative fuel for the heart, brain, liver, muscles, and kidneys (Brooks *et al.* 1999; Wilmore & Costill 1999). Because lactic acid

can experience several metabolic fates, it should be understood that lactic acid levels constantly fluctuate within the muscles and bloodstream. If, then, the serum lactate level is measured in an exercising athlete, it is important to remember that the reported lactate concentration is the net product of lactic acid accumulation and clearance and therefore reflects the metabolic status of other organ systems in addition to skeletal muscle.

Aerobic training enhances the body's oxygen-carrying capacity and utilization, and thereby improves the athlete's ability to rely on the more efficient aerobic metabolism during bouts of intense exercise. Well-trained aerobic athletes typically have a $\dot{V}o_{2max}$ in the range of 55–85 mL · kg^{-1} · min^{-1} (Wilmore & Costill 1999). Elite volleyball athletes appear to generally fall within the range of 55–65 mL · kg^{-1} · min^{-1} (Viitasalo *et al.* 1987). Additional physiological adaptations to aerobic conditioning include increased blood volume and oxygen-carrying capacity, and an increase in skeletal muscle myoglobin content as well as the number and size of mitochondria (Brooks *et al.* 1999; Fleck & Kraemer 1999) (Table 2.1). As a result, the well-trained aerobic athlete is capable of running, cycling, or swimming farther and faster without accumulating large amounts of lactic acid. Conversely, the power athlete trains anaerobically in an effort to increase the rate of ATP production from anaerobic glycolysis, in addition to improving the body's ability to buffer and process the lactic acid produced. Such training may improve anaerobic power by as much as 25% through enhanced glycolytic enzyme activity and an improved tolerance for, and clearance of, lactic acid. The anaerobic (lactate) threshold for well-trained volleyball athletes should be approximately 80% of the $\dot{V}o_{2max}$, e.g. 44–50 mL·kg^{-1}·min^{-1}.

Interplay between the systems

As alluded to earlier, the ATP-CP system, anaerobic glycolysis, and oxidative metabolism do not each function in isolation. Although the three systems have different characteristics in terms of their rate of energy production and energy-generating capacity, the pathways work in concert to meet the athlete's diverse energy needs using the full spectrum of fuel sources available. The relative contribution of each system is dependent upon the duration and intensity of the exercise imposed on the body. For example, a swimmer participating in a 25 km open water challenge event will use fat and glycogen as the primary oxidative fuel sources during the swim. Conversely, a volleyball player will use the high-energy phosphate (ATP-CP) system and glycogenolysis/anaerobic glycolysis to fuel muscle function during work periods, then during recovery periods the athlete will use aerobic pathways to replenish intracellular stores of ATP-CP and oxygenated myoglobin. The longer a particular point is contested, the more likely the athlete will be to rely on anaerobic metabolism for ATP production, thereby generating (and accumulating) lactic acid. During recovery periods, lactic acid is cleared from the tissues. Knowledge of the metabolic demands of the sport and the relative contributions of each energy-producing system therefore allows the exercise physiologist to develop sport-specific programs that develop and train the appropriate energy system(s) (Viitasalo *et al.* 1987).

Recent rule changes (such as the implementation of rally scoring) have decreased the duration of volleyball games and matches and consequently may have altered the metabolic demands of the sport. In 1999, a typical woman's collegiate game played under side out scoring lasted approximately 23 min, with the average match lasting 1 h 46 min. By comparison, the average women's collegiate game played under rally scoring lasts 20 min, with a match

lasting 1 h 38 min on average. In men's collegiate competition played under rally scoring, the average game lasts 24 min and a match approximately 1 h 29 min. Studies have suggested that the periods of exercise in volleyball last from 4 to 30 s (with an average of approximately 9 s), with recovery intervals between points lasting from 10 to 20 s (with an average length of approximately 12 s) (Lecompte & Rivet 1979). Based on this somewhat crude work to rest ratio of 1 : 1.3, and in consideration of the intensity and power demanded during work intervals, a well-trained volleyball athlete can be expected to utilize the high-energy phosphate (ATP-CP) system and anaerobic glycolysis to generate ATP during play. It has been further estimated that the ATP-CP system is used 90% of the time during work periods, with only 10% of the energy needed to perform high-intensity work supplied by anaerobic glycolysis. However, the relatively long time available for recovery between points (as well as during substitutions and time outs) permits the athlete to aerobically replenish intramuscular stores of ATP and phosphocreatine in anticipation of the next bout of high-intensity work. It has thus been estimated that the overall energy demands of the sport of indoor volleyball (including both work and rest periods) are met by a combination of all three energy-producing pathways in the following proportions: ATP-CP system (40%); anaerobic glycolytic system (10%); and aerobic metabolism (50%) (Gionet 1980).

Aerobic conditioning is therefore essential in preparing the volleyball athlete for rigorous training and competition in what is predominantly a power sport. An athlete who possesses a solid aerobic foundation will be capable of generating energy via aerobic pathways at higher intensities, raising the "anaerobic threshold." Furthermore, the well-trained athlete will recover more rapidly during rest intervals both during and between the sets in a match (Fig. 2.2). Note that although no studies have been published investigating the specific energy demands of the discipline of beach volleyball, it is probable that subtle differences exist between the physiological demands of indoor and beach volleyball. For example, recent data from the FIVB indicates that the average beach volleyball point (played under rally scoring) lasts 28 s, with an average men's match lasting approximately 43 min. By

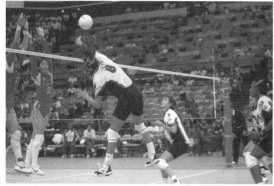

(a)

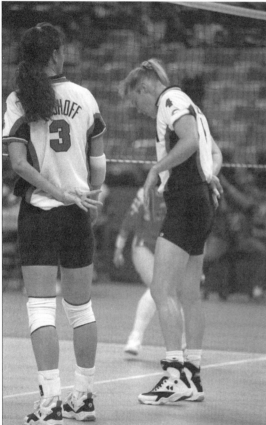

(b)

Fig. 2.2 The duration of the work period in volleyball (a) is typically shorter than the duration of the rest period (b), providing athletes with an opportunity to recover and replenish their pool of rapidly available energy (ATP-CP). (Photos courtesy of Olympic Museum, Lausanne.)

comparison, a men's indoor volleyball match played under rally scoring lasts approximately 90 min, with each point lasting roughly 21 s. Nevertheless, it seems likely that the beach volleyball athlete de-

pends on the same energy systems in roughly the same proportion as does the indoor athlete.

Conclusion

In summary, volleyball athletes generate energy for powerful muscular contraction primarily through the ATP-CP system and anaerobic glycolysis. Their training programs should be designed to enhance these energy systems. In addition, volleyball players must possess a sound aerobic fitness level to ensure appropriate recovery between points and between sets. Indeed, changes in the rules of both indoor and beach volleyball appear to have increased the demand for rapid energy production. As the game of volleyball continues to develop, it seems likely that it will become a game of even greater power. A sound anaerobic system that is grounded in a solid aerobic fitness base is therefore critical to the success of the modern volleyball athlete.

References

Brooks, G.A., Fahey, T.D., White, T.P. & Baldwin, K.M. (1999) *Exercise Physiology: Human Bioenergetics and its Application*, 3rd edn. Mayfield Publications, Mountain View, CA.

Bangsbo, B. (1994) Physiological demands. In: Ekblom, B. (ed.) *Football (Soccer)*, pp. 43–58. Blackwell Scientific Publications, Oxford.

Fleck, S.J. & Kraemer, W.J. (1999) *Designing Resistance Training Programs*, 2nd edn. Human Kinetics, Champaign, IL.

Gionet, N. (1980) Is volleyball an aerobic or an anaerobic sport? *Volleyball Technical Journal* 5 (1), 31–36.

Lecompte, J.-C. & Rivet, D. (1979) Tabulated data on the duration of exchanges and stops in a volleyball Game. *Volleyball Technical Journal* 4 (3), 87–91.

Nelson, D.L. & Cox, M.M. (2000) *Lehninger's Principles of Biochemistry*, 3rd edn. Worth Publications, New York.

Sharkey, B.J. (1997) *Fitness and Health*, 4th edn. Human Kinetics, Champaign, IL.

Stryer, L. (1995) *Biochemistry*, 4th edn. W.H. Freeman, New York.

Viitasalo, J.T., Rusko, H., Pajala, O., Rahkila, P., Ahila, M. & Montonen, H. (1987) Endurance requirements in volleyball. *Canadian Journal of Sport Science* 12 (4), 194–201.

Wilmore, J.H. & Costill, D.L. (1999) *Physiology of Sport and Exercise*, 2nd edn. Human Kinetics, Champaign, IL.

Recommended reading

Denehey, C. & VanHeest, J.L. (2002) *Sport Physiology: a Guide for Practitioners*. Human Kinetics, Champaign, IL.

Gastin, P.B. (2001) Energy system interaction and relative contribution during maximal exercise. *Sports Medicine* **31** (10), 725–741.

Sharkey, B.J. (1997) *Fitness and Health*, 4th edn. Human Kinetics, Champaign, IL.

Shephard, R.J. & Åstrand, P.-O. (2000) *Endurance in Sport*. Blackwell Science, Oxford.

Chapter 3
The biomechanics of jumping

Albert Gollhofer and Sven Bruhn

Introduction

As it is currently played, volleyball is a game in which success depends in large measure on the athleticism of the participants. In particular, the ability to jump high, quickly and explosively is essential to most of the sport's skills, including spiking, blocking, jump serving, and even setting. Thus, it is common for volleyball athletes to place considerable emphasis on jump training. Not surprisingly, overload injuries of the knee and ankle joints, both acute and chronic, occur frequently among volleyball players and are related to the volume of jump training and skill repetition (Watkins 1997). Understanding the biomechanics of jumping is therefore a prerequisite for designing effective training programs which minimize the risk of overuse injuries that may result from excessive jumping, and the repetitive mechanical loading of muscles and joints that is involved in jump training.

Muscles acting about a joint function naturally through a combination of eccentric (lengthening) and concentric (shortening) activations (Komi & Gollhofer 1997; Komi 2000). As will be seen in Chapter 4, advanced volleyball conditioning and strengthening exercises (plyometrics) capitalize upon and train the neuromuscular "stretch–shortening cycle" (SSC). In the lower limb, the SSC is a reflex arc in which the tendomuscular system acting about the knee or ankle is eccentrically preloaded (stretched) in the loading or impact phase of the jump before concentrically shortening in the push-off or take-off phase. In order to achieve a powerful and efficient transition from the lengthening phase to the shortening phase of the SSC, preactivation of the extensor muscles prior to mechanical loading is essential (Fig. 3.1).

The stretch–shortening cycle

All jumps associated with the basic volleyball skills of spiking, blocking, and (jump) serving are characterized by the same general pattern of muscular activation. The concentric action of muscles functioning during the push-off phase is prepared by a preceding eccentric action that occurs during the loading phase. Furthermore, for skills such as the spike in which the athlete follows a more-or-less programed approach to the ball, the extensor muscles are activated in preparation for the loading phase, thereby stiffening the joints of the lower limbs in anticipation of ground contact. Figure 3.2 depicts the sequential activation of the muscles of the lower limb during the SSC.

Following ground contact, the body's center of mass is stabilized and decelerated on its downward movement in the vertical plane. A powerful push off is possible only if the transition phase between eccentric preloading and reflex concentric activation is short and the angular displacement of the knee and ankle joints is small. Figure 3.3 demonstrates the importance of rapid coupling between the eccentric and concentric phases of the jump. Concentric

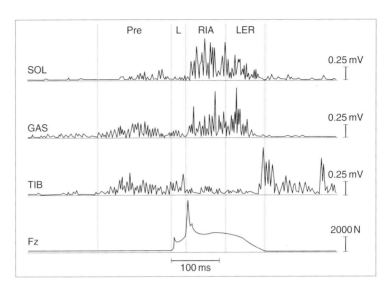

Fig. 3.1 Activity of ankle joint muscles soleus (SOL), gastrocnemius medialis (GAS), and tibialis anterior (TIB) during a drop jump from 90 cm. The muscles are preactivated before ground contact (Pre), and after a latency phase (L) of about 30 ms, reflex-induced activities (RIA) are documented for SOL and GAS. Subsequently, late EMG responses (LER) are recorded during the concentric phase of joint extension. Note the activity of TIB for deceleration of ankle joint dorsal extension after the push off.

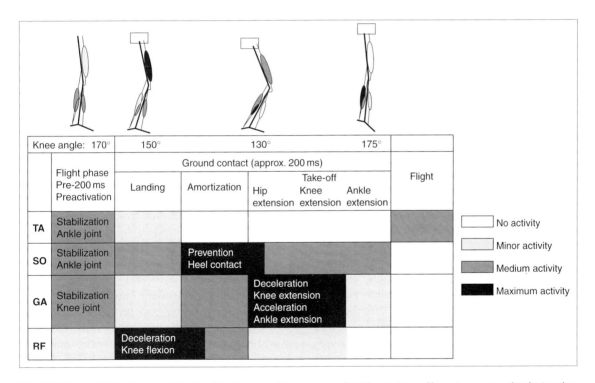

Fig. 3.2 Schematic illustration of the functional role and importance of EMG activition of leg extensor muscles during the stretch–shortening cycle. In the stick figures the grey scale of the muscles indicates the state of activation during a drop jump. The table summarizes the functional importance of each muscle separately. GA, gastrocnemius; RF, rectus femoris; SO, soleus; TA, tibialis anterior. (Modified from Neubert 1999.)

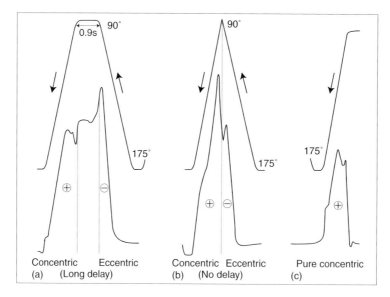

Fig. 3.3 Demonstration of the importance of the short coupling time between eccentric and concentric phases for performance potentiation in the concentric phase of SSC. (a) Longer delay (0.9 s) was allowed between the eccentric and concentric phases. The potentiation effect on the concentric phase was reduced. (b) Concentric action is preceded by eccentric (−) action, but no delay is allowed when contraction type is changed from stretch to shortening. The eccentric (stretch) phase begins in the middle of the movement from the 175° (knee in an extended position) to the 90° position. Note the clear force potentiation in the concentric phase (+) compared with the condition on the right. (c) Pure concentric contraction of the knee extension from 100° to 175°. (From Komi 1983.)

potentiation occurs only if the transition is fast, or "reactive." If the transition is slower or delayed, no enhancement of the concentric phase occurs.

There are three different forms of jumping that have been well investigated biomechanically: the drop jump, the squat jump, and the countermovement jump (Bosco *et al.* 1981; Gollhofer & Rapp 1993). The drop jump, in which the athlete drops from a height and quickly rebounds into the air, is performed most commonly during jump training, but also characterizes the quick repetitive block jumps often required of the middle blocker. The drop jump is considered a reactive jump, with tightly coupled eccentric and concentric phases. Squat jumps are typically performed by blockers, who must react quickly to the opponent's attack. Little preload is possible for this type of jump, in which the athlete remains in a crouched position before jumping. The countermovement jump is typified by the classic spike jump, in which the athlete completes his or her approach with a final closing step, then eccentrically loads the quadriceps

and calves by flexing at the hips, knees, and ankles before pushing off with a concentric activation of those muscle groups. The countermovement jump is a slower, non-reactive jump with little potentiation of the concentric phase.

During a drop jump, the ground reaction force (GRF) rises in proportion to the drop height. Not only does the load/GRF increase with greater drop height, but the athlete's heels also increasingly contact the ground when attempting to rebound rapidly into the take-off phase of the jump. This is exemplified by the shape of the force curve, which changes markedly with varying drop height: the higher the load, the more the maximum force peaks, indicating greater heel strike on the force plate (Fig. 3.4). Conversely, from a lower drop height the athlete is able to perform the drop jump only on the forefoot without their heels touching down.

With higher loads the time of ground contact (heel strike) increases, and consequently an increasing amount of energy is dissipated. The energy lost through heel strike can be compensated for only by

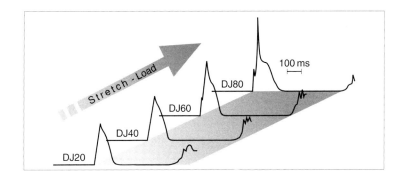

Fig. 3.4 Ground reaction force in dependence of load during the SSC in drop jumps (DJ) of different falling heights (20–80 cm).

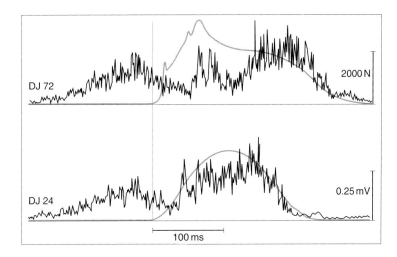

Fig. 3.5 Drop jumps with 24 cm (DJ24) and 72 cm (DJ72) falling height, showing the EMGs of the gastrocnemius medialis muscle (black lines) and ground reaction force (grey lines). The vertical line indicates the landing. Preactivation prior to landing does not alter markedly with the loading condition.

greater concentric phase muscular activation during push off. Increasing heel contact with the floor also results in a progressively passive landing. Rather than absorbing the GRF of landing primarily through eccentric loading of the musculature, more force is transmitted to the bony structures of the lower extremity, potentially increasing the athlete's risk for lower limb injury.

As discussed, in a drop jump (or in the final closing step of a spike approach), some of the lower extremity muscles are activated before ground contact in order to stiffen the joints in preparation for touch down. Neither the timing nor the duration of preactivation is greatly affected by the loading height (Fig. 3.5). Therefore, preactivation depends very little on the loading condition or type of jump performed. Preactivation seems to represent a preprogramed muscular activation functionally necessary for preparation of the landing. As already mentioned, preactivation is also essential for energy potentiation and thus is an important element of a powerful push off. Comparing the activation patterns of selected muscles acting about the ankle and knee joints during different jumping conditions, it is clear that a remarkable amount of muscular preactivation occurs before ground contact.

Stretch reflex contribution to SSC performance

In a drop jump the loading stretch of the muscle–tendon complex is dependent upon the drop height. In addition, touch down induces other involuntary stretch reflexes of the preactivated

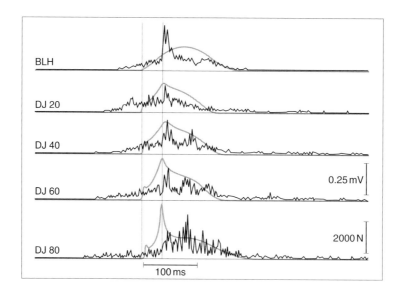

Fig. 3.6 Force–time curves (grey lines) and EMGs of the soleus muscle (black lines) of both leg hopping (BLH) and drop jumps (DJ) with 20, 40, 60, and 80 cm falling heights. The solid vertical line indicates the landing, the dotted vertical line indicates the beginning of the stretch reflex. The highest reflex activity can be detected in the lowest loading condition (BLH). Comparing the lowest loading condition in a drop jump (DJ20) with the next (DJ40), the amount of the reflex contribution gets higher. The highest reflex contribution can be detected in the third condition (DJ60) with a medium stretch load on the muscle–tendon complex, while the amount of the reflex is reduced with the highest loading condition (DJ80).

lower limb muscles. For example, a short latency reflex contribution (SLC) triggered by touch down can be noticed in most of the lower extremity muscles (Gollhofer *et al.* 1990). These reflex responses improve the stiffness of the lower limb musculature. Muscle stiffness and the resultant joint stiffness are prerequisites for a controlled landing in a drop jump, and for a powerful push off. If during the eccentric loading phase the muscle–tendon complex is loaded up to its critical tension, forceful disruption of the actin–myosin sarcomeric cross-bridges may occur. This results in a loss of stored elastic energy within the eccentrically loaded muscle (Rack & Westbury 1974). The critical tension depends in part on the amount of preactivation of the muscle prior to ground contact. Intense muscular preactivation can therefore help prevent cross-bridges from breaking, thereby preserving the potential energy generated by the eccentric loading phase of the SSC, which is then stored within the muscle.

Measurement of muscle fiber length throughout the SSC reveals high-stretch velocities in the early portion of the loading phase (Voigt *et al.* 1998). The maximum stretch velocity achieved is a factor of the load accepted during the eccentric phase. The relationship between the amount of stretch load and SLC contribution is non-linear. The SLC is sensitive to the loading condition during the eccentric phase since the muscle spindle is able to detect the velocity of muscle stretching. Comparing different drop jump conditions, the magnitude of the SLC reflex is smallest from lower drop heights (20 cm), reaches its maximum under medium loading conditions (drop heights of 40 and 60 cm), then decreases again under the highest loading condition (Fig. 3.6). Rather than simply responding in proportion to the magnitude of the load, the SLC reflex contribution to the SSC appears to be unique to each athlete, with an individual optimum loading condition. In practice, the optimum loading condition is largely dependent on the individual athlete's degree of fitness.

There is an ongoing debate regarding the functional significance of such stretch reflex contributions to the SSC. There does appear to be ample evidence that the appropriate reactive movement during the SSC can only be achieved if short latency stretch reflexes are elicited and superimposed on the background activity of the extensor muscles. The SLC reflex appears to influence the degree of tendomuscular stiffness, which in turn is an important factor in energy absorption during the loading phase and in generating force at high rates during the push-off phase (Voigt *et al.* 1998).

The mechanism underlying the observed reduction of short latency reflex activity with increasing preloads beyond the individual optimum level may be decreased facilitation from the muscle spindle and/or increased inhibitory drive from either central or peripheral sources. This reduced reflex activity may serve as a functional protection strategy to prevent muscle or tendon overload injury. If the optimum load is exceeded, the fast reactive SSC turns into a slow non-reactive countermovement-like coupling of an eccentric and a concentric movement, and the immediate transition from eccentric muscle lengthening to concentric shortening disintegrates into its isolated components. The possibility of energy potentiation through the SSC has to be sacrificed to some extent so that the athlete can land safely.

The fact that the SLC reflex decreases with increasing load above the athlete's optimum drop height should therefore be considered when designing training regimens. Two potential hazards occur if the athlete persistently exceeds his or her optimum drop height during jump training. First, the degree of muscle stiffness during the eccentric phase of SSC will be reduced, compromising effective energy potentiation and making an explosive push off during the following concentric phase rather unlikely. Second, reduced muscle stiffness during landing results in reduced joint stability. Consequently, the amount of heel strike/ground contact time increases, meaning that more ground reactive force must be absorbed by the ligaments and bones of the lower limb. These structures are therefore increasingly stressed, placing the athlete at greater risk for overload injuries to the lower limbs.

Movement patterns

This chapter now considers how the biomechanics of the SSC affect the spike, jump serve, and block—the three most jump-intensive volleyball skills.

Jump service

The jump serve has become an increasingly important offensive weapon in volleyball. To execute the jump service, the athlete takes several "approach" steps, tosses the ball upward and in front of them, then takes off from behind the end line—striking the ball while in the air. The player tries to hit the ball at the apex of their jump, imparting to it as much velocity as possible. Performed correctly, the successful jump serve is the product of both a forceful, quick arm swing and a powerful jump permitting the player to hit the ball high above the ground (Fig. 3.7). In order to create a more powerful jump, the last step before the loading phase can be used for energy potentiation as discussed earlier.

The force–time curve (Fig. 3.8) of the jump service reveals a smooth development of the power without a large maximum peak. Ground contact between the final step of the approach and push off lasts about 200 ms. The tibialis anterior muscle is slightly preactivated before touch down (as seen in Fig. 3.1) and remains activated until the eccentric phase of the jump moves into the concentric phase. The vastus lateralis and tibialis anterior muscles are eccentrically activated during the landing phase of the jump, helping to stabilize the knee and ankle joints, respectively. Eccentric activity of the vastus lateralis muscle also acts in the landing phase to decelerate the flexion movement at the knee joint. While the activity of the tibialis anterior disappears in the concentric movement during the push-off phase, the vastus lateralis remains active in order to extend the knee joint. Extension at the ankle joint is realized by the triceps surae (gastrocnemius/soleus complex). The gastrocnemius muscle is active during the concentric phase of push off. There is also slight preactivation before touch down, but only small reflex activity after touch down. Immediately after touch down, the gastrocnemius medialis is reciprocally

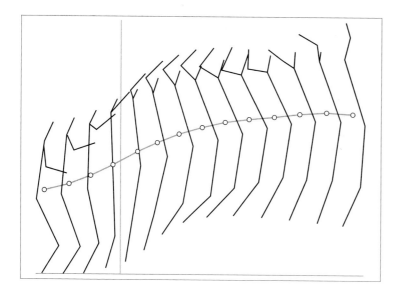

Fig. 3.7 Kinegram of a jump service; the vertical line indicates the push off (end of concentric phase).

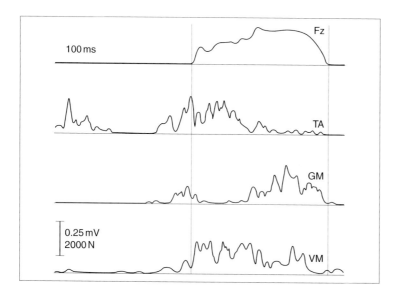

Fig. 3.8 Ground reaction force (F_z), and EMGs of the vastus medialis (VM), tibialis anterior (TA), and gastrocnemius medialis (GM) during service. The left vertical line indicates the landing (beginning of the eccentric phase); the right vertical line indicates the push off (end of the concentric phase).

inhibited by the tibialis anterior, while activation of the gastrocnemius medialis during the concentric phase inhibits the tibialis anterior.

Spike

Most offensive sequences end with a spiked ball. Typically, two or more attackers jump sequentially or simultaneously, thereby providing the setter with tactical options. Therefore, most of the attacks in a match are preceded by a spike jump. The spiker's approach starts from the middle of the court, usually behind the 3 m line in the case of an outside hitter. The spike jump is a countermovement jump, and again the eccentric phase during landing is a prerequisite for energy potentiation and a powerful push off. Weight acceptance during the last step of the athlete's approach can be performed either in a "soft way" on the forefoot, or in a "hard way" on the heel. Because of the shorter ground contact time,

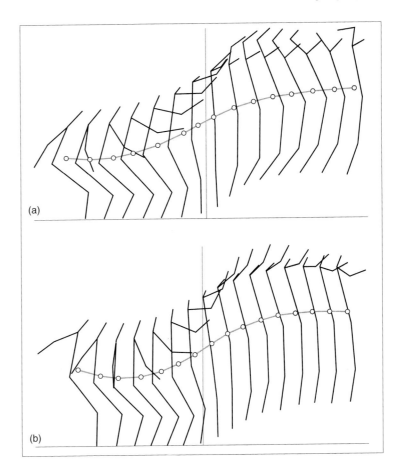

Fig. 3.9 Kinegram of a spike jump:
(a) with soft landing, and (b) with
hard landing. The vertical line
indicates the push off.

the hard landing results in a quicker push off. Consequently, offensive strategy can be designed so that attacks are fast and thus more likely to surprise the defenders, shortening the time available to react to the oncoming spike (Fig. 3.9).

A soft landing on the forefoot attenuates some of the high impact of the landing, resulting in a smoother force–time curve with lower peak forces. The hard landing allows faster push off with shorter ground contact time resulting in pronounced force peaks with higher values (Fig. 3.10). The tactical advantage of a faster spike approach is counterbalanced by the disadvantage of higher stress on the bony and ligamentous structures of the lower limbs.

The electromyographic (EMG) data reflect the different timing and the different dynamics of the two versions of the spike jump. The EMG of the tibialis anterior indicates an earlier beginning and a higher degree of preactivation in the hard landing. Thus it can be suspected that the landing and the following push off is prepared some time before ground contact. Regarding the EMG of the gastrocnemius medialis, it is obvious that there is no substantial activation after touch down in the soft landing. The main activity of this muscle can be observed in the concentric phase of push off. In a hard landing, some phasic EMG contributions are noticed in the gastrocnemius medialis. The activity of this muscle begins and ends much earlier in the hard landing than in the soft landing. Because the EMG of the vastus medialis does not vary with the landing situation, the different jumping conditions mainly affect the lower limb below the knee (Fig. 3.11). It is noteworthy that in both jump modalities the rectified raw EMG traces are nicely reproduced in the tibialis anterior and in the vastus medialis right after touch down.

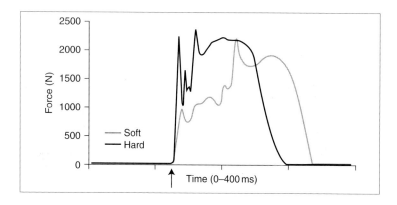

Fig. 3.10 Force–time curve of a spike jump with soft (grey line) and hard (black line) landings. The arrow indicates the landing for both movements.

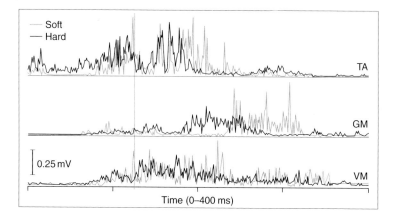

Fig. 3.11 EMG data of the tibialis anterior (TA), gastrocnemius medialis (GM), and vastus medialis (VM) in a spike jump with soft (grey lines) and hard (black lines) landing. The vertical line indicates the landing for both movements.

Block

The block is a defensive movement performed in re-action to the opponent's attack. The blocker has to move laterally and jump vertically very quickly in order to have any chance of successfully blocking the oncoming spike. If the offence surprises the de-fence, there is not enough time to perform signifi-cant preparatory movement, so the blocker is forced to take off immediately—essentially performing a squat jump. If on the other hand the opponent's attack strategy can be anticipated, the blocker can move laterally in order to optimally position him or herself before jumping. The last touch down before the jump push off can be used for energy potentia-tion, as described for the jump service. If the blocker is correctly positioned, she or he can perform a countermovement jump, eccentrically preloading

the hip extensors and knee flexors (Fig. 3.12) and resulting in a higher, more imposing block.

The countermovement can be detected in the force–time curve as a reduction in force (Fig. 3.13). The increasing GRF indicates the subsequent con-centric extension of the lower extremity. The force values again decrease until the push off, when the GRF is zero. The maximum force is a little lower than that produced during a jump service and the rate of force development is slower. The tibialis anterior is most active during the coupling of the eccentric and the concentric movement in order to dynamically stabilize the center of gravity. The gastrocnemius medialis and vastus medialis are most active during the concentric phase of knee and ankle joint exten-sion. None of the muscles show any reflex activity during a countermovement jump.

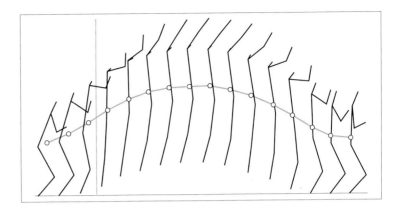

Fig. 3.12 Kinegram of a block; the vertical line indicates the push off (end of concentric phase).

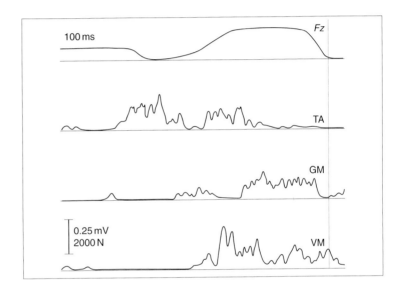

Fig. 3.13 Ground reaction force (F_z), and EMGs of the vastus medialis (VM), tibialis anterior (TA), and gastrocnemius medialis (GM) during a block. The vertical line indicates the push off (end of concentric phase).

Conclusion

The different types of volleyball jumps can be separated into two groups on the basis of ground contact time. A drop jump from low height in which no heel contact occurs results in a fast, reactive form of SSC. A countermovement jump, such as a spike jump, results in a slow, non-reactive type of SSC.

The power output during the concentric phase in the SSC and thereby the performance of jumping is largely dependent on the load accepted during the eccentric phase. With higher loading, the ground contact time is prolonged and thus the whole SSC lasts longer. Since energy potentiation is basically re-

lated to the short range elastic stiffness due to the formed muscle cross-bridges, such a reactive movement is possible only if the ground contact time does not exceed approximately 200 ms. If ground contact is prolonged because of higher loading during the eccentric phase, a fast reactive reversal of the movement is not possible, and the coupling of the movement is divided up into an isolated eccentric landing and a concentric countermovement-like take off. The energy of the eccentric phase cannot be used for the concentric push off, and must be absorbed. Energy absorption is facilitated by strong eccentric muscle contraction. However, if the initial load is too great, the additional GRF is transmitted to bony and ligamentous structures. Proprioceptive training may enhance joint stiffness, thereby reducing the athlete's risk of overload injuries (Bruhn *et al.* 2000). Repeated energy absorption by passive structures increases the risk of overload injury. At the same time, jumping performance decreases, because energy potentiation and thus fast, reactive movement is impossible. The amount of loading within the SSC that can be tolerated by the athlete during the eccentric phase is dependent on the athlete's individual motor performance. Tolerance against eccentric loading allows energy potentiation in a fast, reactive movement reversal in order to perform a powerful concentric push off.

At a given level of motor performance, the eccentric load largely determines the behavior of the leg extensor muscles. The SLC activity varies with the loading height more than the degree of muscular preactivation does. The reflex contribution to the SSC can be enhanced by increasing the load in the eccentric phase up to an individual optimum height. Exceeding the individual optimum loading height decreases the reflex contribution of the leg extensor muscles leading to decreased SSC performance and decreased joint stiffness during landing. Thus, training of jumping performance and the SSC should routinely occur at or below the optimum loading drop height.

Less is more!

One practical method of determining an athlete's individual optimum loading condition is to measure the drop height from which heel strike first occurs. The ground contact time, the shape of the force–time curve, and the amount of reflex contribution are testable parameters that may be useful to the biomechanist in quantifying the athlete's unique optimum loading condition. The coach or trainer should also factor in fatigue when designing training programs. Fatigue can turn a fast SSC into a slow SSC, because muscular reflex activation of the ankle joint muscles is reduced (Avela *et al.* 1999). As a consequence of this reduced reflex activity, for a given loading condition the ground contact time is prolonged and the maximum ground reaction force increases. Fatigue results in a reduction of muscle activity after ground contact, in addition to loss of joint stiffness and decreasing motor performance, culminating in an increased risk of injury to the athlete.

References

Avela, J., Kyröläinen, H. & Komi, P.V. (1999) Altered reflex sensitivity due to repeated and prolonged passive muscle stretching. *Journal of Applied Physiology* **86** (4), 1283–1291.

Bosco, C., Komi, P.V. & Ito, A. (1981) Prestretch potentiation of human skeletal muscle during ballistic movement. *Acta Physiologica Scandinavica* **111**, 135–140.

Bruhn, S., Gollhofer, A. & Lohrer, H. (2000) Functional stability of the knee joint. *Sportorthopädie–Sporttraumatologie* **16** (3), 145–154.

Gollhofer, A., Hostmann, G.A., Schmidtbleicher, D. & Schönthal, D., (1990) Reproducibility of neuromuscular activation patterns in stretch-shortening typed contractions. *European Journal of Applied Physiology* **60**, 7–14.

Gollhofer, A. & Rapp, W. (1993) Recovery of stretch reflex responses following mechanical stimulation. *European Journal of Applied Physiology* **66**, 415–420.

Komi, P.V. (1983) Elastic potentiation of muscle and its influence on sport performance. In: Baumann, W. (ed.) *Biomechanics and Performance in Sport*, pp. 59–70. Karl Hoffmann Verlag, Schorndorf.

Komi, P.V. (2000) Stretch-shortening cycle: a powerful model to study normal and fatigued muscle. *Journal of Biomechanics* **33**, 1197–1206.

Komi, P.V. & Gollhofer, A. (1997) Strech reflex can have an important role in force enhancement in SSC-exercise. *Journal of Applied Biomechanics* **13**, 451–460.

Neubert, A. (1999) *Zur Diagnostik und Trainierbarkeit des reaktiven Bewegungsverhalten*. Sport und Buch Strauß, Köln.

Rack, P.M.H. & Westbury, D.R. (1974) The short range stiffness of active mammalian muscle and its effect on mechanical properties. *Journal of Physiology* **240**, 331–350.

Voigt, M., Dyhre-Poulsen, P. & Simonsen, E.B. (1998) Stretch-reflex control during human hopping. *Acta Physiologica Scandinavica* **163** (2), 181–194.

Watkins, J. (1997) Verletzungen und überlastungsschäden im Volleyball. In: Renström, P.A.F.H. (ed.) *Sportverletzungen und Ärzte,* pp. 310–323. Deutscher Verlag Gmbh, Köln.

Recommended reading

Zatsiorsky, V. (ed.) (2000) *Biomechanics in Sport*. Blackwell Scientific, Oxford.

Chapter 4
Peak conditioning for volleyball

Tudor O. Bompa and Michael C. Carrera

Introduction

Conditioning refers to the process of developing strength, speed, agility, and power. Peak conditioning is essential to achieving optimal athletic performance. The physical demands of different sports vary significantly. Therefore, the athlete who wishes to specialize or excel in a single sport should follow a sport-specific exercise prescription. Volleyball is a sport of power, quickness, and agility, and thus in order to maximize their performance volleyball athletes should follow a conditioning program that develops volleyball-specific neuromuscular abilities.

Volleyball is a sport in evolution. Recent rule changes have altered tactical strategy and this has in turn motivated strength and conditioning specialists to update and adjust strength and conditioning protocols specifically for the modern volleyball athlete. The performance of the volleyball athletes participating in the 2000 Sydney Olympic Games made it clear that elite volleyball players require a greater amount of strength, quickness, and agility than ever before in the history of the sport. Players at all positions are highly taxed during match play, and thus require optimal development of their biomotor abilities in addition to strong overall conditioning (Fig. 4.1).

Critical to the development of these abilities is the trainability of a higher level of strength. Strength training should not be developed independently from other abilities (e.g. agility, quickness, en-

durance), or in disregard of the planned training phases leading to championships or league games. In order to make strength a valuable physiological ingredient of the conditioning program, it has to be trained in such a way that gains in strength lead to enhanced skill performance, which can in turn be applied during competition (e.g. more effective spiking due to more explosive jumping and a higher reach). In order to achieve this, strength training has to be structured into training phases leading into the competitive phase—a concept known as periodization. This chapter will discuss the principles of conditioning as applied to volleyball. The types of strength training required for volleyball will be discussed within the framework of the periodization model.

Goals of strength training

In order to maximize an athlete's potential, gains in strength must lead to sport-specific adaptations. A volleyball player must develop five main abilities:

1 *Strength* (S) is defined as the maximum amount of force that can be generated by a muscle. Strength plays an important role in creating high levels of sport performance.

2 *Power* (P) is defined as the rate at which work is performed (power = force × velocity). When quickness (speed) is integrated with strength, power is the outcome. Power is a determinant quality that is

required in any type of jumping or for a quick change of direction.

3 *Take-off power* is a critical element in volleyball and refers to the ability to project the body to the highest point while spiking or blocking. The greater the force applied against the ground, the higher the jump. The height of the jump is directly proportional to leg power.

4 *Reactive power* refers to the ability to generate force immediately following landing, such as in a drop jump. This kind of power is also necessary to quickly change the direction of motion during a game. The force necessary to adequately perform a reactive jump depends on the height of the jump, and the athlete's body weight and leg power.

5 *Power-endurance* (PE) is defined as the ability to repeat power actions consistently throughout a game. Power development is essential to the success of the elite volleyball player. However, it is endurance that permits the athlete to jump high to spike over the block repeatedly during competition. It has been estimated that the average collegiate volleyball player performs 200 spike or block jumps in a typical match. Unless the athlete has developed excellent

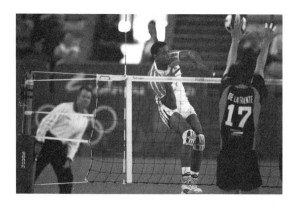

Fig. 4.1 Elite volleyball players possess both power and quickness. (Photo courtesy of Olympic Museum, Lausanne.)

power-endurance, as they fatigue in the latter stages of a match their effectiveness will decline and their risk for incurring a musculoskeletal injury will increase.

Periodization model of strength training

Periodization refers to the process of structuring training over a given period of time in such a way that peak performance will be attained at the time of the main competitions. Most commonly, the period in question (a macrocycle) is 1 year. This year-long macrocycle is subsequently subdivided into phases referred to as mesocycles. As illustrated in Fig. 4.2, the athlete has specific training goals and objectives for each phase.

The above phases of training are manipulated and planned in accordance to the calendar of competitions and the physical abilities of the team or individual player. Figure 4.3 illustrates a more specific model for volleyball, depicting an annualized program that has been utilized by men's volleyball clubs at several Canadian universities and colleges. Figure 4.4 details a periodization model that would be suitable for an elite-level volleyball athlete who must participate in several competitions throughout the year.

As is apparent from these models, the concept of periodization involves the implementation of various phases of training. A discussion of the phases of training inherent to the periodization of strength for volleyball follows.

Phase I: anatomical adaptation (AA)

The AA phase represents the foundation on which the other phases of training are based and is utilized

Preparatory		Competitive		Transition
Anatomical adaptation (AA)	Strength (S)	Conversion to power/power-endurance (P/PE)	Maintenance of power/power-endurance (P/PE)	Transition training (TT)

Fig. 4.2 The main phases for the periodization of strength training for volleyball. Note that the terminology of the various phases is known to differ between Europe and the United States.

Jun	Jul	Aug	Sept	Oct	Nov	Dec	Jan	Feb	Mar	Apr	May
PREPARATORY					COMPETITIVE					TRANSITION	
AA (6 weeks)	S (6 weeks)	P (3 weeks)	S (3 weeks)	Conversion to P/PE (7 weeks)	Maintenance of P/PE					Transition training	

Fig. 4.3 An annual periodization model for college volleyball players. Some conditioning specialists also refer to a week or cluster thereof as a "microcycle."

Jun	Jul	Aug	Sep	Oct	Nov	Dec	Jan	Feb	Mar	Apr	May	Jun	Jul	Aug	Sep	Oct	Nov ⇒
PREPARATORY					COMPETITIVE					T	Special Prep/Comp		W/O	T	PREPARATORY		COMPETITIVE
AA (6 weeks)	S (6 weeks)	P (3 weeks)	S (3 weeks)	Conversion to P/PE	Maintenance of S, P/PE					T T	AA, S (3 weeks)	P/PE (5 weeks)	No Training		AA (3 weeks)	S (3 weeks)	P/PE (3 weeks)	Maintenance of S, P/PE

Fig. 4.4 Periodized training model spanning 18 months for volleyball players involved in national league games (November to April) and World Championship (W) or Olympic (O) games in the month of July. Note the special preparatory and pre-World/Olympic matches for May and June. T, transition; TT, transition training.

during the preparatory phase of training. AA represents the first phase of the periodization model and is organized immediately following the transition phase (the transition phase is occasionally referred to as the "off season"). The name of this phase illustrates the fact that the main objective of strength training is not an immediate overload, but rather a progressive adaptation of the player's anatomy. The objectives of the AA phase are focused around injury prevention and "prehabilitation," with the hope of preventing the need for "rehabilitation." In practical terms, the athlete seeks to build a strong base of both strength and endurance by training with low to medium loads at high volume. As the athlete's muscles, ligaments, and tendons specifically adapt to these imposed demands, the athlete establishes the anatomical and physiological foundation for the more challenging program inherent in the subsequent phases of training. Furthermore, a methodically structured AA phase will aid in the improvement of intermuscular coordination (i.e. balance, coordination, and neural firing patterns), will increase bone mineral content, and will pro-

mote proliferation of the connective tissue that surrounds individual muscle fibers.

Depending on the player's initial level of physical development and strength training experience, the AA phase can be planned for 3–10 weeks. During this long phase the program should be structured to include specific exercises intended to develop the core area of the body and stimulate functional balance among muscular agonists and antagonists. In some cases, balanced development between agonist and antagonist muscles is impossible because some agonist muscles are larger and stronger than others. For instance, the knee extensors (quadriceps) are stronger than the knee flexors (hamstrings). Muscle imbalances that are not identified and corrected during the AA phase will hamper the development of strength and impede performance in the subsequent phases. An injury such as jumper's knee is a good example of how muscle imbalances can lead to chronic symptoms of injury.

When designing an AA program for a volleyball athlete, the easiest method to consider is circuit training (CT). CT represents a good organizational

Training parameter	Novice player	Experienced player
Duration of AA	8–10 weeks	3–5 weeks
Load (if weights are used)	30–40% of 1 RM	40–60% of 1 RM
No. of reps/station (approx.)	15–20	10–15
Repetition tempo	Slow–medium	Slow–medium
No. of stations/circuit	9–12 or 15	6–9
No. of circuits/session	2–3	3–5
Total time of CT/session	20–25 min	30–40 min
Rest interval between exercises	90 s	60 s
Rest interval between circuits	2–3 min	1–2 min
Frequency/week	2–3	3–4

Table 4.1 Suggested training parameters for circuit training (Bompa 1999a).

method that is fun to do and alternates the various muscle groups trained. CT can be used to develop both overall conditioning and combinations of strength. For the purpose of this discussion, a CT program will be presented with the idea of developing AA-specific strength.

A great variety of resistance training equipment can be employed such as body weight, elastic tubing, medicine balls, light implements, dumbbells, and barbells in addition to strength training machines. A circuit may be short (6–9 exercises), medium (9–12 exercises), or long (12–15 exercises) and can be repeated several times depending on the number of exercises. Obviously, the number of sets, repetitions per station, and load must be individualized to meet the needs and work tolerance unique to each athlete. For example, athletes who are injured or who have chronic joint pain should be accommodated with an individualized program that takes their limitations into consideration so as to permit strength gains without further aggravating their symptoms. Adaptations of technique, load, and progression should be considered in these cases (Fees *et al.* 1998). During the AA phase, the total work and intensity of training should not be so high as to push the player to the level of pain or discomfort. CT exercises must be planned in an alternating fashion that will aid in the faster recovery of individual muscle groups. The recommended rest interval between stations is 60–90 s and 1–3 min between circuits.

Considering the scope of the AA phase, exercises should be selected to develop the core area of the body as well as the main muscles used in volleyball. Exercises that train muscles from multiple func-

tional angles should be incorporated along with an overall flexibility program. To select the appropriate load, the player should test for one repetition maximum (1 RM) of the prime movers (muscles primarily involved in the sport movement). Stations are selected in accordance to the equipment available in the gymnasium or fitness facility. It is expected that novice players will experience muscle soreness. Therefore, as a practical consideration, plan two to three sessions that introduce the muscles to the exercises using light loads. This will provide for a more effective means of discovering a player's true 1 RM and training weight.

As illustrated in Table 4.1, training parameters for experienced volleyball players are quite different from those of a novice. A novice player should undergo a longer AA phase since they generally require a longer timeframe for anatomical adaptation to occur. By comparison, an AA phase of 3–5 weeks should suffice for the experienced, well-conditioned player. Table 4.1 lists the suggested average duration of an AA phase, the recommended frequency of training sessions per week, and other parameters for CT programs for both younger and more mature athletes. Representative examples of possible circuits utilizing various forms of equipment are presented in Box 4.1.

Every player regardless of the sport in question should complete an AA phase of training. The strength training experience of the player will ultimately determine the duration of this phase. Once completed, the AA phase of training is followed by a strength phase.

Phase II: strength (S)

The main objective of the strength (S) phase of training is to develop the highest possible level of muscular force production, which will aid in the development of power and power-endurance. The level of strength affects each of these types of power. Without a high level of strength, maximum power cannot be attained. Since power is the product of speed and strength, it is logical to first develop strength and then convert it to power.

Strength training plays an important role in optimizing volleyball-specific conditioning. The more important the role of strength training, the longer this phase of training should last. A player's ability to

increase strength depends on the cross-sectional area of the muscle involved, the capacity to recruit fast-twitch muscle fibers, and the ability to synchronize all the muscles involved in the action. The capacity to recruit fast-twitch muscle fibers is developed through the use of increasing loads and explosive power exercises. Strength training represents the only means of activating the powerful fast-twitch motor units.

Strength improves as a result of creating high tension in the muscle, which is directly related to the training method employed. A player does not have to increase body weight as a function of strength training. Volleyball players do not require a large, hypertrophic muscle mass; however, they do rely on an enormous amount of strength for maximum performance. The ability to increase strength without a concomitant increase in muscle mass has led to characterizing the strength phase of training as "nervous system" training. Strength training improves links with the central nervous system, thus promoting both the improvement in intermuscular coordination (i.e. activation of synergists and cocontraction of antagonists) and intramuscular coordination (i.e. recruitment and firing rate of motor units, reflex response, and motor unit synchronization).

Unfortunately, relatively little is known about the involvement of the nervous system in developing strength. However, small amounts of empirical evidence and large amounts of anecdotal evidence collected from coaches, trainers, and athletes suggest that strength training is the most effective method of improving maximal muscular force production.

Maximum load method

Absolute strength is defined as the greatest amount of weight a player can lift in a specified movement irrespective of body weight. Relative strength is defined as the greatest amount of weight a player can lift and is expressed as a function of body weight. In other words, building upon the previous point, players who desire an increase in strength in the absence of greater body weight, require an increase in relative strength. The following discussion will provide an overview of methods of improving relative strength that can be applied during the strength phase of training.

The maximum load method (MLM) is probably the most efficient means of developing volleyball-specific strength. The MLM positively influences speed and power by increasing the diameter of fast-twitch muscle fibers and by recruiting more fast-twitch motor units. The MLM method can result in strength gains that are up to three times greater than the proportional increase in muscle size (hypertrophy). Although increases in muscle size are possible for players who are just starting to use the MLM, muscular hypertrophy is less visible in players with a longer training background.

Program design

The MLM should be reserved for more mature athletes who have completed at least 2–3 years of moderate general strength training. Novice athletes should focus on the use of lower loads ranging from 60 to 80% 1 RM during this phase of their strength training program. Highly trained players with 3–4 years of MLM training are so well adapted to such training that they are able to recruit some 85% of their fast-twitch muscle fibers. The remaining 15% represent a latent reserve that is not easily activated through training.

Creating the highest tension possible in the muscle develops strength. According to the size principle, motor units are recruited in sequence beginning with the recruitment of slow-twitch motor units followed in turn by fast-twitch motor units. Therefore, in order to recruit the most powerful fast-twitch motor units, loads greater than 85% of 1 RM are required. The MLM should employ exercises that specifically emphasize the prime movers, including the squat, calf raise, dead lift, bench press, shoulder press, and other multijoint movements. Exercises should be ordered in a way that alternates muscle groups and facilitates local muscle recovery between sets. The player's classification, training background, and phase of training, along with the number of exercises employed, will determine the number of repetitions performed per exercise. MLM training sessions should demand the greatest number of sets that the athlete can tolerate, ranging from four to six or more. One to four repetitions are rec-

Table 4.2 MLM training parameters (after Bompa 1999a).

Training parameters	Regimen
Duration of phase	3–4 weeks
Load	85–100%
No. of exercises	3–5
No. of reps per set	1–4
No. of sets per session	6–10 or 12
Rest interval	3–6 min
Speed of execution	Fast
Frequency per week	2–3 or 4

ommended per set, with 15–18 repetitions per exercise per training session. A 3–6 min rest interval between sets is recommended given that MLM training involves the central nervous system, which takes longer to recover than does muscle. A shorter rest interval could potentially compromise the nerve impulse to the muscle and will negatively impact the restoration of ATP-CP. Accordingly, due to the high demand placed on the neuromuscular system, the frequency of MLM training should be increased to no more than 2–3 times per week.

The speed of contraction plays a very important role in MLM training. To achieve explosive force, the player must concentrate on activating the muscles quickly even though the barbell is moving slowly. Only high speed contraction performed against maximum load will successfully recruit the fast-twitch fibers needed to increase strength and power. Suggested training parameters for the MLM are provided in Table 4.2, while Fig. 4.5 gives a sample 6-week strength training program for the volleyball athlete.

A player must be physiologically and developmentally prepared before participating in the strength phase. Similarly once a high level of strength has been developed, a player is physiologically prepared to further develop power and power-endurance.

Phase III: conversion to power

Power is the ability of the neuromuscular system to produce force quickly and is defined as the product of muscle force (F) produced and the velocity (V) of movement: $P = F \times V$. Therefore, improvements in

No.	Exercise	Dates					
		May 13–19	May 20–26	May 27–June 2	June 3–9	June 10–16	June 17–23
1	Squats/leg presses	$\frac{70}{8}$3	$\frac{70}{8}$1 $\frac{80}{6}$2	$\frac{80}{8}$1 $\frac{90}{3}$2	$\frac{70}{10}$3	$\frac{80}{8}$1 $\frac{90}{3}$2	$\frac{90}{3}$1 $\frac{95}{2}$2
2	Sit ups	3 × 15	3 × 18	3 × 20	3 × 15	3 × 18	3 × 20
3	Military presses	$\frac{70}{8}$3	$\frac{70}{8}$1 $\frac{80}{6}$2	$\frac{80}{8}$1 $\frac{90}{3}$2	$\frac{70}{10}$3	$\frac{80}{8}$1 $\frac{90}{3}$2	$\frac{90}{3}$1 $\frac{95}{2}$2
4	Leg curls	$\frac{50}{12}$1 $\frac{60}{10}$2	$\frac{60}{10}$3	$\frac{60}{10}$2 $\frac{70}{8}$1	$\frac{60}{10}$3	$\frac{60}{12}$1 $\frac{70}{10}$2	$\frac{70}{10}$3
5	Calf raises	$\frac{70}{8}$3	$\frac{70}{8}$1 $\frac{80}{6}$2	$\frac{80}{8}$1 $\frac{90}{3}$2	$\frac{70}{10}$3	$\frac{80}{8}$1 $\frac{90}{3}$2	$\frac{90}{3}$1 $\frac{95}{2}$2
6	Front lateral pull downs	$\frac{70}{8}$3	$\frac{70}{8}$1 $\frac{80}{6}$2	$\frac{80}{8}$1 $\frac{90}{3}$2	$\frac{70}{10}$3	$\frac{80}{8}$1 $\frac{90}{3}$2	$\frac{90}{3}$1 $\frac{95}{2}$2
7	Simple dead lifts	$\frac{50}{12}$1 $\frac{60}{10}$2	$\frac{60}{10}$3	$\frac{60}{10}$2 $\frac{70}{8}$1	$\frac{60}{10}$3	$\frac{60}{12}$1 $\frac{70}{10}$2	$\frac{70}{10}$3

Fig. 4.5 Example of a 6-week strength training program for volleyball. The coach or athlete may choose to add 1–2 more exercises for the arms and legs. The numbers in each cell refer to the percent of the 1 RM the athlete should be lifting, the number of repetitions, and the number of sets. For example, 70/8 3 means 70% 1 RM, 8 reps, 3 sets.

the athlete's strength or speed will improve their ability to generate power. A player may possess a very lean muscle mass and a tremendous amount of strength, yet lack the ability to contract those strong muscles quickly. To overcome this deficiency, a player must undergo training that will improve the rate of force development (power). In general, power training for volleyball employs methods of moving objects such as medicine balls, shot puts, heavy bags (10–30 kg bags) and plyometric training. Power training exercises are designed to recruit motor units more quickly, resulting in nervous system adaptation. Power training, then, is mainly focused on improving the rate of force development. Strength training increases the number and frequency of motor units discharged, while power training increases the rate at which the same motor units are recruited. Power-endurance involves the repeated performance of powerful jumps and bounds. In volleyball, players are required to repeat a strenuous activity only after a few seconds of game interruption. To be successful, players should have a high power output and have the ability to repeat this output a

minimum of 20–30 times per set. Players with a high level of power-endurance will have the capacity to maintain their jump height and stride quickness throughout the duration of a match.

Neuromuscular adaptation to power training leads to improved intermuscular coordination, which may be defined as the ability of agonist and antagonist muscles to cooperate and perform a movement efficiently. In order to make the movements even more effective, exercises employed in the power training phase should utilize or closely mimic the movement patterns most used in volleyball. In other words, power training should be as sport-specific as possible.

The ballistic method

The ballistic method of power training involves the use of weighted objects such as medicine balls that the athlete dynamically propels through a full range of available motion. Plyometric training represents a good example of ballistic training.

Ballistic exercises can be planned at the end of a

Table 4.3 Training parameters for the ballistic method (after Bompa 1999a).

Training parameters	Regimen
Load	Standard
No. of exercises	2–5
No. of reps per set	10–2
No. of sets per session	3–5
Rest interval	2–3 min
Speed of execution	Explosive
Frequency per week	2–4

training session or following the warm up depending on the training objectives. The fast, ballistic application of force is possible as a result of quick recruitment of fast-twitch muscle fibers and effective intermuscular coordination of the agonist and antagonist muscles. Therefore, it is necessary that the player be alert, rested, and motivated prior to performing the movements, since a rested central nervous system can transmit more powerful nerve impulses to the working muscles for quick contractions. The speed of contraction is the key to utilizing the benefits of this method, as the player must attempt to increase the speed constantly up to the release of the object. The number of repetitions is dependent on the speed of movement achieved. The number of exercises should remain low and the number of sets for each exercise should be set relatively high. The training load is dictated by the weight of the implements. Furthermore, as in any other power training method, the exercises selected should attempt to reproduce the movement patterns inherent in volleyball-specific skills. Table 4.3 lists the suggested training parameters for the ballistic method.

Power training for volleyball involves a vast array of methods and suggested programs, which seem to span an endless continuum. Like any other training method, a power training program must be individualized to meet the needs and strength abilities of a player. A variety of factors, including nutritional status, level of fatigue, and injury history should be considered before designing a power training program. What works for one athlete may not work, or may even be detrimental, for another athlete.

Plyometric training

Plyometric training is an extremely successful method of transforming strength into power. Only those who are extremely fit and have completed several years of strength training should perform plyometric exercises. As with most types of exercise, plyometric exercises range from those that are easy to perform to those that are extremely difficult to perform. This permits the athlete to progress through a program of progressive overload in order to promote neuromuscular adaptation to the demands of training and, with that, improved sporting performance.

Plyometric training consists of exercises in which muscle is loaded eccentrically (lengthening activation) followed immediately by a concentric (shortening) activation. Research has demonstrated that a muscle stretched prior to a shortening activation will contract forcefully and rapidly. This stretch–shortening cycle (Chapter 3) forms the physiological basis for plyometric training. While plyometric training is employed most commonly to train the lower body—particularly in jump training—the method can also be adapted to train the upper body in general and the shoulder girdle in particular. For example, medicine balls can be useful in improving the power of a volleyball player's spike or jump service.

Plyometric action relies on the muscle stretch reflex, which is mediated by the muscle spindle located in the muscle belly. The main purpose of the stretch reflex is to monitor the degree of muscle stretch and prevent overstretching. A plyometric exercise such as a drop jump requires a quick, reactive body movement to attain the power required for the action. Similarly, the quick backward action of an overhead throw provides the necessary muscle energy needed to propel the medicine ball forward.

Plyometric training causes muscular and neural changes that facilitate and enhance the development of rapid and powerful movements. Eccentrically loading a muscle stores potential energy within the series elastic component of the muscle. Similar in concept to a loaded spring, when released during the subsequent concentric muscular activation, this energy augments that energy generated by the contractile apparatus of the muscle fibers. A muscle will

Table 4.4 The five levels of intensity for plyometric exercises (Bompa 1996)

Intensity level	Type of exercises	Intensity of exercises	No. of reps and sets	No. of reps per training session	Rest interval between sets
1	Shock tension, high reactive jumps >60 cm	Maximum	8–5 × 10–20	120–150	8–10 min
2	Drop jumps 80–120 cm	Very high	5–5 × 5–15	75–150	5–7 min
3	Bounding exercises (on one or two legs)	Submaximum	3–25 × 5–15	50–250	3–5 min
4	Low reactive jumps 20–50 cm	Moderate	10–25 × 10–25	150–250	3–5 min
5	Low-impact jumps/throws (on spot or with implements)	Low	10–30 × 10–15	50–300	2–3 min

therefore contract more forcefully and quickly from a prestretched position. Furthermore, the more rapid the prestretch, the more forceful the concentric action. This forms the basis of plyometric training. Correct technique is essential. The shortening action should occur immediately after completion of the prestretch phase. The transition from the prestretch phase should be as smooth, continuous, and as swift as possible.

It is essential that the athlete have a solid base of strength training prior to adding plyometric training into their conditioning program. As a child must learn to walk before he or she runs, an individual must be strong before he or she is fast. Strength is simply the foundation of power. When introduced at the proper time in a training program, plyometric training will improve a player's muscular dynamics, reflex control, and neuromuscular potentiation.

Intensity levels for plyometric exercises
Five intensity levels can be applied in a plyometric training program. Table 4.4 illustrates the five intensity levels as previously described by Bompa (1996).

As the intensity "level" progresses from level 1 to 5 the intensity of exercises correspondingly decreases. The intensity of exercise is directly proportional to the height of the jump, the size of the load, and the length of the exercise. The higher the intensity the greater the neuromuscular response required to perform the movement. Furthermore, there is an inverse relationship between the numerical intensity level and the recommended rest interval between sets. In other words, the greater the neuromuscular

response required of the exercise, the longer the rest interval.

Plyometric exercises are fun to perform but because they demand a high level of concentration they are both vigorous and taxing. Impatience and the lack of discipline required to wait for the right moment for each exercise might prompt the athlete to incorporate high-impact exercises into their training program before they are physically ready to withstand the stress of such training. As with any training program, injury prevention and safety considerations should be foremost in the coach's or trainer's thoughts. Knowledge of the five levels of intensity will help in the selection of appropriate exercises and rest interval. The suggested number of repetitions and sets in Table 4.4 is for advanced athletes. The coach should resist the temptation to demand the same number of repetitions and sets from beginners, or from athletes with an inadequate foundation of strength. Progression through the five stages of intensities is a long-term proposition. The incorporation of low-impact exercises into the training program of young athletes for 2–4 years provides needed time for the progressive adaptation of ligaments, tendons, and the bony structure of the limbs involved. It also allows for the gradual preparation of the shock-absorbing sections of the body, such as the hips and spine (Fig. 4.6).

Microcycle training programs
A coach or trainer who is experienced and well versed in plyometric training should have the ability to prepare effective weekly plans, or "microcycles."

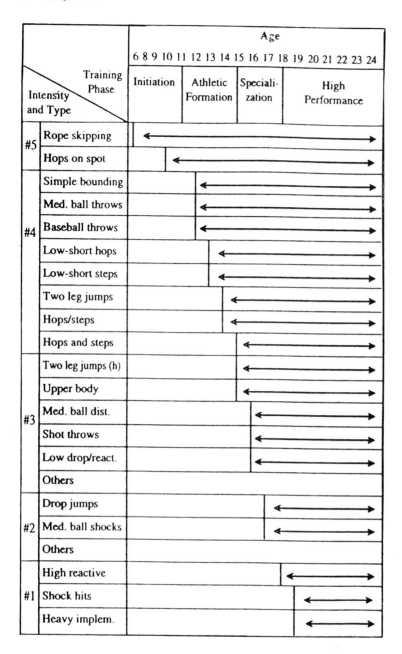

Intensity and Type	Training Phase	Age 6 8 9 10 11 12 13 14 15 16 17 18 19 20 21 22 23 24			
		Initiation	Athletic Formation	Speciali-zation	High Performance
#5	Rope skipping	←—————————————————————→			
	Hops on spot	←————————————————→			
#4	Simple bounding	←————————————→			
	Med. ball throws	←————————————→			
	Baseball throws	←————————————→			
	Low-short hops	←————————————→			
	Low-short steps	←————————————→			
	Two leg jumps	←——————————→			
	Hops/steps	←——————————→			
#3	Hops and steps	←————————→			
	Two leg jumps (h)	←————————→			
	Upper body	←————————→			
	Med. ball dist.	←——————→			
	Shot throws	←——————→			
	Low drop/react.	←——————→			
	Others				
#2	Drop jumps	←————→			
	Med. ball shocks	←————→			
	Others				
#1	High reactive	←——→			
	Shock hits	←——→			
	Heavy implem.	←——→			

Fig. 4.6 Long-term planning: recommended progression of plyometric exercises during athlete development. (From Bompa 1996.)

Figures 4.7–4.9 suggest three different volleyball microcycles. The type of training proposed reflects the need to alter the type of activities performed and the energy systems trained in order to achieve positive adaptations to training (for more information see Bompa 1999a).

Plyometric exercises
See Figures 4.10–4.21 for different plyometric exercises (note that the numbers in parentheses represent the intensity level, with 5 being the least difficult and 1 the most difficult).

MaxEx training

The development of strength should not be pursued in strict isolation from other methods of conditioning, particularly in volleyball where power development is the predominant goal of training. MaxEx training (maximum tension plus explosiveness) represents a dynamic combination of strength training loads and exercises intended to develop power. MaxEx training focuses on increasing the recruitment and discharge rate of the fast-twitch muscle fibers and on improving the player's ability to perform the explosive movements demanded by the sport of volleyball.

The exercises suggested below need not be performed year round. They can be planned at the end of the preparatory phase or, in the case of several strength phases, during the last phase. The incorporation of power training during the strength phase

Mon	Tues	Wed	Thurs	Fri	Sat	Sun
T S	T/TA	TA S	T	T/TA S	?	Off

Fig. 4.7 A suggested microcycle plan for the preparatory phase. T, technical training; TA, tactical training; ?, your choice to train on this day.

enhances speed and explosiveness to prepare athletes for the competitive phase. Combining strength with power must be done carefully and conservatively. Although many combinations are possible, remember that training has to be simple so athletes can focus on the main task of the workout or training phase.

A variation to the exercise in Fig. 4.22 is illustrated in Fig. 4.23. The player performs a drop jump (barbell on shoulders) with a quick concentric contraction followed by box plyometrics. A drop jump from 25 to 40 cm (10–15 inches) is maintained for 2 s. Once the spotters remove the barbell, the jumper performs plyometrics on and off a set of boxes or benches of the same height (Fig. 4.24).

Figures 4.25–4.28 give examples of other exercises employed in MaxEx training.

Strength training during the competitve phase

The strength and power derived from a comprehensive volleyball conditioning program can be maintained as long as the neuromuscular system retains the adaptations induced by the program. However, once strength training ends, the gains in strength,

Mon	Tues	Wed	Thurs	Fri	Sat	Sun
T P: 2 sets, 3–4 exercises	T/TA S: 1 set, 3 exercises P: 1–2 sets, 3–4 exercises	T PE: 2 sets, 4–5 exercises	Same as Tues	T Same as Wed	?	Off

Fig. 4.8 A suggested challenging late preparatory/competitive phase microcycle for elite-class volleyball players (note: no games are scheduled for the end of the week).

Mon	Tues	Wed	Thurs	Fri	Sat	Sun
Recovery Low-intensity, short workout	T P: 2 sets, 3–4 exercises	T/TA S: 1 set, 3–4 exercises PE: 1 set, 3–4 exercises	T/TA P: 2 sets, 3–4 exercises	Unloading Low-intensity TA training	Game	Off

Fig. 4.9 A suggested microcycle for the competitive (league games) phase with a scheduled game on the weekend. Note the importance of low-intensity training for Monday and Friday as a means of recovery and unloading, respectively. If the team travels on Friday, a 20–30 min warm up after arrival is strongly recommended.

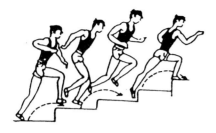

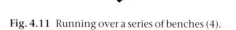

Fig. 4.11 Running over a series of benches (4).

Fig. 4.10 Running up two stairs (4).

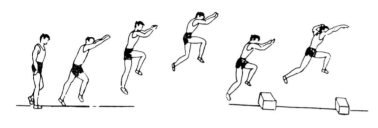

Fig. 4.12 Alternate- and single-leg jumps (1).

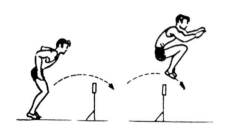

Fig. 4.13 Reactive jumps over hurdles (1).

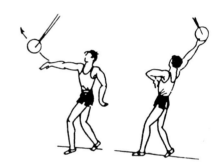

Fig. 4.14 One-arm overhead toss (3).

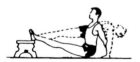

Fig. 4.15 Hip thrusts (3).

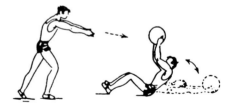

Fig. 4.16 Seated sit-up throw (2).

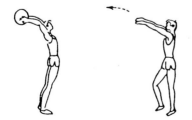

Fig. 4.17 Standing overhead throw (4).

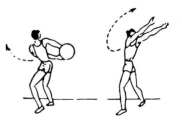

Fig. 4.18 Two-hand side throw (4).

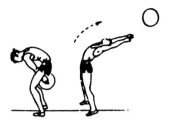

Fig. 4.19 Back throw (3).

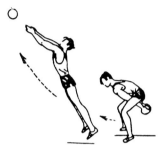

Fig. 4. 20 Scoop throw (3).

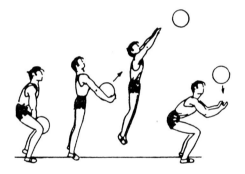

Fig. 4.21 Forward shot throw (3).

endurance, and power rapidly begin to dissipate as the athlete enters into a detraining state. A noticeable decrease in the contribution of strength to athletic performance may result. In order to avoid detraining during the competitive phase, the coach and athlete should plan a volleyball-specific strength-maintenance program. The maintenance of strength and other physiological gains during the competitive phase is a critical element to the success of any sport-specific training program. The coach must design a maintenance program that is once again synchronized with the physiological demands of the sport. For instance, since volleyball requires elements of strength, power, and power-endurance,

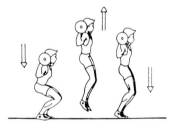

Fig. 4.22 Slow eccentric action of a half squat followed by an upward explosive concentric action. It is suggested that inexperienced players use dumbbells when performing this exercise. Experienced players may use a barbell. The suggested program for this variation is: load, 40–60%; number of reps, 4–6; number of sets, 1–4; rest interval between sets, 2–3 min. Be sure to keep the upper body vertical with the barbell tight on the shoulders. Place a heavy towel on the shoulders to avoid bruising. Absorb the shock of landing by contacting the ground first with the toes and balls of the feet, then the heels.

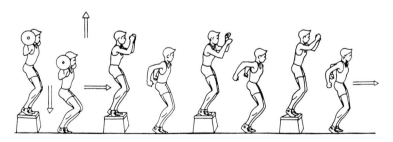

Fig. 4.23 A drop jump from 25 to 40 cm (10–15 inches) is maintained for 2 s; as soon as the spotters take the barbell off the shoulders, the player does plyometrics on and off a set of boxes or benches at the same height. Note that the use of dumbbells is suggested over barbells for the exercise. The suggested program is as follows: load, 40–80%; number of reps, 4–8; number of sets, 2–4; rest interval between sets, 2–4 min.

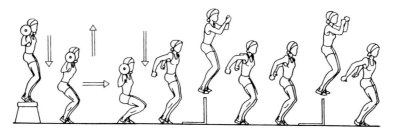

Fig. 4.24 A drop jump with a quick concentric action and slow eccentric action followed by bounding or jumping over objects. Note that dumbbells or heavy vests can replace the use of barbells. The suggested program is: load, 110–140% of 1 RM for one leg; number of reps, 2–4 with each leg, followed by 8–10 plyometrics; number of sets, 2–3; rest interval between sets, 2–4 min.

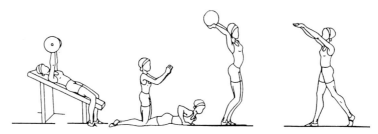

Fig. 4.25 Example of MaxEx training in which incline bench and drop push ups are combined with medicine ball overhead throws. Suggested program: load, 70–90%; number of reps, 2–4 for bench press, 8–10 for push ups, and 10–12 for medicine ball overhead throws.

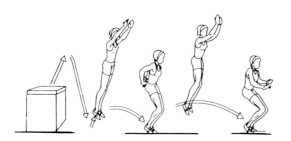

Fig. 4.26 Exercise for reactive power followed by several double-speed hops.

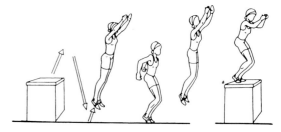

Fig. 4.27 Reactive jumps from a high box onto a high box.

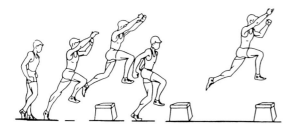

Fig. 4.28 One-leg reactive jumps over several boxes or benches.

the most important decision for designing the program is not which of the three elements should be maintained, but rather in what proportion and how to best integrate them into ongoing training.

In volleyball, where power is the dominant goal of training, both strength and power should be maintained. As far as power-endurance is concerned, the specific training of repetitive spiking and blocking, in addition to power training in the gym, should suffice to meet the particular power-endurance demands of volleyball. Therefore, a volleyball strength training maintenance program should emphasize strength and power in a ratio of 1:4. It is especially important to appreciate that the composition of the maintenance program depends on the duration of the competitive phase. The longer the competitive phase, the more important it is to emphasize strength so as to maintain the element of power. Detraining of strength will negatively impact on both power and power-endurance.

During the maintenance phase, one should apply the same training methods as previously suggested. The number of exercises performed must be minimal and address the specific prime movers and skills that are used in volleyball. Two or three, 20–30 min strength training sessions per week should be planned. Obviously, the frequency of strength training sessions will depend on the competition schedule. If no games are scheduled on the weekend, one may perform two or possibly three strength training sessions. If a game is planned on the weekend then one (maximum two) short strength training sessions can be planned, normally in the early part of the week.

The number of sets performed per exercise usually falls between one and four depending on whether power or power-endurance is being trained. For power and strength, 2–4 sets are possible due to the low number of required repetitions. The rest interval should be longer than normally suggested, primarily because the athlete should recover almost entirely during the break. The intent of the maintenance phase is stabilization and retention of performance and not aggravation of fatigue. Therefore, a longer rest interval is required for full recovery.

Strength training during the transition phase

The transition phase, which is often inappropriately called the "off season," represents a linkage between two annual cycles. The major objectives of this phase are to facilitate psychological rest, relaxation, and biological regeneration as well as to maintain an acceptable level of general physical preparedness. Therefore, the duration of this phase cannot be

longer than 4–6 weeks otherwise athletes will inevitably enter a state of detraining. During the transition phase, athletes should train two or three times per week. Maintaining an adequate level of fitness will make the start of training camp more efficient and will permit athletes to quickly resume normal "in season" training patterns.

During the transition phase, it is recommended that the player engage in exercises that work the entire body. The emphasis of transition training (or compensation training) is on recovery, which is achieved by reducing the number of repetitions (8–10) and sets (2–3), in addition to the load (50–60% IRM) during strength training. If indicated the athlete should also perform prescribed rehabilitation (or prerehabilitation) exercises. Transition training is not meant to be stressful; indeed it should be relaxed in order to promote both physical and psychological recovery and avoid overtraining.

Aerobic conditioning

This chapter has focused primarily on strength training, which by nature taxes and develops the power and anaerobic glycolytic energy systems. As discussed in Chapter 2, volleyball athletes will benefit from a sound aerobic conditioning base. However, studies have shown that training both systems during a given mesocycle may prove counterproductive and may even predispose the athlete to overtraining. It would therefore seem advisable to emphasize power development throughout the majority of the training program, while relying on "on court" activities or periodic aerobic conditioning sessions (1–2 times per week) to build and maintain the athlete's aerobic fitness level. Aerobic conditioning may also assume greater importance during the transition phase, and on days of scheduled recovery or "active rest" during the competition phase.

Conclusion

Conditioning for peak volleyball performance requires a systematic approach using a periodized training methodology that is planned around preparatory and competitive phases. The complexities of the sport of volleyball demand a year-round training and conditioning program. The physical attributes of strength, power, power-endurance, agility, and speed can be effectively trained through a periodized training program. The application of a periodized model for all aspects of volleyball including the physical, technical, tactical, and psychological elements of the sport, will further the development of the athletes and the team as a whole, producing a more dynamic and spectacular sport.

References

Bompa, T. (1996) *Power Training for Sport: Plyometrics for Maximum Power Development.* Mosaic Press/Coaching Association of Canada, Oakville, WA.

Bompa, T. (1999a) *Periodization Training for Sports: Program for Peak Strength in 35 Sports.* Human Kinetics, Champaign, IL.

Bompa, T. (1999b) *Periodization: Theory and Methodology of Training.* Human Kinetics, Champaign, IL.

Fees, M., Decker, T., Snyder-Mackler, L. & Axe, M.J. (1998) Upper extremity weight-training modifications for the injured athlete. *American Journal of Sports Medicine* **26** (5), 732–742.

Recommended reading

American College of Sports Medicine (2001) The team physician and conditioning of athletes for sports: a consensus statement. *Medicine and Science in Sports and Exercise* **33** (10), 1789–1793.

Kraemer, W.J. & Häkkinen. K. (eds) (2002) *Strength Training for Sport.* Blackwell Science, Oxford.

Chapter 5
Optimal nutrition and hydration for the volleyball athlete

D. Enette Larson-Meyer

Introduction

A proper diet and adequate hydration are essential to optimal training and athletic performance, as well as to good health in general. Volleyball athletes at all levels—from secondary school to Olympic calibre alike—require a diet that provides adequate energy, carbohydrate, protein, fat, vitamins, minerals, and fluid. Although the composition of an athlete's diet may vary based on several factors (including the metabolic demands of the sport and the level of competition) most athletes can satisfy their nutritional requirements by consuming a diet rich in a variety of plant products including grain products, fruits, vegetables, and protein-rich plant foods. In order to provide variety or satisfy personal preferences, the diet may also contain several servings per day of meat or fish, low-fat dairy products, and small amounts of nuts. This chapter will review the energy, micronutrient, and vitamin, mineral, and fluid requirements of the volleyball athlete and provide tips for maintaining nutrition and hydration status during heavy training and competition. The chapter will also briefly discuss weight reduction and the special nutritional concerns of the female volleyball athlete.

Energy and macronutrient requirements

Energy

Daily energy or caloric needs vary considerably among individual volleyball athletes, depending on the athlete's body size, body composition, gender, training regimen, and general activity pattern. The energy cost of volleyball play has been estimated at $0.142 \, \text{kcal} \cdot \text{kg}^{-1} \cdot \text{min}^{-1}$ $(0.596 \, \text{kJ} \cdot \text{kg}^{-1} \cdot \text{min}^{-1})$ for vigorous play and $0.064 \, \text{kcal} \cdot \text{kg}^{-1} \cdot \text{min}^{-1}$ $(0.269 \, \text{kJ} \cdot \text{kg}^{-1} \cdot \text{min}^{-1})$ for moderate recreational play (calories are mainly used in this chapter, but these can be converted to joules using the formula: $1 \, \text{kcal} = 4.2 \, \text{kJ}$). When coupled with the metabolic demands of strength training and conditioning, it is reasonable to conclude that the daily energy requirement for a volleyball athlete is considerably higher than for a more sedentary individual. Furthermore, a small female setter would be expected to have a lower daily energy expenditure than a large male middle blocker. Unlike several other sports, the total daily energy expenditure of volleyball athletes has not been measured by accurate, free-living techniques (e.g. doubly labelled water). Nevertheless, the average daily energy expenditure for female volleyball players can be estimated to be between 2,400 and 4,200 kcal (10,080–17,640 kJ) and between 2,800 and 5,000 kcal (11,760–21,000 kJ) for male players. Of course, more elite-level athletes are likely to have

Box 5.1 Estimation of daily energy expenditure of a 70 kg student volleyball athlete (20% body fat) who practices for 90 min and weight trains for 30 min daily. Lean body mass = 70 kg × (1 − 0.20) = 56 kg.

Energy expenditure	Formula	Example
Resting energy expenditure (REE)	REE = 22 × Fat Free Mass (kg)	22 × 56 = 1,232 kcal
Energy expenditure during non-training physical activity (NTEE)	Light activity = 1.3 × REE Moderate activity = 1.5 × REE Heavy activity = 1.5 × REE	Assume light occupational activity (student): 0.3 × 1,232 kcal = 370 kcal
Energy expenditure during training regimen (TEE)	Use energy expenditure of physical activities chart (found in many nutrition or exercise physiology texts)	A 70 kg athlete uses $10.1\,kcal\cdot min^{-1}$ for vigorous volleyball practice and $8.1\,kcal\cdot min^{-1}$ for weight training: $10.1\,kcal\cdot min^{-1} \times 90\,min = 909\,kcal$; $8.1\,kcal\cdot min \times 30\,min = 243\,kcal$
Total daily energy expenditure (DEE)	DEE = REE + NTEE + TEE	$1,232 + 370 + 909 + 243 = 2,754\,kcal\cdot day^{-1}$

higher energy demands. As a comparison, energy expenditure assessed by doubly labelled water is shown to vary from $2,600\,kcal\cdot day^{-1}$ in female swimmers to approximately $8,500\,kcal\cdot day^{-1}$ in male cyclists participating in the Tour de France (Goran 1995).

Daily energy expenditure (DEE) can be approximated by directly estimating total DEE, or by estimating the individual components of DEE including energy expenditure at rest (REE), as well as energy expenditure during training (TEE) and during non-training (NTEE) activities. For example, figures from the American Heart Association can be used to directly estimate that athletes who perform moderate activity (weekend recreational athletes) need approximately $33\,kcal\cdot kg^{-1}\cdot day^{-1}$ to maintain body mass whereas very active individuals (exercising three times per week) need $35\,kcal\cdot kg^{-1}\cdot day^{-1}$. By this method, competitive athletes need approximately $37.5\,kcal\cdot kg^{-1}\cdot day^{-1}$, or more. For athletes, however, the component method is the preferred and more accurate means of estimating DEE and is shown in Box 5.1.

Meeting energy needs is the first nutritional priority for all athletes. Energy balance is achieved when energy intake (the sum of energy from food, fluids, and supplements consumed) equals energy expenditure (the sum of energy expended for resting metabolism, activities of daily living, and training and competition). While some athletes may need to tilt the energy balance one way or the other to gain

or lose body mass, it is particularly important that athletes maintain adequate energy intake during periods of high-intensity training or competition to permit adequate tissue repair and remodeling. Sufficient energy consumption is important for maximizing the effect of training, maintaining body mass, and maintaining good health. Inadequate energy intake can result in loss of muscle mass, menstrual dysfunction, loss of or failure to gain bone density, and an increased risk of injury, illness, and fatigue.

It should be noted that some athletes have trouble meeting energy needs. This may be due to excessively high energy requirements, food choices that are bulky or too high in fiber, or hectic schedules that do not allow the athlete enough time to eat. Striving for 6–8 meals or snacks per day and executing adequate planning ("brown bag" lunches, snacks packed in the gym bag, etc.) may help remedy this situation. When appropriate, athletes can increase energy intake and decrease fiber by consuming one-third to one-half of their cereal/grain servings from refined rather than whole grain sources and by replacing some high-fiber fruit/vegetable servings with juice servings. The Food Guide Pyramid developed by the United States Department of Agriculture (USDA), Modified Food Guide Pyramid developed by Applegate (Figs 5.1 and 5.2), or eating plans, such the one developed by Houtkooper (1992), may be helpful for educating athletes to meet their energy and other nutrient needs.

Carbohydrate

Carbohydrates should make up the bulk of the volleyball athlete's nutritional regimen. While carbohydrate, fat, and, to a lesser extent, protein can be used to fuel the activities of volleyball, carbohydrate is the only fuel that can sustain high-level activity such as continuous jumping and intense court play, and which can also be used by the central nervous system. Carbohydrate (glycogen) stores in the muscle and liver are limited and become depleted during intense intermittent activities common to both training and competition. Depleted muscle and liver glycogen stores correlate with muscle and whole-body fatigue.

Diets high in carbohydrate are important because

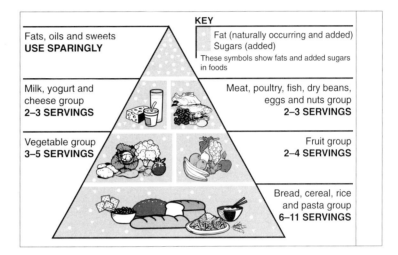

Fig. 5.1 The USDA food guide pyramid.

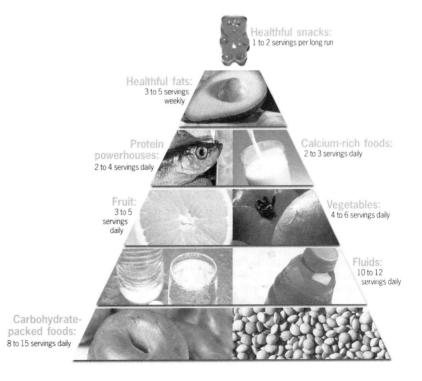

Fig. 5.2 The Runner's Food Guide Pyramid. (Courtesy of Liz Applegate and reprinted with permission of Runner's World magazine.)

they maintain muscle and liver glycogen stores and thereby optimize performance during intermittent and short-duration, high-intensity exercise. For the volleyball athlete, this translates into a longer playing (or training) time before fatigue, and, most likely, the maintenance of jumping potential towards the end of a long match or tournament. Also of interest to volleyball players is the ability of carbohydrate (vs fat) to delay the onset of fatigue by preserving the bioenergetic state of exercising muscle (the ratio of creatine phosphate, CP, to inorganic phosphate) (Larson *et al*. 1994). This could ultimately effect regeneration of adenosine triphosphate (ATP) for the ATP-CP system, which (as discussed in Chapter 2) is the energy system used primarily for power and speed activities lasting less than 10 s, e.g. jump serving, spiking, blocking, or digging.

Volleyball athletes at all levels may benefit from education on carbohydrate utilization, recommended daily carbohydrate consumption, and

dietary sources of carbohydrate. The recommended dietary intake of carbohydrate is from 6 to 10 g per kilogram of body mass per day (American College of Sports Medicine 2000). Players with higher energy demands, such as collegiate or Olympic-level athletes in heavy training, may benefit from a higher carbohydrate intake and should strive for the upper range of close to $9-10 \, g \cdot kg^{-1} \cdot day^{-1}$ g. Conversely, smaller female athletes and those participating at a level that demands less training, e.g. at the recreational, club, or secondary school level, may require only $6-7 \, g \cdot kg^{-1} \cdot day^{-1}$.

A general understanding of the carbohydrate content of foods and beverages (Table 5.1) combined with information provided on the food label (which in the United States lists the carbohydrate content of most foods in grams per serving) should help the volleyball athlete meet their recommended carbohydrate intake. Knowledge of carbohydrate sources is also useful in assuring adequate carbohydrate

Selected foods	Portion	Carbohydrate (g)
Breakfast cereal, cold	1/3–1/2 cup (varies)	15–20
Breakfast cereal, hot	1/2 cup	15
Grits, plain	1/2 cup	15
Pancake	12.5 cm, thin	15
Bun or English muffin	1/2	15
Bagel	60–85 g	30–45
Bread, sliced	1 slice	15
Roll	1 small (30 g)	15
Rice	1/3 cup	15
Corn	1/2 cup	15
Pasta, cooked	1/2 cup	15
Potato, mashed	1/2 cup	15
Potato, baked	1 medium	30
Legumes (black-eyed peas, pinto and kidney beans, etc.)	1/3 cup	15
Fruit, all	1/2 cup	15
Orange, peach, pear	1 medium	15
Apple or banana	1 large	30
Fruit, dried	1/3–1/2 cup	60
Vegetables (non-starchy)	1/2 cup	6
Milk	1 cup	12
Yogurt, fruited	1 cup	40–45
Fluid replacement beverages	1 cup	15–19
Fruit juice or lemonade	1 cup	30
Soda	355 mL (12 oz)	40–45
Sports bar	1 bar	40–60
Sugar	1 tsp	4
Jam, jelly, honey, syrup	1 tsp	15

Table 5.1 Approximate carbohydrate content of selected foods and beverages.

intake before, during, and after exercise. Occasionally counting carbohydrate intake at a meal, snack, or over the course of a day may further assist athletes in meeting these guidelines. When combined with a training log or performance feedback from a coach, this activity should make the athlete aware of the connection between carbohydrate intake and performance. For example a low carbohydrate intake on a particular day may have been associated with light-headedness or "dead" legs after a training session.

Protein

The protein needs of athletes vary according to the type of activity and the level of training. The protein needs of the recreational or club volleyball athlete who plays several times a week are most likely met by the recommended daily allowance (RDA, as established by the United States Food and Drug Administration) of 0.8 g of protein per kilogram of body mass per day. The protein requirements of more heavily trained athletes, however, are higher than the RDA. According to a recent joint position statement from the American College of Sports Medicine (ACSM), the American Dietetic Association, and the Dietitians of Canada (2000), endurance athletes need $1.2–1.4 \, g \cdot kg^{-1} \cdot day^{-1}$, whereas resistance and strength-trained athletes may require as much as $1.6–1.7 \, g \cdot kg^{-1} \cdot day^{-1}$. The rational for the additional required protein during training results from the need to repair exercise-induced microdamage to muscle fibers, the small use of protein for fuel during exercise, and the need for additional protein to support muscle development. Thus, the protein needs of volleyball athletes in heavy training are likely to be somewhere in the range of $1.2–1.7 \, g \cdot kg^{-1} \cdot day^{-1}$, and may vary depending on training periodization.

Providing the diet is adequate in energy intake, protein requirements can generally be met through diet alone without supplements such as protein or amino acid powders, bars, shakes, or tablets. This is true for both omnivorous as well as vegetarian athletes. Athletes who prefer to eat little or no animal products can obtain adequate protein by meeting energy needs and consuming a variety of plant-based protein-rich foods such as legumes, grains, nuts, and seeds. Table 5.2 provides a general

Table 5.2 Approximate protein content of selected foods and beverages.

Food	Portion	Protein (g)
Beef	28 g	7
Egg, whole	1 large	7
Fish	28 g	7
Lamb	28 g	7
Pork	28 g	7
Cheese, medium and hard	28 g	7
Cheese, cottage	1/4 cup	8
Milk, all	1 cup	8
Yogurt, all	1 cup	8
Legumes (most beans and peas)	1/2 cup cooked	7
Tofu, firm	1 cup	20
Tofu, soft	1 cup	10
Vegetarian 'burgers'	1 patty	8–16
Peanut butter	2 tbsp	7
Nuts, most	2 tbsp	7
Bread, grains, rice, pasta	1 serving	2–3
Vegetables, most	1/2 cup cooked	2–3

list of protein-rich foods. Although surveys have shown that most athletes easily meet their protein requirements, this list can be used as a reference by athletes concerned about their dietary protein intake (in conjunction with food label information).

Fat

Fat is a necessary component of the diet, providing essential components of cell membranes, essential fatty acids, and associated nutrients such as vitamins E, A, and D. Dietary fat should make up the remainder of energy intake after the athlete's carbohydrate and protein needs are met. A general guideline is that fat should provide approximately 20–30% of the athlete's daily energy intake. However, the point should be made that athletes with high-energy needs can still meet their carbohydrate and protein requirements on a diet that provides 30–35% of energy from fat (ACSM 2000). For example, a 70 kg athlete expending 5,000 kcal meets carbohydrate and protein needs on a diet which provides approximately 35% of their energy from fat (70 kg × 10 g carbohydrate/kg = 700 g or 2,800 kcal from carbohydrate; 70 kg × 1.5 g protein/kg = 119 g or 476 kcal from protein; 5,000 kcal minus 2,800 kcal from carbohydrate and 476 kcal from protein = 1724 kcal from fat; 1724 kcal from fat divided by 5,000 total kcal × 100 = 34.5% of calories from fat). In this particular case, however, it is recommended that the athlete consume foods that are high in mono- and polyunsaturated fatty acids such as nuts, seeds, nut butters, tahini, avocados, olives, olive oil, sesame oil, and canola oil, and that they avoid foods high in saturated fatty acids such as fatty meats, lard, butter, full-fat dairy products, and most processed "fast food" products.

On the other hand, the volleyball athlete should understand that their diet should not be too low in fat. Recent studies have noted that diets too low in fat (in which fat comprises less than 15% of the total daily energy consumed) may elevate serum triglycerides, compromise the immune function, contribute to exercise-induced amenorrhea, and possibly impair performance by reducing intramuscular fat deposits that are crucial for supplying free fatty acids to skeletal muscle during endurance exercise. It is a misconception that calorically balanced diets which contain dietary fat promote weight gain, increasing adiposity or obesity.

Micronutrients: mineral and vitamin requirements

Vitamins and minerals, while not energy sources themselves, play an important role in energy production, synthesis of hemoglobin (the oxygen-carrying component of red blood cells), maintenance of bone health, immune function, and protection of cells and tissues from oxidative damage. They also assist in the building and repair of muscle tissue following exercise. Most athletes can meet their need for vitamins and minerals from a diet providing adequate energy and consisting of a variety of wholesome foods. Due to hectic training and work/school schedules, however, athletes may be prone to making poor dietary choices — resulting in a deficient intake of many vitamins and minerals. Surveys of various groups of athletes have suggested that intake of iron, calcium, and zinc is often insufficient, particularly among female athletes. While food choice is important, the athletes at greatest risk

for poor vitamin and mineral status are those who restrict energy intake, employ severe weight-loss practices, consciously eliminate one or more food groups from their diet, or consume excessive quantities of processed foods that are low in vitamins and minerals. Volleyball athletes participating in these types of practices should be encouraged to improve their eating habits, but may also need to use a multivitamin and mineral supplement to improve their overall micronutrient status.

Because it is always preferred that athletes improve their nutritional status through better food choices, the remainder of this section will briefly discuss the micronutrients that tend to be low in athletes as a group.

Calcium

Regular exercise has not been shown to increase calcium requirements above that of the general population. Thus, adult volleyball athletes should strive for the recommended intake of 1,000 mg of calcium per day, and those under 18 should strive for 1300 mg · day. Evidence suggests that amenorrheic athletes (those not experiencing a menstrual cycle for at least 3 months) may require an intake of 1500 mg · day to retain calcium balance. Low calcium intake has been associated with an increased risk of stress fractures, decreased bone mineral content, and decreased bone density, particularly in anemorrheic athletes.

Eumenorrheic (regularly menstruating) athletes can meet calcium requirements by including several servings of dairy products and/or calcium-containing plant foods daily. Plant foods that are rich in absorbable calcium include low-oxalate green leafy vegetables (collard, mustard, and turnip greens), calcium-set tofu, fortified soymilk, textured vegetable protein, tahini, certain legumes, and fortified orange and other fruit juices. The approximate calcium content of selected calcium-containing foods is presented in Table 5.3. Depending on their energy intake and food choices, amenorrheic female athletes may need to use fortified foods or calcium supplements to meet calcium requirements. Calcium carbonate and calcium citrate are both well-absorbed sources commonly used in supplements, but calcium carbonate is generally

Table 5.3 Calcium content of selected foods and beverages (Vegetarian Nutrition Dietetic Practice Group 1995; Pennington 1998).

Food	Portion	Calcium (mg)
Milk	1 cup	300
Yogurt	1 cup	400
Cheese, cheddar	28 g	200
Soymilk, fortified	1 cup	200–500
Bok choy	1/2 cup, cooked	79
Collard, dandelion, mustard, turnip greens and kale	1/2 cup, cooked	70–100
Almonds	1/4 cup	94
Tahini (sesame butter)	2 tbsp	128
Juice, calcium fortified	1 cup	100–300 (varies)
Cereal, calcium fortified (e.g. Total)	28 g	200–250

less expensive. Recent evidence has suggested that long-term supplementation with calcium carbonate does not compromise iron status in iron-replete adults (Minihane & Fairweather-Tait 1998), but studies have also indicated it is preferable to ingest calcium supplements at bedtime rather than with iron-containing meals. Because vitamin D is also required for adequate calcium absorption, regulation of serum calcium levels and promotion of bone health, a calcium supplement that also contains vitamin D is advised. In general, indoor volleyball athletes may be at risk of poor vitamin D status if exposure to the sun is limited (especially in northern climates).

Iron

All athletes, and female athletes in particular, are at risk of iron depletion and iron deficiency anemia. Iron loss is increased in some athletes due to gastrointestinal bleeding (perhaps stemming from the regular use of antiinflammatory medications), heavy sweating, and destruction of red blood cells due to the stress of repetitive foot strikes from running and jumping. However, the two most common causes of iron deficiency among athletes are insufficient dietary iron intake or reduced absorption. Iron is found in both animal and plant foods, but the form found in most animal foods (heme iron) is better absorbed than that found in plant foods (elemental iron). Iron deficiency can lead to impaired performance, fatigue, anemia, abnormal temperature regulation, and decreased resistance to infection.

Table 5.4 Iron content of selected foods (Graig 1994; Pennington 1998).

Food	Portion	Iron (mg)
Beef, ground, extra lean	100 g	2.4
Beef tenderloin	100 g	3.4
Chicken, white	100 g	1.2
Chicken, dark	100 g	1.4
Fish, cod	85 g	0.3
Fish, trout	85 g	1.6
Fish, tuna, light	85 g	1.3
Lamb, leg	100 g	2.1
Pork loin	100 g	1.3
Soybeans	1/2 cup cooked	2.7
Lima beans	1/2 cup cooked	2.0
Red kidney beans	1/2 cup cooked	1.8
Lentils	1/2 cup cooked	1.6
Peas	1/2 cup cooked	1.5
Oatmeal	1 cup cooked	1.7
Pasta, enriched	1 cup cooked	1.4
Brown rice	1 cup cooked	0.8
Whole-wheat bread	1 slice	0.8
Collard greens	1/2 cup cooked	1.0
Tomato	1 medium	0.8
Potato	1 medium	0.8
Sunflower seeds	28 g	2.2
Almonds	28 g	1.3
Peanuts	28 g	1.0
Prunes	5 large	1.7
Watermelon	1 slice	1.5
Strawberries	5 large	1.0
Raisins	28 g	1.0

Volleyball athletes can meet iron needs by regularly including iron-rich foods in the diet. The approximate iron content of selected iron-rich foods is presented in Table 5.4. Iron absorption from plant sources can be enhanced by concurrently consuming foods containing vitamin C (citrus fruit or juice, tomatoes, melon, etc.). Iron absorption from plant sources, however, can be inhibited by excessive intake of tea, coffee, milk, or soda. Volleyball athletes concerned about dietary iron intake may want to take a multivitamin and mineral supplement containing iron. An athlete should not take iron supplements alone unless prescribed or monitored by his/her physician. In fact, since the Food and Drug Administration (FDA) and other governmental agencies do not regulate the manufacture of dietary supplements, it is advisable for athletes to inform their team physician of all supplements they may be consuming.

Zinc

Several studies have reported altered zinc status in athletes during heavy training. This finding, coupled with the reportedly low zinc intake among athletes, has prompted concern that some athletes may be at risk for compromised zinc status. Although more research is needed in this area, published studies have reported that zinc supplementation does not influence zinc levels during periods of heavy training, and results in no apparent improvement in athletic performance during these intervals. Food sources of zinc include meat, poultry, fish, legumes, hard cheeses, milk, whole grain products, wheat germ, fortified cereals, nuts, tofu, and miso.

Antioxidants

Mounting evidence suggests that vitamins C and E, in addition to β-carotene and other phytochemicals, may protect against exercise-induced "oxidative stress." Supplementation with antioxidants appears to reduce oxidative damage to cell membranes (lipid peroxidation) but has not been shown to enhance exercise performance. Theoretically, dietary antioxidants should be expected to enhance recovery, and attenuate the oxidative damage that occurs with heavy training. While it remains controversial whether recreational or elite athletes might benefit from antioxidant supplementation, there is little doubt that athletes should ingest foods rich in antioxidants. An abundance of natural antioxidants are readily obtained from a diet containing a variety of fruits, vegetables, whole grains, legumes (particularly soy foods), nuts, and seeds.

Fluid requirements

Adequate fluid intake during exercise is required to optimize performance and reduce the risk of heat-related illness. In active individuals, the total daily fluid requirement must replace fluid lost via the urinary, gastrointestinal, and respiratory tracts as well as that lost via the skin due to sweating and insensible losses. Sweat rates will vary depending on variables such as body size, exercise intensity, ambient temperature, humidity, and acclimatization (well-trained individuals sweat more), but can exceed $1.8 \, L \cdot h^{-1}$. In addition to water, sweat also contains significant amounts of sodium (approximately $1 \, g \cdot L^{-1}$) and potassium, and small amounts of iron, calcium, copper, magnesium, and zinc.

Exercise performance is optimal when athletes maintain fluid balance during exercise and is conversely impaired with progressive dehydration. Generally, it is recommended that athletes attempt to remain well hydrated before, during, and after exercise. Both water and "sport drinks" such as Gatorade and PowerAde can replace fluid losses. However, the ACSM recommends that the fluids consumed during exercise be cool and flavored (to enhance palatability and increase voluntary fluid intake), contain carbohydrate to enhance performance, and include sodium chloride to promote rehydration (American College of Sports Medicine 1996). Certainly, the promotion of voluntary fluid intake is one of the most important factors in ensuring adequate hydration in individual athletes. In an interesting study of elite Australian basketball, netball, and soccer athletes, Broad *et al.* (1996) found that the factors influencing fluid replacement during exercise included provision of an individual water bottle to each athlete, proximity to water bottles during training sessions, encouragement to drink, duration and number of breaks or substitutions, rules of the game, and the athlete's awareness of their own sweat rate. These findings should be helpful to volleyball coaches at all levels and may help to optimize fluid intake in volleyball athletes.

Nutrition before, during and after exercise

Before exercise

The meal before a competition or training session should provide carbohydrate and adequate fluids in order to prevent both hunger and gastrointestinal distress. Studies have shown that consumption of between 1 and 5 g of carbohydrate per kilogram body mass 1–4 h before endurance exercise has the potential to improve endurance performance by as much as 14%, and is also thought to benefit high-intensity athletic activity lasting up to several hours. General guidelines are to consume $1–2 g^{-1} \cdot kg$ between 1 and 2 h before exercise or $3–4 g \cdot kg$ approximately 4 h before exercise. Volleyball athletes can prepare their pregame meal from a list of recommended menus according to their game or match times and individual preferences or tolerances. Boxes 5.2 and 5.3 give specific suggestions and ideas for pre-event breakfasts, lunches, and dinners. Within these guidelines, athletes should consume familiar, well-tolerated, high-carbohydrate meals that are relatively low in sodium, fat, simple sugars, and fiber. Some athletes report reflux or other gastrointestinal problems with milk, raw sulfur-containing vegetables, onions, garlic and spicy condiments. In addition, the ACSM and National Athletic Trainers Association recommend drinking 400–600 mL of fluid 2–3 h before a bout of exercise. Guidelines for special circumstances such as nausea and rebound hypoglycemia are also presented in Box 5.4.

Supplementation during exercise

Carbohydrate ingestion at a rate of between 30 and $60 g \cdot h^{-1}$ has been shown to benefit performance during intermittent, high-intensity activities such as sprinting and soccer. While studies specific to volleyball have not been conducted, it is speculated that carbohydrate consumption should prevent fatigue in the latter part of a match or long practices. This is particularly important during tournament play for those athletes who play the majority of each match. Consumption of fluids during matches is a key to preventing dehydration. Dehydration can drastically impair performance and can also have serious health consequences. To prevent dehydration, the ACSM recommends that athletes drink enough fluid during exercise to replace that which is lost through sweating (American College of Sports Medicine 1996). A typical sweat rate is between 1 and $1.5 L \cdot h^{-1}$, and is even higher during workouts in a hot and humid gym. Ingestion of a sports drink containing the recommended concentration of 6–8% carbohydrate by volume $(g \cdot mL^{-1})$ easily meets carbohydrate requirements while simultaneously meeting fluid needs. Alternatively, solid foods rich in carbohydrate work equally well providing they are ingested with sufficient quantities of water. For example, an athlete who prefers water over sports drinks should consume approximately 240 mL (8 ounces) of water with every 15 g of carbohydrate ingested (producing, in effect, a 6% solution). Box 5.5 provides a list of nutritious foods that make great snacks during and between matches.

Postexercise nutrition

Glycogen stores can be completely depleted at the end of a hard match or practice. Consumption of carbohydrate within 20–30 min of the completion of exercise is essential to begin replenishing muscle glycogen stores. Research has shown that muscle glycogen can be replenished within 24 h, providing the postevent intake and overall diet is high in carbohydrate. Low muscle glycogen stores can impair subsequent performance. The current recommendation to replace muscle glycogen and ensure rapid recovery is to consume 1.5 g of carbohydrate per kilogram of body mass within the first 30 min after exercise, and again every 2 h over a 4–6 h period. Since hard exercise and competition often impairs appetite, it is often easier for the athlete to consume fresh fruit and/or carbohydrate-containing beverages. This regimen will allow athletes to begin replenishing their muscle glycogen while the team showers and travels to the postgame meal. The regimen is imperative when the team is playing matches spaced 24–48 h apart (see Box 5.3). To replace lost body fluids during this period, athletes should consume at least 1 L (preferably closer to 1.5 L) of fluid for every kilogram of body mass lost. Volleyball

Box 5.2 Pre-event meal guidelines and suggestions.

Morning matches. Players should eat a hearty, high-carbohydrate dinner and a bedtime snack the night before the match. Breakfast should provide approximately 1–2 g of carbohydrate per kilogram of body mass and should be consumed approximately 1.5–2 h prior to warm-up time. Thus for athletes weighing 60–90 kg the breakfast should contain at least 60–90 g of carbohydrate (1 g · kg^{-1}) and c.250–400 kcal. Higher amounts of carbohydrate (2 g · kg^{-1}) are for longer events (tournaments) and athletes with higher energy needs.

Afternoon matches. Players should eat a hearty, high

carbohydrate dinner and a bedtime snack the night before the match. A carbohydrate-filled breakfast up to 500–600 kcal. and a light lunch that provides approximately 1 g carbohydrate · kg^{-1}. The pre-event lunch should be consumed approximately 4 h after breakfast and 1.5–2 h before warm-up time.

Evening matches. Athletes will need a carbohydrate-rich breakfast and lunch. A light snack that provides close to 1 g carbohydrate · kg^{-1} should be consumed close to 1.5 h before warm-up time.

Pre-event breakfast meal ideas containing 60–90 g carbohydrate

1	1-11/2 cups of oatmeal*	30–45	*Optional:	1 tsp sugar
	1/2 cup fruit	15–30		1/4 cup milk
	1/2 cup fruit juice	15		1 tsp margarine
	2–2.5 cups water			
2	2 slices of toast*	30	*Optional:	2 tsp jelly
	1 tsp margarine (1/2 tsp each)			additional 1 tsp margarine
	Banana or 1 cup fruit	30		
	1 cup fruit juice	30		
	2 cups water			
3	Bagel, large*	45	*Optional:	2 tsp jelly
	1/2–1 cup fruit	15–30		1 tsp margarine
	2–2.5 cups water			
4	1 cup grits, no pepper	30		
	1–2 slices toast	15–30		
	1/2–1 cup fruit juice	15–30		
	2–2.5 cups water			

Pre-event lunch meal and snack ideas containing 60–90 g carbohydrate

1	2–3 slices of bread	30–45	Optional:	mustard or light
	28–57 g lean meat			mayonaise if tolerated
	1–1 1/2 cups fruit juice	30–45		
	2–2.5 cups water			
2	Fruited yogurt	40–45		
	1/2–1 bagel	22–45		

Hearty, carbohydrate-rich breakfast ideas

1 Three or 4 small pancakes (or 1 waffle) topped with fruit and/or yogurt and limited (2–3 tbsp) syrup, 235–355 mL (8–12 oz) glass of fruit juice, water.
2 Bowl of oatmeal topped with fruit and 2–3 tsp brown sugar, 2 slices of toast or 1 English muffin spread with a thin layer of margarine (1 pat), 235–355 mL (8–12 oz) glass of fruit juice, water.
3 Two scrambled eggs or 1 cup of milk or fruited yogurt, toasted bagel or English muffin with 2 tsp of honey or jelly, fresh fruit and/or fruit juice, water.

500–600 kcal lunch ideas

1 Sandwich made with 55–85 g turkey, lean ham or lean roast beef on a bulky roll, bagel or three pieces of bread (no salad mixes with mayonnaise; mustard and light mayo or 1 slice of cheese if tolerated), large piece of fruit (apple, banana or 2 oranges), 2 Fig Newtons or 1 low-fat granola bar, water.

2 Two cups pasta salad made with light dressing (no onions or garlic), French roll, large piece of fruit or 355 mL (12 oz) bottle of lemonade or fruit juice, water.

Hearty dinner ideas (dinner the evening before or evening after the match)

1 Garden salad with 1–2 tbsp regular salad dressing (2–4 tbsp light)
  Pasta with marinara sauce
  Cooked vegetables
  French or garlic bread, lightly buttered
2 Chicken or vegetable stir-fry (order extra rice)
  Sweetened beverage
3 Baked turkey, chicken or fish in a low-fat sauce
  Large serving of steamed rice or large baked potato (limit to 2–3 tsp pats or 4–5 tbsp sour cream)
  Cooked vegetables
  Bread or rolls, lightly buttered

Nutrition and hydration 55

Box 5.3 Tournament nutrition

Sample tournament A
Game times: 5:00 p.m. Friday, noon Saturday, 5 p.m. Saturday

- Hearty high-carbohydrate dinner the evening before
- 7:00–8:00 a.m. breakfast providing 90 g carbohydrate
- Post-practice lunch providing 500–600 kcal
- 3:15–3:30 p.m. snack or fluid replacement beverage (FRB) providing 30–60 g carbohydrate (if needed)
- Carbohydrate supplementation at 30–60 g · h^{-1} during the 5:00 p.m. match
- 2–4 cups of water or FRB immediately following the 5:00 p.m. match
- Hearty high-carbohydrate dinner, limited added fats (pasta, rice)
- 7:00 a.m. 500–600 kcal high-carbohydrate breakfast
- 10:30 a.m. snack providing 30–60 g carbohydrate and fluids (if needed)
- Carbohydrate supplementation at 30–60 g · h^{-1} during the noon match
- 3:15 p.m. snack providing 60–90 g carbohydrate and fluids, i.e., 1/2 sandwich, fruit, water
- Carbohydrate supplementation at 30–60 g · h^{-1} during the 5:00 p.m. match

- Hearty high-carbohydrate dinner post-tournament (perhaps even dessert)

Sample tournament B
Game Times 10:00 a.m., 2:00 p.m. and 6:00 p.m. Friday, Saturday to be determined

- Hearty high-carbohydrate dinner the evening before (pasta)
- High-carbohydrate bedtime snack 30–45 g carbohydrate
- 6:45–7:00 a.m. breakfast providing 90 g carbohydrate
- Carbohydrate supplementation at 45–60 g · h^{-1} during first match
- Snack providing 60–90 g carbohydrate and fluids immediately following the 10:00 match, i.e., sports bar, piece of fruit, c.3–4 cups of water
- Carbohydrate supplementation at 45–60 g · h^{-1} during 2:00 p.m. match
- Snack providing 60–90 g carbohydrate and fluids immediately following the 2:00 p.m. match, i.e., 1/2–1 sandwich, piece of fruit, c.3–4 cups of water
- Carbohydrate supplementation at 30–60 g · h^{-1} during 6:00 p.m. match
- 2–4 cups of fluid immediately following the 6:00 p.m. match
- Hearty high-carbohydrate dinner, limited added fats (pasta, rice), plentiful fluids assuming a Saturday match

Box 5.4 Special concerns for pre-event meals

- *Nausea.* Pre-event emotional tension or anxiety may delay digestive time and contribute to nausea and even vomiting before practice or game time. Research has suggested that liquid meals are more easily tolerated and digested under these conditions. Specifically, the player should attempt consuming 1–2 liquid supplements or smoothies as tolerated. A few soda crackers or piece of dry toast are also an option. Water should also be consumed as tolerated.
- *"Hypoglycemia."* Although rare, some athletes will experience a condition called "rebound hypoglycemia" when carbohydrate foods are consumed within 20–60 min of exercise. Symptoms include fatigue, tiredness, heaviness, lightheadedness, etc., associated with carbohydrate consumption as suggested above. In this setting, the pre-event meal should be consumed 90–120 min

before exercise. If necessary, 1–2 cups of a carbohydrate-containing fluid replacement beverage can be consumed 10 min before exercise.
- *Hunger.* Fluid replacement beverage consumed 10 min before exercise (practice or conditioning) may delay feelings of hunger and acts similarly to consumption during exercise (i.e., it is readily absorbed and appears in the bloodstream with 5–10 min of ingestion and does not contribute to "rebound hypoglycemia" in sensitive athletes).
- *Multimatch weekends.* On weeks with two scheduled matches, i.e., Friday night and Sunday afternoon, athletes need to focus on consuming adequate carbohydrate Friday night and all day Saturday to avoid being glycogen depleted at the start of the second match.

athletes participating in heavy, prolonged workouts should also make an effort to include sodium and potassium in the recovery meal(s). Excellent sources of potassium include fresh fruit, vegetables (particularly potatoes), and low-fat dairy products. Sources of sodium include table salt, salted foods, and

processed foods. Overall, the postevent meal should contain ample carbohydrate for glycogen replacement, provide fluids, contain a good-sized serving of a protein-rich food (lean meat, legumes, dairy products, etc.), and contain a little more fat and sodium as required by the individual athlete.

Box 5.5 Suggestions for snacks during and between matches.

Water
Sports drink
Fruit juice
Lemonade
Limeade
Fresh fruit in season
Dried fruit (raisins)
Bagels
Bread slices
FigNewtons
Healthier oatmeal cookies
Muffins (low-fat)
High-carbohydrate sports bar
Low-fat and non-fat yogurt
individual puddings
Sandwiches or sandwich fixings (turkey, chicken, tuna with low-
   fat mayo, lean ham peanut butter for peanut butter and banana
   or jelly sandwiches)
Dutch-style pretzels
Soda crackers
Graham crackers
Boxes of ready-to-eat cereal
Skim milk or soy milk

Special concerns for the volleyball athlete requiring weight reduction

As in all sports, certain individual athletes may be more predisposed to weight gain due to genetic factors or environmental influences (sedentary off the court lifestyle or overeating). College-level coaches may notice that freshmen athletes gain weight during their first year—possibly because they play less during matches yet still eat as much as their junior and senior classmates. In one study of National Collegiate Athletic Association (NCAA) Division I female basketball, softball, and volleyball players, significantly more volleyball players (71%) than softball players (32%) or basketball players (11.3%) reported using weight-reduction products, diuretics, or laxatives. Close to 27% of the volleyball players reported using diuretics and 19% reported using laxatives to keep weight down, particularly during the season (Martin *et al*. 1998). While many athletes do struggle with legitimate weight issues, it is also possible that many normal or even underweight athletes struggle with the perceived notion (theirs or

their coach's) that reducing body mass will improve vertical jump performance and quickness on the court. In any case, it is imperative that volleyball players, particularly females, be educated on sensible weight-management practices.

When weight reduction is required, weight loss should be accomplished slowly and not during the competitive season. The general recommendation is to reduce energy intake by approximately 500 kcal to no more than 1,000 kcal $\cdot$ day^{-1} to promote a weight loss of 2–4 kg $\cdot$ week^{-1}. Weight reduction in athletes, however, can be somewhat problematic because the diminished energy intake can compromise exercise performance and nutrient intake. Consultation with a registered dietician trained in sports nutrition can help athletes at all levels maintain a healthy diet while reducing total energy intake to promote gradual weight loss. Low carbohydrate and/or high protein diets (such as the zone diet) that have been recently popularized are not appropriate for athletes and may result in fatigue, dehydration and nutritional deficiences (ACSM 2001, Manore 1999). Furthermore, these diets offer no performance advantage (Jarvis *et al*. 2002).

Special concerns for the female volleyball athlete

The prevalence of amenorrhea among exercising women is reported to be between 3.4 and 66% (Otis 1992) with a higher prevalence in runners as opposed to cyclists and swimmers. The prevalence among volleyball athletes has not been reported. The cause of this secondary hypothalamic amenorrhea is unknown, but may be related to training level, nutritional status, body composition changes, stress, and/or hormone changes due to exercise. Several studies involving predominately endurance runners have documented reduced intake of total calories, protein, fat, and zinc, and higher intake of fiber and vitamin A in amenorrheic athletes when compared with eumenorrheic athletes. Female volleyball athletes should understand that loss of the menstrual cycle is unhealthy and is not a normal part of training. Low circulating estrogen levels associated with the loss of monthly cycles can predispose the athlete to reduced bone density and increased risk of stress fractures and other overuse injuries. Volleyball athletes experiencing amenorrhea should see their team or personal physician for a thorough evaluation.

Conclusion

By following the guidelines discussed in this chapter, the volleyball athlete should be able to choose a diet that is adequate in energy, carbohydrate, protein, vitamins, minerals, and fluids. A good sports diet is rich in a variety of grain products, fruits, and vegetables, contains several servings of meat or protein-rich plant foods, small amounts of added nuts and vegetable oils, and low-fat dairy products (or other calcium-containing foods). Sound dietary practices should help volleyball athletes at all levels perform and train optimally and avoid the negative health consequences associated with making poor food choices.

References

American College of Sports Medicine (2001) Position stand. Appropriate intervention strategies for weight loss and prevention of weight regain for adults. *Medicine and Science in Sports and Exercise* **33** (12), 2145–2156.

American College of Sports Medicine (1996) Position stand. Exercise and fluid replacement. *Medicine and Science in Sports and Exercise* **28** (1), i–vi.

American College of Sports Medicine, American Dietetic Association & Dietitians of Canada (2000) Nutrition and athletic performance. Joint position statement. *Medicine and Science in Sports and Exercise* **32** (12), 2130–2145.

Broad, E.M., Burke, L.M., Cox, G.R., Heeley, P. & Riley, M. (1996) Body weight changes and voluntary fluid intakes during training and competition sessions in team sports. *International Journal of Sport Nutrition* **6** (3), 307–320.

Goran, M. (1995) Variation in total energy expenditure in humans. *Obesity Research* **3** (1), 59–66.

Graig, W. (1994) Iron content of plant foods. *American Journal of Clinical Nutrition* **59** (Suppl.), S1233–S1237.

Houtkooper, L. (1992) Food selection for endurance sports. *Medicine and Science in Sports and Exercise* **24** (9), S349–S359.

Jarvis, M., McNaughton, L., Sedelon, A., Thompson, D. (2002) The acute one-week effect of the Zone Diet on body composition, blood lipid levels and performance in recreational endurance athletes. *Journal of Strength and Conditioning Research* **16** (1), 50–57.

Larson, D.E., Hesslink, R.L., Hrovat, M.I., Fishman, R.S. & Systrom, D.M. (1994) Dietary effects on exercising muscle metabolism and performance by P-MRS. *Journal of Applied Physiology* **77** (3), 1108–1115.

Manore, M. (1999) Low-carbohydrate diets for weight loss are back. Do they work any better this time? *A CSM's health and Futness Journal* **3** (5), 41–43.

Martin, M., Schlabach, G. & Shibinski, K. (1998) The use of nonprescription weight loss products among female basketball, softball, and volleyball athletes from NCAA Division I institutions: issues and concerns. *Journal of Athletic Training* **33**, 41–44.

Minihane, A. & Fairweather-Tait, S. (1998) Effect of calcium supplmentation on daily nonheme-iron absorption and long-term iron status. *American Journal of Clinical Nutrition* **68**, 96–102.

Otis, C.L. (1992) Exercise-associated amenorrhea. *Clinics in Sports Medicine* **11** (2), 351–362.

Pennington, J.A.T. (1998) *Bowes and Church's Food Values of Portions Commonly Used.* Lippincott, New York.

Vegetarian Nutrition Dietetic Practice Group (1995) *Calcium in Vegetarian Diets.* American Dietetic Association, Chicago.

Recommended reading

Clark, N. (1997) *Nancy Clark's Sports Nutrition Guidebook,* 2nd edn. Human Kinetics, Champaign, IL.

Manore, M. & Thompson, J. (2000) *Sport Nutrition for Health and Performance.* Human Kinetics, Champaign, IL.

Maughan, R.J. (ed.) (2000) *Nutrition in Sport.* Blackwell Science, Oxford.

PART 2
THE VOLLEYBALL
MEDICAL PROFESSIONAL

Chapter 6
The role of the volleyball medical professional: the preparticipation examination

William W. Briner Jr.

Introduction

The role and responsibilities of the sports medicine practitioner caring for volleyball athletes may vary depending upon several factors, including the nature of their professional qualifications. While a physician with expertise in treating musculoskeletal sport-related injuries should supervise the medical care and rehabilitation of the injured volleyball player, an athletic trainer or a physiotherapist experienced in treating athletes may provide most of the day to day ongoing management of the athlete's injury-related concerns. Ideally, athletes should be cared for by a team of medical professionals collaborating together to provide comprehensive, subspecialty-level care. In addition to physicians and therapists/trainers, the team of volleyball medical professionals might also include a dentist, optometrist, podiatrist, massage therapist, chiropractor, exercise physiologist, biomechanist, nutritionist, strength and conditioning specialist, and/or a sports psychologist. A familiarity with the sport itself, an understanding of the risk factors for injury inherent to the sport, and a familiarity with the most common injuries encountered by volleyball athletes are all critical components of providing effective, expert care to the volleyball player. The medical team may attend to only a few volleyball players among numerous other athletes treated during the course of a season or year, or alternatively the medical staff may be responsible for covering several teams of volleyball athletes over the course of a mul-

tiday tournament. The role of the tournament medical director is addressed in Chapter 7. This chapter will discuss some of the duties of the volleyball medical professional, with particular emphasis on the preparticipation examination.

Over the course of a season, the volleyball medical professional will develop a unique relationship with each volleyball athlete for whom they provide medical care. The availability of the physicians, trainers, and other medical consultants to promptly see and evaluate an athlete who may have suffered an injury is a key element of this relationship. By gaining the trust and confidence of not only the players but also of the coaches, positive physician–athlete and physician–coach relationships will build naturally. Optimally, regular and timely interaction between the athlete and members of the medical team will help to facilitate identification of injury and illness early in its course, so that therapeutic intervention can occur before there are long-term detrimental effects to the athlete or the team. Ideally, a member of the medical team (preferably a trainer or physician) should attend team practices and competitions. This will help establish and maintain open lines of communication between the athlete(s), coach(es), and the team of involved volleyball medical professionals.

The role of the team physician is not always an easy one. The athletes are aware that the physician is usually responsible for making decisions regarding return to play following an injury, or for otherwise certifying an athlete's eligibility for competition. There may be instances where a potential conflict exists between the short-term benefits to the team and the long-term health of an individual athlete, complicating the decision to clear the athlete for participation. In some situations, the medical professional may be the only person (coaches, athletes, and parents included) who keeps the overall health of the athlete as their highest priority. The volleyball team physician who has demonstrated a sincere interest in the success of the team and its athletes, and who has experience treating volleyball-related injuries, will be more likely to gain the confidence of all parties involved, making it somewhat easier to handle these difficult situations fairly and effectively when they arise.

Preparticipation sports examination

When should sports preparticipation examinations be performed?

As a discipline, sports medicine has evolved rapidly over the last several decades. Technological advancement, combined with both clinical and basic science research, have advanced our understanding of the pathophysiology of musculoskeletal injuries and consequently sports medicine professionals have an unparalleled ability to diagnose and treat such conditions. However, the ultimate goal of sports medicine should be injury prevention. One mechanism by which early stage (perhaps subclinical) injuries might be more easily diagnosed, and by which risk factors for injury or illness can be detected, is the preparticipation physical examination.

Preparticipation physical examinations are performed differently in different parts of the world. In the United States, nearly every state has a law that mandates yearly exams for adolescent athletes during their secondary school years. Ironically, it could be argued that adolescence might not actually be the most appropriate time to carry out such examinations. Since most of the data on presport examinations suggests that injury incidence rises with increasing length of sporting involvement/participation, it may therefore be more reasonable to defer annual examinations until the athlete reaches young adulthood. This may particularly hold true

for the recreational athlete. Conversely, it could be argued that earlier examinations are entirely appropriate in light of the increasing prevalence of early sports specialization and year-round training programs for aspiring young athletes. Nevertheless, once players have had a comprehensive initial exam, a briefer examination can be performed in successive years with attention to any recent injuries or changes in the medical history. Sports preparticipation examinations should be performed at least 4–6 weeks prior to the start of the competitive season. This allows the physician and athlete time to investigate and, if possible, treat any abnormalities detected on the exam that might jeopardize the athlete's ability to participate.

History

Perhaps the most important component of the preparticipation examination is the athlete's medical history. The vast majority of conditions that may impact upon an athlete's fitness for competition will be evident from a thorough history. Only rarely are new or unsuspected diagnoses discovered on the physical examination. There are a few medical conditions for which it is especially important to screen volleyball athletes. With respect to injuries, the most important risk factor for any type of injury is a history of similar injury. For example, the most common ankle injury in volleyball is the recurrent inversion sprain injury involving the previously injured ankle. A standardized form (Fig. 6.1) may help the clinician and athlete identify potential problems that should be addressed before the season starts. If the athlete conscientiously completes a form like this one, most important medical issues should be identified. Note that young athletes should have a parent or responsible adult complete the form to ensure the greatest accuracy of historical information.

Cardiovascular concerns

The American Heart Association (AHA) has recommended that clinicians obtain a thorough history in an effort to detect any significant cardiovascular disease or conditions that might predispose an athlete to sudden death. The AHA has suggested that the

Athletic Physical – Lutheran General Sports Medicine

Examining Physician _____ Date of Exam _____

Athlete's Name _____ Age _____

Date of Birth _____ Parent Name(s) _____ Sport(s) _____

Address _____ Phone _____

Family Doctor _____ Phone _____

1. **Have you ever had any of the following problems during or after exercising:**
   - Chest pain/discomfort .... ☐ Yes ☐ No
   - Passing out .... ☐ Yes ☐ No
   - Severe lightheadedness/dizziness .... ☐ Yes ☐ No
   - Coughing .... ☐ Yes ☐ No
   - Wheezing .... ☐ Yes ☐ No
   - Extreme shortness of breath .... ☐ Yes ☐ No
   - Excessive fatigue .... ☐ Yes ☐ No

2. **Have you ever had any of the following problems**
   - Concussion/knocked out .... ☐ Yes ☐ No
   - Neck pain/injury .... ☐ Yes ☐ No
   - Back pain/injury .... ☐ Yes ☐ No
   - Broken bone .... ☐ Yes ☐ No
   - Joint injury .... ☐ Yes ☐ No
   - Ligament/muscle injury .... ☐ Yes ☐ No
   - Sprains/strain .... ☐ Yes ☐ No

3. **Has anyone in your family (including grandparents, aunts uncles, cousins) ever died suddenly before age 50?** .... ☐ Yes ☐ No
   Has anyone in your family (that you know of) been diagnosed with:
   - Hypertrophic cardiomyopathy .... ☐ Yes ☐ No
   - Dilated cardiomyopathy .... ☐ Yes ☐ No
   - Long QT syndrome .... ☐ Yes ☐ No
   - Marfan syndrome .... ☐ Yes ☐ No
   - Arrhythmias .... ☐ Yes ☐ No

4. **Do you worry about your weight often** .... ☐ Yes ☐ No

5. **Allergies** _____
   _____ ☐ None

6. **Do you avoid eating meat?** _____ ☐ Yes ☐ No
7. **Do you avoid eating dairy food?** _____ ☐ Yes ☐ No
8. **Have you had medical problems such as:** ☐ Yes ☐ No
   - Heart murmur .... ☐ Yes ☐ No
   - High blood pressure .... ☐ Yes ☐ No
   - Heat stroke/heat exhaustion .... ☐ Yes ☐ No
   - Diabetes .... ☐ Yes ☐ No
   - Mononucleosis .... ☐ Yes ☐ No
   - Bleeding problems .... ☐ Yes ☐ No
   - Bruise easily .... ☐ Yes ☐ No
   - Eye problems .... ☐ Yes ☐ No
   - Absence of one kidney .... ☐ Yes ☐ No
   - Absence of one testicle .... ☐ Yes ☐ No
   - Hernia .... ☐ Yes ☐ No
   - Seizures .... ☐ Yes ☐ No
   - Bee sting allergy .... ☐ Yes ☐ No

9. **List any medications you take regularly:** _____
   _____ ☐ None

10. **List any other chronic illness or medical problems:** _____
    _____ ☐ None

11. **List any hospitalizations you have had:** _____
    _____ ☐ None

12. **Females:**
    Menstrual period frequency:
    During competitive sports season, every ...... days

    During off-season, every ...... days

All "Yes" anwers, describe: _____
_____
_____

The above information is correct: _____   _____
                                        Signed (athlete)   Parent

Fig. 6.1 An example of a comprehensive preparticipation exam form used to document the athlete's history (*above*) and physical exam (*opposite*).

EXAM (to be completed by Physician)

BP_____   P_____   Ht _____   Wt_____   Glasses/Contacts _____   Pupils: R ____ L ____   Vision: R ____ L ____

	NL		**NL**

Upper Limb: .... | **Heart:** Supine ....

ROM .... | Standing ....

Symmetry .... | Murmur? .... ☐ Yes ☐ No

Spine/neck .... | If 'Yes', is there change with standing?   ☐ Increase ☐ Decrease
                                ☐ No change

Scoliosis .... | **Lungs** ....

Lower Limb: .... | **Skin** ....

Gait .... | **Abdomen** ....

Squat .... | **Testicles** ....

Duck walk .... | **Hernia** ....

ROM .... | **Other** ....

Femoral pulses palpable?   ☐ Yes ☐ No

If there is a history of joint injury, perform exam and describe: _____

_____

_____

_____

Findings/Recommendations: _____

_____

_____

_____

_____

_____ **Preventive issues addressed (as appropriate):** _____ ETOH, _____ Smoking, _____ Drugs (steroids)
                                           _____ Safe sex, _____ Seat belts, _____ Firearms,
                                           _____ Bike helmets

_____ Females: Regular Pap smear, Breast exam discussed
_____ Males: Self-testicular exam reviewed

CLEARANCE (circle A, B, C)

    A – CLEARED FOR: ☐ Collision Sports   ☐ Contact Sports   ☐ Non-Contact Sports
    B – NOTIFY (prior to clearance):   ☐ Family Doctor   ☐ Coach
    C – CLEARANCE DEFERRED DUE TO: _____

_____

Physician's signature _____
physical/wwb/mm

Fig. 6.1 Continued.

preparticipation history include the following 13 questions to help rule out such conditions:

1 Is there a history of exercise-associated chest pain/discomfort?

2 Is there a history of exercise-associated near-syncope (severe dizziness/light-headedness)?

3 Is there a history of exercise-associated syncope (transient loss of consciousness/fainting)?

4 Is there a history of exercise-associated shortness of breath (worse than that experienced by other athletes engaged in the same activity)?

5 Is there a history of exercise-associated fatigue?

6 Has the athlete ever been diagnosed with a heart murmur?

7 Has the athlete ever been diagnosed with systemic hypertension (high blood pressure)?

8 Is there a family history of premature death in close relatives younger than age 50?

9 Is there a known history of hypertrophic cardiomyopathy?

10 Is there a known history of dilated cardiomyopathy?

11 Is there a known history of long QT syndrome?

12 Is there a known history of significant arrhythmia (abnormal heart rhythm)?

13 Is there a known history of Marfan syndrome?

Marfan syndrome

Flo Hyman of the United States National Team was widely regarded as the best female volleyball player in the world when she collapsed and died on court during a volleyball competition in 1986 (Fig. 6.2). On autopsy, it was discovered that she had dissected her ascending aorta, secondary to aortic root dilatation stemming from Marfan syndrome. Although she exhibited many of the stigmata of Marfan syndrome, she had never been diagnosed with the condition. The untimely and tragic death of this elite athlete should serve as a constant reminder to volleyball medical professionals to maintain a high index of suspicion for Marfan syndrome during preparticipation physical examinations, since many of the traits of the condition are generally regarded as desirable among volleyball players. Physical characteristics common among individuals with Marfan syndrome that, if present, should alert the

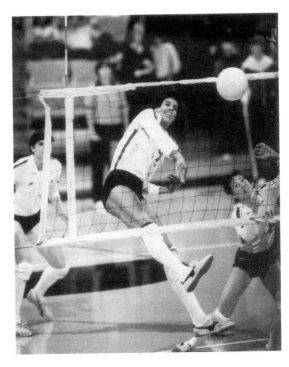

Fig. 6.2 Flo Hyman of the USA was considered one of the best female volleyball players in the world when she died from complications of Marfan syndrome. (Courtesy of USA Volleyball.)

astute clinician to the possibility of the diagnosis include:

• Arachnodactyly: long, thin fingers—also referred to as "spider fingers."

• Pectus abnormalities:

   Pectus excavatum: a "scooped out" indentation in the region of the sternum or breastbone.

   Pectus carinatum: "pigeon breast"—a sternum that protrudes outward.

• Arm span that exceeds height.

• Lower limb length (measured from the pubic symphysis) that is greater than 50% of height.

• Mitral valve abnormalities, including mitral valve prolapse.

• The "Steinberg thumb sign"—the ability to passively bend the thumb backwards so that it touches the radial aspect of the forearm.

Athletic heart syndrome

Athletic heart syndrome is a benign condition that is

quite common among individuals who follow a dedicated exercise program, occurring in up to 50% of athletes. Two-dimensional (surface) echocardiography reveals four-chamber hypertrophy secondary to relative volume overload. The athlete's electrocardiograph may demonstrate changes consistent with left ventricular or right ventricular hypertrophy. Most sports medicine professionals are familiar with the resting bradycardia (slow heart rate, <60 beats·min^{-1}) that occurs in athletes. A resting heart rate of 40 beats·min^{-1} or slower is not uncommon among well-trained endurance athletes. Cardiac auscultation may reveal an extra heart sound, such as an S3 or S4, that should be considered normal in this setting. Frequently, there is a systolic ejection murmur as the result of increased stroke volume with each beat of the heart. This flow murmur decreases with standing or with the Valsalva maneuver. The point of maximal impulse, or apex of the heart, may also be laterally displaced on palpatory examination. No further diagnostic evaluation is indicated once the athletic heart syndrome is recognized.

Other medical conditions

Special attention should be paid to a prior history of heat stroke, heat cramps, or heat exhaustion. Athletes who have suffered from these conditions in the past are probably more likely to have similar problems in the future. They should be counseled regarding acclimatization to exercise in conditions of high heat and humidity, and should be instructed to consume adequate fluids before, during, and after competition (see Chapters 5 and 9 for additional information).

Reactive airways disease (asthma) can impair delivery of oxygen to the tissues, thereby adversely affecting performance. In severe cases, asthma can be life threatening. The most sensitive screening question for exercise-induced asthma is, "Do you cough after exercise?" Players with positive responses should be evaluated and, if indicated, treated for this potentially dangerous condition.

It is important to obtain a menstrual history from postmenarchal female athletes. Athletes whose menses become less frequent during intense training and competition may be at risk for the "female athlete triad," a condition consisting of oligomenor-

rhea, disordered eating, and osteoporosis. It is now clear that competing athletes with this condition are at increased risk for stress fractures, secondary to structural insufficiency as the result of bone demineralization. Careful attention should be given to the female athlete's dietary history. It may be reasonable to involve a dietician to take a complete diet history and make specific recommendations for adequate energy, vitamin, and mineral intake (see Chapter 5). Menstruating female athletes with a thin body habitus may have inadequate dietary intake of several nutrients, including iron. Those athletes at risk for the female athlete triad should have their hemoglobin, hematocrit, and ferritin levels evaluated, especially if they are vegetarians.

An analysis of every medical condition that might impact on an athlete's fitness for volleyball competition is beyond the scope of this chapter. Suffice it to say that chronic medical conditions ought to be thoroughly assessed and should be clinically stable prior to competition. When indicated, regular follow-up visits with the athlete should be arranged to insure that the demands of athletic participation are not adversely affecting their chronic health condition.

Prior injuries

Athletes who have been previously injured, whether playing volleyball or while participating in another sport, should be carefully examined to insure that the injury has been appropriately diagnosed, treated and rehabilitated, and fully healed. The ankle sprain, for example, is the most common acute injury among volleyball players, as it is among athletes participating in most other sports. In addition to examining the ankle for excessive residual ligamentous laxity, swelling, or other evidence of inadequate healing, the athlete should be tested functionally to insure that he or she can adequately withstand the demands of volleyball training and competition. If the athlete has recently suffered an ankle sprain injury, they should complete a 10-week neuromuscular/proprioceptive rehabilitation program in order to decrease the chance of reinjury (see Chapter 10). Players with a history of ankle sprain may also reduce their risk of recurrent injury by wearing an ankle orthosis such as an air stirrup or other similar devices for up to 6 months following injury. While this type of ankle brace has been demonstrated to be effective for secondary prevention of ankle sprains, there is no compelling evidence that braces decrease the chance of a first-time injury to an ankle that has not been sprained before. The volleyball medical professional should also confer with the coach or trainer to determine if flaws in the athlete's technique may be predisposing the player to specific types of injury. Again, using ankle sprain injury as an example, athletes with a history of ankle sprain should have their hitting approach analyzed to determine whether they are "problem attackers." These attackers typically start their attack jump too far away from the net and must therefore jump forward to contact the ball. This makes them more likely to penetrate the centerline and make contact with the opposing blockers, thereby increasing the risk of ankle injuries for both the attacker and the blockers. By working in cooperation with the appropriate members of the medical team, the team physician can hope to not only treat injuries but also potentially reduce the incidence of recurrent injuries through a combination of interventions.

Physical examination

Vital signs are an important part of the physical examination in athletes. The heart rate (pulse) is a good measure of aerobic fitness, with a lower resting pulse generally consistent with a higher level of aerobic fitness. Blood pressure should be assessed, although it is rarely so high as to contraindicate sports participation. When present, hypertension should be treated in athletes using the same guidelines as in any patient. Height and weight, which may be used to calculate body mass index, may help to give an idea of the athlete's fitness level as well.

Brief examination of the skull, eyes, ears, nose and throat, and palpation for lymphadenopathy and thyromegaly in the neck is usually adequate for a presports exam of the head and neck. Vision should be assessed in all athletes, as this is one aspect of the physical exam where a known deficit can be effectively corrected and can result in improved performance. The heart and lungs should be carefully auscultated in both the supine and standing positions. A benign systolic ejection murmur consistent with athletic heart syndrome will diminish upon standing, as this reduces venous return to the heart and thus decreases flow through the affected cardiac structure. Any heart murmur that increases on standing warrants consideration of hypertrophic cardiomyopathy, which is the leading cause of sudden death in exercising individuals. Athletes thought to be at risk for hypertrophic cardiomyopathy on screening examination should have a two-dimensional echocardiogram to confirm or rule out the suspected clinical diagnosis. The femoral pulses should be palpated, since a decreased or delayed femoral pulsation may be a clue to coarctation of the aorta. This condition can result in lower extremity pain with exercise (vascular claudication).

Musculoskeletal examination

A major goal of the screening musculoskeletal examination should be to identify those volleyball athletes who are at increased risk of injury as the result of a functional deficit or an imbalance of strength or flexibility. All athletes should undergo a screening exam that assesses range of motion and motor function of the upper and lower limbs and the trunk. Functional motor tests are preferable to isolated manual muscle testing in this setting since functional tests, such as heel and toe walking, and deep knee bending provide simultaneous information regarding the athlete's coordination and balance in addition to motor function and control. Gross motor function and active range of motion of the upper limbs can be evaluated using the Apley scratch test (Fig. 6.3) Gross motor function and active range of motion of the lower limbs can be evaluated by having the athlete squat and "duck walk" (Figs 6.4 and 6.5). For volleyball players, it is also reasonable to have them squat and then jump up, in addition to hopping repeatedly on each foot—thereby grossly assessing neuromuscular control of the lower limbs, pelvis, and spine. For a volleyball player with no prior history of illness or injury, this brief screening functional physical exam is probably adequate for the musculoskeletal portion of the preparticipation evaluation. If the athlete has a history of prior injury, however, or if the screening examination reveals evidence of abnormality, the affected body part should be carefully examined. The following describes several techniques used in the physical evaluation of the volleyball athlete with a complaint

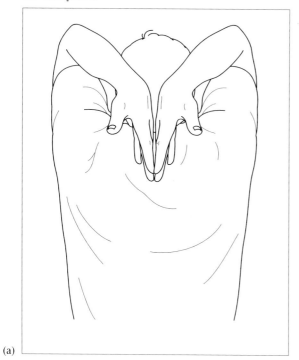

(a)

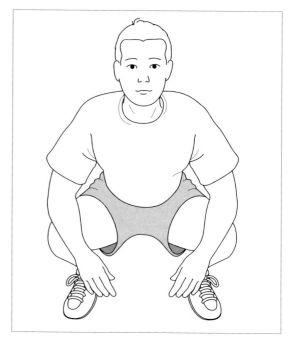

Fig. 6.4 The squat.

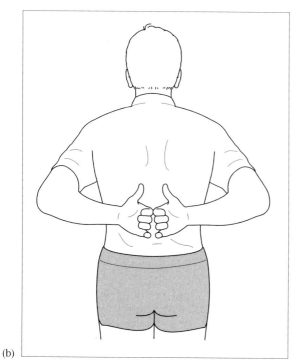

(b)

Fig. 6.3 Apley's scratch test: (a) abduction, flexion, and external rotation; (b) extension and internal rotation.

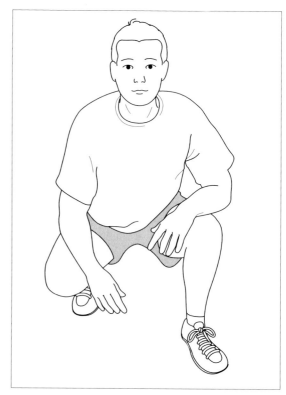

Fig. 6.5 The duck walk, which evaluates the functional weight-bearing range of motion of the ankles, knees, and hips.

of shoulder pain. For details regarding the examination of other structures, the interested reader is referred to Magee's (1997) excellent textbook.

Athletes who repetitively perform overhead skills such as spiking or serving may develop altered mechanics of the dominant shoulder. On testing shoulder range of motion at 90° of abduction, internal rotation is often decreased, while external rotation is typically increased. Thus, the normal 180° range of motion may be preserved albeit with abnormal end points. This condition may predispose the overhead athlete to rotator cuff tendinopathy and should therefore be addressed with an appropriate flexibility and strengthening program.

Volleyball athletes with a history of shoulder pain often have a positive "scapular slide test," suggestive of scapular dysfunction. The test is simple to perform. The athlete is observed from behind, with the arms initially hanging at the sides at rest. The athlete then places their hands on their hips before abducting the upper limbs to 90° in the coronal plane. The test is positive if significant asymmetry of scapular protraction is detected through the range of motion (this is defined as a difference of 1.5 cm or more, when measured from the spinous processes to the inferomedial angle of the scapula (Fig. 6.6). A positive scapular slide suggests scapular dysfunction due to chronic overload, and is commonly associated with anterior shoulder pain/rotator cuff tendinopathy in the dominant (hitting) arm of volleyball athletes. When inspecting the scapulae, the astute volleyball clinician should also note any atrophy of the infraspinatus fossa suggestive of entrapment of the suprascapular nerve—an often painless condition for which volleyball athletes appear to be at particular risk (discussed in greater detail in Chapter 12).

Athletes with a history of shoulder pain with overhead activity should be evaluated for signs of impingement syndrome. Hawkin's test (Fig. 6.7a) is performed with the humerus abducted to 90° in the plane of the scapula and internally rotated as far as possible. Neer's maneuver (Fig. 6.7b) involves forward flexion of the humerus as far as possible in the scapular plane. Anterior shoulder pain with either of these maneuvers is considered a sign of impingement of the rotator cuff tendons. This condition can be addressed with an exercise program emphasizing scapular stabilization and strengthening of the rotator cuff.

Injury to the glenoid labrum can result in a functionally unstable shoulder, which may predispose the volleyball athlete to shoulder pain with overhead activity. The glenoid labrum and the glenohumeral ligaments serve as the principal static stabilizers of the shoulder joint. The labrum is vulnerable to attritional injury through chronic overuse and to acute injury when the athlete falls on an outstretched arm. Historical details suggestive of labral injury include pain and palpable "clicking" in the shoulder joint with active range of motion. Multiple clinical tests designed to detect labral pathology have been described. Although perhaps best performed in combination to increase the sensitivity of detecting a labral tear, many clinicians feel that the O'Brien maneuver is the best single test for detecting a tear of the superior labrum. The O'Brien test is performed with the involved shoulder forward flexed to 90°, then horizontally adducted past the midline. The examiner has the athlete place their upper extremity in a pronated (internally rotated) position with the little finger up, then has the athlete forward flex the upper limb upward against resistance (Fig. 6.8a). This maneuver is then repeated with the involved limb in a supinated (externally rotated) position with the thumb up (Fig. 6.8b). O'Brien's test is considered positive if the athlete complains of pain in the internally rotated position that is relieved in the externally rotated position. If a glenoid labral tear is diagnosed as the aetiology of shoulder girdle pain that limits athletic performance, a course of rehabilitation should be attempted before considering surgical repair.

Diagnostic testing

In general, diagnostic testing should be dictated by the clinical scenario. Testing should be performed if the diagnosis is in question, or if the result of the test will influence the athlete's treatment plan or training program. This axiom applies to both laboratory/chemistry tests and to radiographic imaging tests such as standard X-ray and advanced cross-sectional imaging including magnetic resonance imaging (MRI). Screening blood tests, such as determination of the athlete's lipid profile, should be left for the

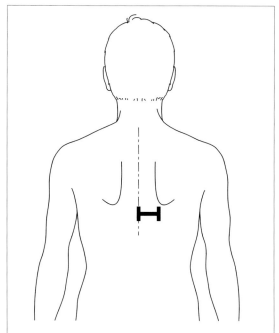

(a)

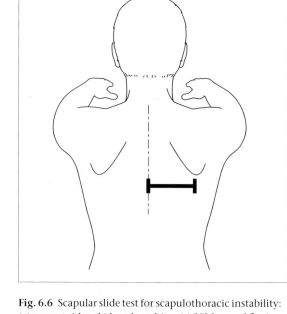

(c)

Fig. 6.6 Scapular slide test for scapulothoracic instability: (a) arms at sides; (b) hands on hips; (c) 90° forward flexion of the shoulders. In all three positions measure the distance from midline to the inferior angle of the scapula. A difference of 1.5 cm or greater in scapular abduction on the involved side (as compared to the uninvolved side) constitutes a positive scapular slide.

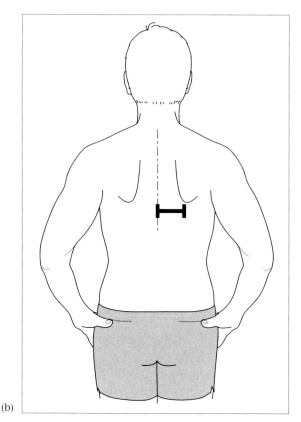

(b)

athlete's primary care physician to direct. Hemoglobin concentration is often found to be below the lower limit of the normal adult reference range in athletes, secondary to athletic "pseudoanemia." With training, red cell mass typically increases, but due to a larger relative increase in plasma volume, the athlete's hemoglobin and hematocrit may be effectively "diluted" and therefore appear falsely low. Menstruating female athletes may be transiently anemic, and as mentioned earlier females suspected of disordered eating are at risk for developing chronic anemia. Team physicians may wish to consider routine drug testing at the time of the preparticipation exam to identify athletes who are using banned substances. Note that while the presence of blood or protein in the urine may signal abnormalities of kidney function, both can occur benignly as the result of strenuous exercise.

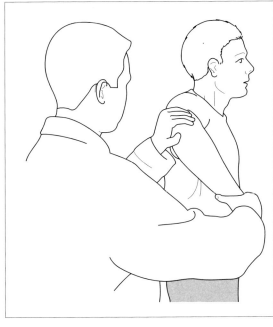

(a)

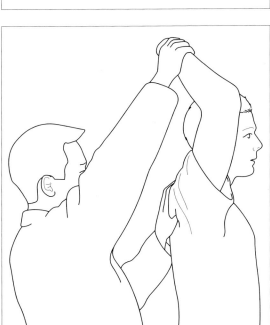

(b)

Fig. 6.7 Impingement maneuvers often cause pain in athletes with rotator cuff or biceps tendonitis. (a) Hawkin's test: internal rotation of the shoulder at 90° abduction in the plane of the scapula; (b) Neer's test: external rotation of the shoulder at the limit of forward flexion.

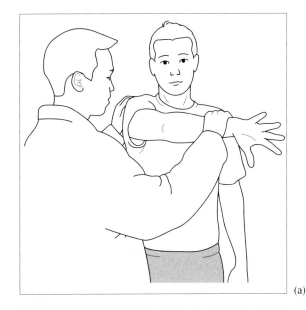

(a)

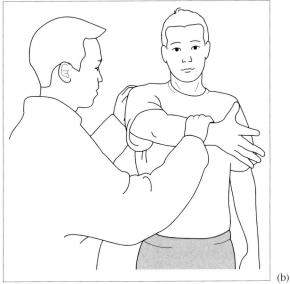

(b)

Fig. 6.8 O'Brien's test for a tear of the superior glenoid labrum from anterior to posterior, the SLAP lesion. (a) In forward flexion, horizontally adduct the arm past midline, place the little finger up, then resist as the patient tries to forward flex upward against the examiner's pressure. This causes pain with a SLAP lesion. (b) Same position and examination technique, but the patient places their thumb up, in pronation. This results in no pain or much less pain than with the little finger up.

Preventive measures

Since the preparticipation exam may be the only contact that healthy athletes will have with a physician during the course of the season, age-appropriate preventive measures should be addressed at this time. For adolescent athletes, risky behaviors such as smoking, drinking alcohol, and drug use, as well as unsafe sex practices should be discussed as appropriate. The physician should review any medications the athlete may be using, both by prescription and "over-the-counter," to insure that none of the medications contains chemicals on the IOC list of banned substances. The presports exam is also a good time to ask athletes whether they are currently using or have used legal or illegal supplements. This is a difficult issue to tackle during the brief time period often allotted for these exams. However, the health risks of such compounds as anabolic steroids and human growth hormone should be reviewed with athletes who are considering their use. The fact that such compounds are prohibited by the IOC and that their use is contrary to the ideal of fair play should be emphasized (see Chapter 19). Unfortunately, athletes will almost certainly have been exposed to anecdotal evidence that supplements are effective in enhancing volleyball sports performance. It is important for the volleyball sports medicine professional to provide as much factual information to athletes as possible in order to facilitate reasonable, informed decision making on these issues.

Reference

Magee, D.J. (1997) *Orthopaedic Physical Assessment.* W.B. Saunders, Philadelphia.

Recommended reading

American College of Sports Medicine (2000) Team physician consensus statement. *Medicine and Science in Sports and Exercise* **32** (4), 877–878.

Kibler, W.B. (1996) *ACSM's Handbook for the Team Physician.* Williams & Wilkins, Baltimore, MD.

Kurowski, K. & Chandran, S. (2000) The preparticipation physical examination. *American Family Physician* **61** (12), 2683–2690.

Chapter 7
Medical coverage of volleyball events

Fernando Pena and Elizabeth Arendt

Introduction

Volleyball competitions may take many forms, from single matches between two teams to single-day multiteam tournaments to multiday multiteam events. Thus, organizing the medical services for a volleyball event may assume varying degrees of complexity and may require different levels of infrastructure depending on several factors, including the number of teams and athletes participating, the location of the event, and the level and type of the competition. Regardless of the competition format, however, it is important to insure that the medical needs of the athletes and other participants have been accounted for and that all potential medical emergencies have been anticipated and planned for accordingly.

Medical supervision of single matches is usually routinely provided by one of the medical professionals working with the host volleyball club. The "home" team will, of course, have access to its own training room and the standard complement of facilities and personnel to which it is accustomed, both before and after the match. Visiting teams may or may not travel with their own medical personnel and equipment. Access to the host facilities may be requested depending on need, and should (at the very least) be made available in the case of an emergency. For events larger in scope than a single match, more advanced planning is typically involved and it is advisable to designate a "tournament medical director" to coordinate medical care during the event.

The tournament medical director should be an individual with training in sports medicine and with experience in working with volleyball athletes. The medical director needs to have his or her responsibilities well outlined. Typically, the medical needs of spectators and of the general public should be provided by separate medical teams — particularly during larger events. However, this "division of responsibility" needs to be clearly established well in advance so that the necessary arrangements can be made to insure adequate care is provided to all. The number and type of medical personnel required to staff an event depends on the number of participating athletes and support staff, the anticipated number of spectators, the demands of the sport, and the level of competition. In general, one physician and four paramedics per 250 participants, and one physician and one to two paramedics per 10,000 spectators represent a minimum standard. For larger tournament events, an adequate number of paraprofessionals, including massage therapists, should be available to assist athletes who depend on such services.

The tournament medical director should know in advance the type of medical personnel traveling with each team, and whether any team will require special services that may not be routinely provided. For teams traveling with their own medical physician and athletic trainer/physiotherapist, the tournament medical director should consult with the visiting medical team and provide them with detailed instructions on how and when they can access host medical facilities and how they can

Table 7.1 Medical equipment usually provided by the event hosts.

- Blankets
- Adjustable crutches
- Knee immobilizer
- Rigid plastic cervical collars
- Spine back board
- Ice/small plastic bags
- Drinking water and paper cups
- Telephone service (frequently mobile)
- An equipped examination room

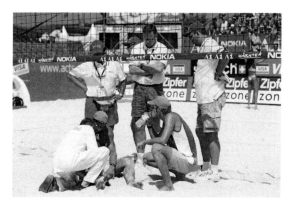

Fig. 7.1 Tournament medical personnel should be prepared to provide courtside attention to injured athletes if necessary.

contact host medical personnel. The visiting team physician and/or athletic trainer need to be informed regarding what resources are available to them. Table 7.1 lists the medical equipment usually supplied by the event host.

For those teams not traveling with medical personnel, the host medical team may be agreeable to providing coverage. Unlike the dedicated team physician, the event health care professional will, in most instances, have no prior knowledge of most of the athletes for whose care he or she is potentially responsible during the event. Thus, the event medical and paramedical staff must establish open communication with the members of the teams to whom they will be attending. Elite teams often have the luxury of traveling with an athletic trainer, physiotherapist, and/or physician who takes primary responsibility for their care throughout the event. Nevertheless, the event medical staff should be briefed at the outset by each team's trainer (or physician or coach) regarding any individual currently receiving treatment for an injury or other medical condition that might potentially increase their risk of additional injury or harm. In addition, it is important to identify players who have medical conditions that may require special attention, such as diabetes, asthma, or epilepsy.

Personnel

The role of the volleyball medical professional is discussed in Chapter 6. Ideally, the medical care of

any athletic team is supported by a team of medical professionals collaborating together to provide subspeciality-level care for the athletes. However, one principal team physician is usually responsible for coordinating these efforts. The role of team physician is frequently one of communicator or triage director between the team and its other associated medical professionals, including other subspecialty physicians who assist in caring for the athletes.

During an event, the primary responsibility of the team physician is to care for the acutely injured athlete. In addition to evaluating the nature and extent of the injury and then providing appropriate treatment, it is usually the responsibility of the team physician to determine if an injured athlete can return to play in the contest (Fig. 7.1). In the absence of a team physician, this responsibility will rest with the tournament medical director. The core principle governing such decision making must be the health and well being of the individual athlete. Factors influencing return to play decisions include:

1 Whether the injury could potentially worsen with further exposure.

2 Whether the injury (or the consequences of the injury and treatment) might pose a safety hazard to other competitors.

Open communication between the medical team, the coach, and the athlete will facilitate the best care of the injured athlete. In the event of an injury limiting or preventing ongoing participation, such communication will also help the coach plan and develop an alternative team strategy.

Often, more elite teams have a certified athletic trainer or physiotherapist to coordinate the athlete's day to day medical care and rehabilitation programs. This individual reports directly to the team physician(s) and works daily with the team to assess the progress made in treating current injuries. Typically, the athletic trainer or physiotherapist attends all practice sessions and competitions, and is certified in cardiopulmonary resuscitation in addition to having knowledge of first aid and medical triage plans. In fact, the National Collegiate Athletic Administration (NCAA) requires certification in cardiopulmonary resuscitation for all athletic personnel associated with competitions or practices, including strength and conditioning training.

Emergency medical services (EMS) should be "on call" and have ready access to the sporting event in the case of a medical emergency. The tournament medical director should decide whether EMS personnel should be present "on site" during the event. This decision may be made after evaluating both the anticipated demand for medical services and the location of the event. If, for example, the competition venue is located within minutes of an emergency medical facility then the on-site presence of an ambulance or other EMS personnel may not be necessary. If, on the other hand, the venue is remote from an emergency care facility, the presence of an EMS unit might be considered advisable.

Prior to the event, a meeting with tournament medical personnel should be scheduled to direct and clarify the role of each member of the team in the event of an emergency. If the EMS unit is not on site, they should be familiar with the most efficient routes into the venue. Proper accreditation should be issued to the EMS team to guarantee prompt access to the sporting event. An emergency care triage plan is necessary and should include the presence of a physician, or at a minimum planned access to a physician "on call" or at a nearby medical facility. Furthermore, the availability of subspecialty-level care on an urgent/as needed basis should be confirmed in advance. All medical staff should be familiar with the location and operation of basic EMS equipment. Routes for emergency evacuation with or without the participation of paramedics should be clearly marked and understood, and in some occasions rehearsed, to guarantee a maximum level of efficiency during critical situations.

Immediate access to a telephone or some other telecommunication device is vital to activating the EMS if and when it is needed. In addition, supervising medical personnel should promptly alert and debrief the medical professionals involved in transporting an injured athlete to facilitate and coordinate optimal acute care. In this regard, the medical professionals associated with a team should have ready access to the pertinent medical history of each athlete, including present and prior injuries, medical conditions, known drug allergies, current medications, insurance information, and emergency contact phone numbers.

Referees should be included in all event planning and precautions without underestimating their importance and role. In particular, it is useful to review with the referees the proper procedure for attending to a player injured during competition.

Facilities, equipment, and procedures

The equipment present at an athletic facility can vary tremendously, and may be influenced by the nature of the sport and the level of competition. In the case of volleyball, the inventory of equipment and supplies required also depends on whether the event is held indoors or outdoors. At the most basic level, it is essential that an examination room guaranteeing privacy is available. The medical examination room should be accessible to all medical personnel involved with the athletic event. For events within the USA, these facilities should also meet standards for the prevention of disease transmission through exposure to blood and body fluids as adopted by the United States Occupational Safety and Health Administration (e.g. pertaining to disposal of sharps, soiled dressings, etc.). These guidelines are available online at www.osha.gov. Outside the United States, team medical personnel should be sensitive to guidelines specific to each country.

Equipment needed to initially stabilize a seriously injured athlete (including, but not limited to, airway management tools, splints, and bandages) should be present at the site and quickly accessible. All staff present should be familiar with their use and location. Although the team physician medical bag typically carries medications and some diagnostic equipment, it is helpful to have the host facility provide larger items that are typically more difficult to transport (for example, these items might include splints for upper and lower extremity fractures—see Table 7.1). The new generation of automatic external defibrillators (AEDs) that administer an appropriate electric shock for the treatment of cardiac dysrhythmias may also be included. If an AED is available at an event, make sure that it (and other electrical or battery-powered equipment) is properly charged and that there are on-site medical personnel trained in its use should the need arise.

A physical examination by an experienced sports medicine physician is an indispensable tool to help establish an accurate diagnosis. Basic diagnostic equipment to enable a thorough physical exam should be readily available to the volleyball medical professional. Indeed, many of these items are found routinely within the "physician's black bag." Important items include a stethoscope, a sphygmomanometer for measuring blood pressure, an otoscope, an ophthalmoscope, a flashlight or disposable penlight, tongue blades, a reflex hammer, and an oral thermometer. When covering larger participatory events, additional equipment might include a glucometer, and a rectal thermometer to measure core body temperature. All equipment should be checked prior to the event to make sure that it is operational. Some sporting venues may be equipped with on-site radiographical imaging services, depending on the size and importance of the event. Although expensive to staff and operate, on-site radiology facilities certainly maximize the efficiency of athlete care.

Volleyball athletes occasionally suffer lacerations, and the event medical staff should be prepared to treat the wound on site. Preprepared "laceration kits" are a useful item to have readily available. Such kits include a sterile set up that permits lavage of the laceration, debridement, and, if indicated, closure of the wound. A variety of needle types and suture sizes would be preferred, with smaller gauged sutures for facial lacerations and larger gauge sutures for extremity lacerations. Steristrips, "butterfly"-type ban-

dages, and/or skin "glue" are also useful to have on hand for quick, efficient care of skin abrasions/lacerations.

The medical professional assigned to work with a team may have available several different classes of pharmaceutical agents that can be dispensed to treat symptoms of pain, inflammation, nausea, diarrhea, fever, headache, and insomnia. The trade names of these different medications vary between countries and therefore will not be listed here. In the United States, individual states regulate the prescription and distribution of such medication within the state. Local regulations should be checked in advance to assure compliance. Typically, the tournament medical director can serve as the local prescribing physician should the use of a specific medication prove necessary. Before administering or prescribing any medication, medical personnel should confirm that the agent is not on the IOC list of prohibited substances.

If it is anticipated that at some point during the course of the event selected athletes will be asked to undergo doping control, the event organizers should provide acceptable facilities to carry out such testing. The organization sponsoring the competition (IOC, FIVB, NCAA, etc.) will typically have well-outlined procedures for performing such controls, and care should be taken to meet appropriate standards so as not to invalidate any testing performed. Note that referees for international competitions sponsored by the FIVB are subject to mandatory pregame breath testing to detect intoxicating levels of alcohol that would impair their performance.

Outdoor events may be subject to weather extremes. Beach volleyball events held in conditions of high temperature and humidity may result in dehydration or heat illness (see Chapter 9). Adequate supplies of oral and intravenous (IV) fluids should be available to rehydrate the symptomatic athlete. Supplies needed to obtain IV access, listed in Table 7.2, should be available on demand. Tournament officials should monitor the wet bulb globe temperature (calculated as WBGT = 0.7 [wet bulb temperature] + 0.2 [black globe temperature] + 0.1 [ambient temperature]) and if it exceeds 28°C consideration should be given to postponing play or canceling the competition outright.

In the case of an advancing thunderstorm, the

Table 7.2 Equipment needed for IV access.

- Rubber tourniquet
- Non-sterile gloves
- Sterile gloves in a variety of sizes
- Tegaderm and/or tape
- IV tubing
- Alcohol preparatory pads
- Lactated ringers, 500 mL
- Normal saline, 500 mL
- Butterfly infusion set (23 gauge/19 gauge)
- Gelco angiocatheters (18 gauge/16 gauge/14 gauge)
- Gauze pads/dressings

most basic first aid care. Before the visiting teams depart, plans for the continuing care of injured athletes should be agreed upon by the responsible parties.

Once concluded, it is recommended that the tournament medical director go over the details of the medical care provided during the event, gathering input from the staff and volunteer members involved. Suggestions for improvements should be noted, to help in planning for the next event. In this way, the athletes, coaches, officials, and spectators can be assured that they will be receiving the finest medical care possible.

tournament medical director may be asked to decide if the event can safely continue. One method for determining the distance of a lightning strike is to monitor the "flash to bang count." Using this method, the number of seconds between the flash of lightening and the subsequent thunderclap (bang) divided by 5 estimates the distance in miles. The United States National Severe Storms Laboratory recommends that all individuals should evacuate an outdoor competition venue by the time the "flash to bang count" reaches 15 s (which would suggest that the lightning is 4.8 km or 3 miles away).

Postevent management

The event medical staff should document all encounters with athletes. The record should be kept on file with other event-related documents. The name of the volleyball medical professional caring for the athlete should be included as well. A copy of any report should be given to the athlete and their team physician or trainer (if one exists). Note that informed parental consent must be obtained before treating minors, or before providing more than the

Recommended reading

American College of Sports Medicine (2001) Sideline preparedness for the team physician: consensus statement. *Medicine and Science in Sports and Exercise* **33** (5), 846–849.

Green III, J.R. & Burns, S. (1999) Event coverage. In: Arendt, E.A. (ed). *Orthopaedic Knowledge Update: Sports Medicine 2*, pp. 85–91. American Academy of Orthopaedic Surgeons, Rosemont, IL.

Jones, B.H. & Roberts, W.O. (1991) Medical management of endurance events. In: Cantu, R.C. & Micheli, L.J. (eds). *ACSM: Guidelines for the Team Physician*, pp 266–286. Lea & Febiger, Philadelphia.

Kujala, U.M., Heinonen, O.J., Lehto, M., Jarvinen, M. & Bergfeld, J.A. (1998) Equipment, drugs and problems of the competition and team physician. *Sports Medicine* **6**, 197–209.

Laird, R.H. (1989) Medical care at ultra endurance triathlons. *Medicine and Science in Sports and Exercise* **21** (Suppl. 5), S222–S225.

Monto, R.R., Bassett III, F.H. & Hardaker Jr, W.T. (1990) Team physician no. 9: the role and responsibilities of the competition physician. *Orthopaedic Review* **19**, 1015–1020.

Painter, J. (ed.) (2001) *2001–2002 NCAA Sports Medicine Handbook*, 14th edn. National Collegiate Athletic Association, Indianapolis, IN.

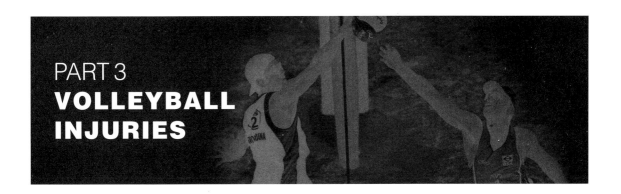

PART 3
VOLLEYBALL INJURIES

Chapter 8
Volleyball injury epidemiology

Jonathan C. Reeser

Introduction

Sports injury epidemiology is the discipline of understanding the kinds of injuries that befall athletes and the risk factors that predispose athletes to injury. Research has demonstrated that the injuries suffered by athletes in one sport tend to differ from those incurred through participation in other sports. These sport-specific "injury patterns" are thought to result from the interplay between the risk factors that are inherent to the athlete (intrinsic risk factors) and those that are inherent to the sport and the sporting environment (extrinsic risk factors). The study of volleyball injury epidemiology should therefore permit insight into those risk factors that predispose volleyball athletes to injury. Unfortunately, due to methodological limitations of the studies that exist in the literature, the scientific foundation of volleyball injury epidemiology and sports science is not as sound as would be optimal.

Variation in the methodology of the studies in the literature that have investigated the epidemiology of volleyball injuries hampers comparison between those studies and therefore limits the ability to make inferences about risk factors. Table 8.1 summarizes data on volleyball injury patterns from selected studies. Methodological and design considerations that limit the power of the published investigations include whether the data were collected prospectively or retrospectively, the demographics of the population studied (particularly in terms of gender and skill level), and the definition of injury employed. Clearly, studies that define an injury as any complaint for which an athlete seeks treatment cannot be compared without some degree of caution to studies that consider only those injuries resulting in a specified amount of time lost from training or competition. Nevertheless, it is important that volleyball coaches, trainers, therapists, and team physicians attempt to understand what is known so that injuries can be appropriately treated and rehabilitated or, ideally, avoided altogether.

The epidemiology of volleyball injuries

Cross-sectional population studies

The study population, or cohort being investigated, inevitably introduces bias into the data collected during epidemiological research. In general, what might be referred to as "population" studies provide information about injury incidence among a wide cross-section of the population at large. The studies of this type in the volleyball literature, while tending to focus on recreational athletes, permit comparison of the injury patterns characteristic of volleyball with injury patterns of other sports. Unfortunately, not all population studies collect data on the number of athlete exposures, making it difficult to calculate injury rates—a statistic by which the risk of injury in different sports can be compared more quantitatively. Furthermore, even when injury rates are reported, use of variable denominators

Table 8.1 Summary data from selected studies investigating the most commonly occurring injuries among competitive volleyball players. As discussed in the text, the comparison between existing epidemiological studies is difficult due to variation in design, methodology, and the definition of injury.

	NCAA (1999–2000)	Schafle *et al.* (1990)	Aagaard & Jørgensen (1996)	Bahr & Bahr (1997)
Diagnosis				
First most common	Sprain	Strain	Acute injury	Acute injury
Second most common	Strain	Sprain	Overuse injury	
Third most common	Tendinopathy	Inflammation		
Affected area				
First most common	Ankle	Ankle	Digits	Ankle
Second most common	Shoulder	Low back	Ankle	Low back
Third most common	Knee	Knee	Knee	Knee/shoulder
Time loss injury rate	4.2 per 1,000 AE	2.3 per 1,000 h	3.8 per 1,000 h	1.7 per 1,000 h

AE, athlete exposures; h, hours of athlete participation.

often precludes direct comparison between studies. For example, injury rates may be reported in terms of injuries per hours of competition, per number of athlete "exposures," or per year. Finally, although these studies may allow some inference about risk factors (depending on the type of data collected), the design of these observational studies typically does not permit determination of cause and effect relationships.

Chan and his group in Hong Kong have published two population studies analysing sports injury data collected prospectively over nearly 7 years. Among athletes presenting to an emergency room for evaluation of sport-related injuries, volleyball ranked behind soccer and basketball and was comparable to cycling (Chan *et al.* 1993). Volleyball athletes injured their knees more often than other body parts, with shoulders, ankles, and lower backs ranking second through fourth, respectively. Among athletes 16 years of age or younger, volleyball ranked fifth among sporting activities causing injury (Maffulli *et al.* 1996). In a retrospective analysis of the Finnish national sports injury insurance registry data, Kujala *et al.* (1995) found that volleyball had the lowest overall injury rate of any sport (60 injuries per 1,000 person-years). Ankle sprains were the most common injury for which treatment was sought. A similar analysis of Swiss military insurance registry data (deLoës 1995) found that males and females aged 14–20 years experienced similar (low) rates of injury over a 3-year period: 3.0 and 3.8 injuries per 10,000 h participation, respectively.

Event—specific studies

More detailed sport-specific information on volleyball injury risk factors has been derived from studies which prospectively catalogue injuries occurring at a specific event, such as the United States Open volleyball tournament or the volleyball competition at the US Olympic Festival. Collecting data at these venues permits computation of accurate injury rates for the specific populations studied based upon the hours of athlete participation. Schafle *et al* (1990) examined the incidence of injury at the 1987 US Open and reported an injury rate of 1.97 per 100 h of participation—of which 0.23 per 100 h were time-loss injuries. Males and females had roughly comparable injury rates, but the authors noted that males competing in the most skilled division experienced the highest incidence of injury. Ankle injuries predominated, and middle blockers and strong side attackers (the positions required to jump most often at the net) were most frequently injured. Briner and Ely (1999), on the other hand, found that patellar tendinopathy ("jumper's knee") was the most common injury reported by athletes at the 1995 US Olympic Festival. The overall injury rate reported was 1 per 25 h of competition, with no significant difference detected between males and females. While valuable, and generally more informative than the wider population-based studies considered earlier with respect to risk factors for injury, these studies provide only a "snap shot in time," and therefore provide no information about the effect of season-long training on injury incidence.

The NCAA injury surveillance system

Perhaps the best data on injury incidence among volleyball players comes from the Injury Surveillance System (ISS) database maintained by the National Collegiate Athletic Association (NCAA, Indianapolis, IN USA). Since the 1984–85 season, the ISS has been prospectively collecting data on time-loss injuries sustained by athletes competing in women's volleyball at over 100 participating institutions across all three NCAA divisions. Volleyball has one of the lowest injury rates of the 15 sports for which data are collected (American football has the highest). Over the years, the pattern of injuries in women's volleyball has remained remarkably constant. For the 1999–2000 season, ankle injuries comprised roughly 23% of all the injuries recorded, with shoulder (13%) and knee (11%) injuries ranking second and third, respectively. Low back injuries ranked fourth. Over the past decade, sprains and strains have been the most common acute injury, while tendinopathy represents the most common overuse injury. Spiking and blocking are the skills most often associated with injury. The highest injury rate typically occurs in Division I (NCAA Division I universities are generally larger and attract the more talented athletes), with a higher rate of injury during competition than during practice. The overall injury rate for the 1999–2000 season was 4.2 per 1,000 athlete exposures (defined as either a practice or game in which the athlete participates). For the 1999–2000 season, the practice injury rate was comparable to the game injury rate (4.2 vs 4.3 per 1,000 athlete exposures, respectively). However, over the preceding two seasons the injury rate during competition exceeded the practice rate by a greater margin (4.2 vs 3.2, respectively). Bahr and Bahr (1997) have also documented a higher injury rate during competition than during training, particularly with regard to ankle sprain injuries. Most of the injuries recorded by the NCAA ISS during the 1999–2000 season were relatively minor: 71% resulted in 6 or fewer days off from training or competition. Approximately 5% of injuries required surgical intervention. Unfortunately the NCAA ISS does not track men's intercollegiate volleyball, but Lanese et al. (1990) found no significant gender difference in either the rate or severity of injuries over a 1-year period among a cohort of male and female volleyball athletes competing for a major Midwestern university.

The elite volleyball athlete

The studies reviewed so far vary in their target population, ranging from recreational to collegiate athletes. Very few investigations have focused on the elite volleyball athlete specifically. Aagaard and Jørgensen (1996) catalogued injuries sustained by elite Danish volleyball athletes over one competitive season and found an overall injury rate of 3.8 injuries per 1,000 h of participation. A rather broad definition of injury was employed; participating players were instructed to self-report any condition which impaired their play or required "special treatment." Although males spent more time training, males and females had equivalent injury rates. Ankle sprains and finger trauma accounted for the majority of acute injuries, while knee and shoulder injuries were the most common overuse injuries. When the authors compared their results with those from a similar study conducted 10 years previously, the overuse injury rate had increased threefold. Not insignificantly, the number of training hours for male athletes had increased by 50%. Further study would appear to be needed to identify what constitutes safe and effective training volumes for the elite athlete so that overload injuries can be avoided. Bahr and Bahr (1997) conducted a prospective study recording the acute time-loss injuries sustained by a cohort of elite Norwegian volleyball athletes over one season. They found an acute injury rate of 1.7 per 1,000 h, without significant variation between men and women. Ankle sprains were by far the most common injury. Importantly, over half of the ankle sprains occurred as the result of contact with an opponent under the net (Fig. 8.1). Furthermore, 79% of the ankle sprains were recurrent, suggesting that prior injuries may have been inadequately rehabilitated. The long-term functional consequences of recurrent ankle sprain among volleyball athletes are not well understood, but at least one study has suggested that repeated ankle sprain injury may increase risk of developing osteoarthritis of the affected ankle joint (Gross & Marti 1999).

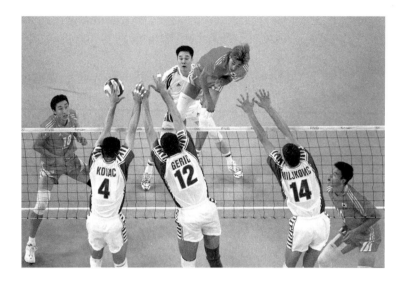

Fig. 8.1 Studies have shown that ankle sprains (the most common volleyball injury) occur most frequently as a consequence of net play. (© Allsport/ Michael Steele.)

The young volleyball athlete

Volleyball is a sport which can be enjoyed by all generations, and at the US Open tournament participants well into their seventies can be found competing out of a love for the game. At the other end of the age spectrum, there are an ever-increasing number of opportunities for young people to become involved in volleyball. There is reason for concern that engaging young athletes in competitive and overly structured volleyball programs may increase their risk of injury. For example, in their 1991 study Backx *et al.* found that although volleyball ranked fourth overall among the sports surveyed in injury rate, volleyball athletes aged 8–17 years actually experienced the highest practice injury rate. The authors concluded that volleyball and other high "jump rate" sports should be considered high risk for injury among young athletes. In a 1998 study in Germany, Von Wrende and Pforringer reported that the injury rate among youth rose with increasing age. Since most of the injuries occurred during training/practice, it would seem reasonable to conclude on the basis of these two studies that training volume in developing athletes should be limited so as to reduce the risk of developing overuse injuries due to chronic overload. In fact, the American Academy of Pediatrics Committee on Sports Medicine and Fitness (2000) recently au-

thored a position paper on intensive training and sports specialization in which "specialization in a single sport before adolescence" was discouraged. Unfortunately, no studies have been done to quantify appropriate training volumes that would serve to reduce the risk of injury, and therefore the burden of responsibility rests with parents, coaches, and the athletes themselves to recognize the signs and symptoms of overuse injury (among them, pain and deteriorating performance).

Injuries in beach volleyball

Beach volleyball, although growing in worldwide popularity, has not been well studied. However, based on the different environmental factors, tactics, and rules it would be reasonable to hypothesize that the injury patterns among beach volleyball players might differ from their indoor counterparts. Indeed, in their 1997 study Aagaard *et al.* demonstrated that beach players were more likely to develop overuse shoulder pathology than were indoor players. Nevertheless, the overall injury rate was comparable between indoor and outdoor volleyball athletes in that study. Bahr and Reeser recently conducted a study of the injuries occurring among the athletes participating in the 2001 FIVB World Tour (Bahr & Reeser, in press). The data collected suggest that overuse injuries affecting the low back, knees, and shoulder represent a significant source of disability and impaired performance for professional beach volleyball athletes. The study also estimated the rate of acute time-loss injuries among beach volleyball players at 3.1 per 1,000 h of player exposure, roughly comparable to that for indoor volleyball.

Specific injury conditions

While the population and event studies considered above provide useful information about injury patterns, case series may in some instances permit more careful analysis of the factors influencing those patterns. Ferretti (1986; Ferretti *et al.* 1992) has written extensively on knee injuries in volleyball, publishing case series of both knee ligament injuries and jumper's knee. From his work it became apparent that the volume of jump training and the firmness of the playing surface were both risk factors for volleyball-related knee injuries. Briner and Ely (1999) estimated that athletes training and competing on hard, unforgiving surfaces suffer five times the rate of time-loss lower limb injuries than do those athletes playing outdoors in the sand. Ferretti *et al.* (1998) has also published a large case series investigating the natural history of suprascapular neuropathy. This condition, which results in shoulder weakness but curiously does not seem to impair performance to a great extent, is so specific to volleyball that it has been termed "volleyball shoulder."

As mentioned, ankle sprain injuries are the most common acute volleyball-related trauma. Through Bahr's elegant work (Bahr *et al.* 1994) we know that ankle sprains most commonly occur when a blocker lands on the foot of an opposing attacker whose foot penetrates the centerline. Perhaps not surprisingly, given the different tactics employed in beach volleyball and the less congested area around the beach volleyball net, Aagaard *et al.* (1997) found that beach volleyball players experienced fewer acute ankle injuries than their indoor counterparts, a finding confirmed by the FIVB beach volleyball injury study (Bahr & Reeser, in press). Bahr and Bahr (1997) have also calculated that an ankle sprain within the past 6 months significantly increases a volleyball athlete's risk of incurring a sprained ankle (risk ratio 9.8 compared with uninjured ankles). These findings have important implications for athlete training, injury rehabilitation, and decisions regarding return to play following injury.

Conclusion

From the studies reviewed we may conclude that volleyball athletes are in general at greatest risk for non-surgical injuries to ligaments (sprains) and muscles (strains) as the result of acute dynamic overload, and to tendons as the result of chronic overuse (tendinopathies). The most frequently injured body parts are the ankle, knee, shoulder, and low back. Spiking and blocking, in part because these skills demand repeated jumping at the net, should be considered "high-risk" activities. The injury patterns observed between beach and indoor volleyball differ slightly, reflecting the different competitive environments and tactics of the two disciplines. Although volleyball in general should probably be considered a relatively "safe" sport when compared with other sporting activities, elite or more skilled athletes appear to have an increased risk of injury—particularly overuse injuries. These studies also suggest that there is probably no statistically significant difference between the injury rates for male and female volleyball players, although several of the studies did identify a slightly higher injury rate among young male athletes during competition.

Volleyball is a sport in evolution, particularly over the past several years as new rules and strategies have quickly been assimilated into the game. How these changes will effect the injury patterns associated with the different disciplines of the sport remains to be seen. It is apparent, however, that Cherebetiu's (1980) contention that "great results in sports are the result of a team effort" remains true. Over the past several decades, a new paradigm has developed in which athletic success has come to depend on more than simply great individual talent and effort. While victory in the arena ultimately depends on the athlete, the groundwork for success is prepared by a dedicated support staff of coaches and sports medicine personnel all striving to help the athlete run faster, jump higher, become stronger, and play smarter. Therefore, it is important for volleyball coaches and athletes, in addition to team physicians and trainers, to understand the basics of injury treatment and prevention (Schafle 1993; Briner & Kacmar 1997; Briner & Benjamin 1999; Schutz 1999). Injury epidemiology provides the foundation of our understanding of sport-specific risk factors. Although based on imperfect studies, we appear to have a reasonable appreciation of several intrinsic and extrinsic risk factors for injury in volleyball. Through further research, our knowledge base and understanding of volleyball injury epidemiology will undoubtedly be refined and deepened in the years ahead.

References

Aagaard, H. & Jørgensen, U. (1996) Injuries in elite volleyball. *Scandinavian Journal of Medicine and Science in Sports* 6, 228–232.

Aagaard, H., Scavenius, M. & Jørgensen, U. (1997) An epidemiological analysis of the injury pattern in indoor and in beach volleyball. *International Journal of Sports Medicine* 18 (3), 217–221.

American Academy of Pediatrics (2000) Intensive training and sports specialization in young athletes. *Pediatrics* 106 (1), 154–157.

Backx, F.J.G., Beijer, H.J.M., Bol, E. & Erich, W.B.M. (1991) Injuries in high-risk persons and high-risk sports. *American Journal of Sports Medicine* 19 (2), 124–130.

Bahr, R. & Bahr, I.A. (1997) Incidence of acute volleyball injuries: a prospective cohort study of injury mechanisms and risk factors. *Scandinavian Journal of Medicine and Science in Sports* 7, 166–171.

Bahr, R., Karlsen, R., Lian, Ø. & Øvrebø, R.V. (1994) Incidence and mechanism of acute ankle inversion injuries in volleyball. *American Journal of Sports Medicine* 22 (5), 595–600.

Bahr, R. & Reeser, J.C. (2002) The FIVB beach volleyball injury study: injuries among professional beach volleyball players. *American Journal of Sports Medicine*, in press.

Briner, W.W. & Benjamin, H.J. (1999) Volleyball injuries. *Physician and Sports Medicine* 27 (3), 48–60.

Briner, W.W. & Ely, C. (1999) Volleyball injuries at the 1995 United States Olympic festival. *International Journal of Volleyball Research* 1 (1), 7–11.

Briner, W.W. & Kacmar, L. (1997) Common injuries in volleyball. *Sports Medicine* 24 (1), 65–71.

Chan, K.M., Yuan, Y., Li Pg, C.K., Chien, P. & Tsang, G. (1993) Sports causing most injuries in Hong Kong. *British Journal of Sports Medicine* 27 (4), 263–267.

Cherebetiu, G. (1980) Cooperation among the doctor, the coach, and player. *Volleyball Technical Journal* 5 (2), 5–11.

deLoës, M. (1995) Epidemiology of sports injuries in the Swiss organization 'Youth and Sports' 1987–89. *International Journal of Sports Medicine* 16, 134–138.

Ferretti, A. (1986) Epidemiology of jumper's knee. *Sports Medicine* 3, 289–295.

Ferretti, A., DeCarli, A. & Fontana, M. (1998) Injury of the suprascapular nerve at the spinoglenoid notch. *American Journal of Sports Medicine* 26 (6), 759–763.

Ferretti, A., Papandrea, P., Conteduca, F. & Mariani, P.P. (1992) Knee ligament injuries in volleyball players. *American Journal of Sports Medicine* 20 (2), 203–207.

Gross, P. & Marti, B. (1999) Risk of degenerative ankle joint disease in volleyball players: study of former elite athletes. *International Journal of Sports Medicine* 20, 58–63.

Kujala, U.M., Taimela, S., Antti-Poika, I., Orava, S., Tuominen, R. & Myllynen, P. (1995) Acute injuries in soccer, ice hockey, volleyball, basketball, judo, and karate: analysis of national registry data. *British Medical Journal* 31, 1465–1468.

Lanese, R.R., Strauss, R.H., Leizman, D.J. & Rotondi, A.M. (1990) Injury and disability in matched men's and women's intercollegiate sports. *American Journal of Public Health* 80 (12), 1459–1462.

Maffulli, N., Bundoc, R.C., Chan, K.M. & Cheng, J.C.Y. (1996) Paediatric sports injuries in Hong Kong: a seven year survey. *British Journal of Sports Medicine* 30, 218–221.

Schafle, M.D. (1993) Common injuries in volleyball. *Sports Medicine* 16 (2), 126–129.

Schafle, M.D., Requa, R.K., Patton, W.L. & Garrick, J.G. (1990) Injuries in the 1987 National Amateur Volleyball Tournament. *American Journal of Sports Medicine* 18 (6), 624–631.

Schutz, L.K. (1999) Volleyball. *Physical Medicine and Rehabilitation Clinics of North America* 10 (1), 19–34.

Von Wrende, A. & Pforringer, W. (1998) Traumatologie biem Volleyball in Jugend- und Kindersalter. *Sportverletzung   Sportschaden* 12, 39–41.

Recommended reading

Ferretti, A. (1994) *Volleyball Injuries*. Federation Internationale de Volleyball, Lausanne, Switzerland.

International Olympic Committee Medical Commission (2000) *Sport Medicine Manual*. International Olympic Committee, Lausanne, Switzerland.

Chapter 9
Environmental concerns in volleyball

William W. Briner, Jr.

Introduction

The sporting environment in which the volleyball athlete trains and competes clearly influences performance and risk of injury. Although in a broad sense, the "environment" can be considered to include the court or playing surface and other equipment of the game, in addition to the presence (or absence) of spectators, the principal focus of this chapter will be on weather- and temperature-related concerns. In this regard, the most important environmental concern pertaining to the sport of volleyball is exertional heat illness. Obviously, heat illness is likely to occur more frequently during outdoor competitions, such as beach volleyball and park volley. However, symptoms of heat illness can occur during any sporting event contested in conditions of high heat and ambient humidity

Heat illness

Humans can tolerate a wide range of environmental temperatures, but ultimately cellular viability is affected by temperature extremes. At 1°C ice crystals form in the tissues; at 45°C cellular proteins begin to denature. The human body can withstand temperatures of 41.1°C for only brief periods of time without sustaining potentially fatal tissue damage.

The heat load on an athlete may be defined as the sum of the heat produced by the athlete's basal metabolism, combined with the heat absorbed through environmental exposure and that generated by exercise. Active muscles are capable of generating heat at a rate 100 times greater than inactive muscles. During intense exercise, the rate of heat production may exceed $15\,kcal \cdot min^{-1}$ ($63\,kJ \cdot min^{-1}$). Because the body is only 25% efficient, only one-quarter of the energy expended during exercise results in useful work. The other 75% results in heat production that must be dissipated if the athlete is to continue functioning.

There are four processes by which heat may be gained from or lost to the environment: radiation, conduction, convection, and evaporation. Radiation refers to heat lost to the ambient air via electromagnetic waves. Heat is lost most efficiently if the air in contact with the skin is significantly cooler than the body's core temperature. Conduction is the transfer of heat through direct contact; usually, this represents only about 2% of body heat loss. Convection is loss of heat via the movement of ambient air. On a windy day, heat will be lost more effectively through convection. Evaporation results in heat loss because of the conversion of liquid (sweat) to gas on the surface of the skin. Evaporation is the body's most effective mechanism for heat loss. However, it may be necessary to employ techniques based on each of the methods of heat energy transfer when treating an athlete with acute exertional heat illness.

Thermoregulation is the process by which the body maintains its core temperature (normal body temperature is 37°C or 98.6°F). Heat may be retained to raise the body temperature or heat may be lost to the environment in order to lower the core temperature. This process is controlled by the central nervous system's temperature regulatory center, located in the anterior hypothalamus. Afferent receptors (sensors) are found in the skin and body core, and efferent nerve fibers transmit the autonomic nervous system response that results in thermoregulation. The sympathetic nervous system regulates vascular constriction and dilatation, while the parasympathetic system controls sweating.

Sweating begins within 30s to 3min after the onset of exercise. The sweat rate usually increases for the next 10min and then levels off. Sweating is the body's adaptive response to exercise in heat. The average runner will sweat $1 L \cdot h$. An athlete acclimatized to exercising in hot climates, however, may generate up to 2L of sweat per hour. The evaporation of 1mL of water dissipates approximately 0.6 kcal (2.5kJ) of heat energy. Thus, a well-trained athlete who is acclimatized to exercising in the heat is capable of transferring heat energy to the environment at a rate of greater than $1,000 kcal \cdot h$ ($4,200 kJ \cdot h$). Note that sweat contains small amounts of electrolytes, including sodium, chloride, and, to a lesser extent, potassium and magnesium. As an athlete becomes more acclimatized and sweat volume increases, the concentration of electrolytes in the sweat is reduced. Athletes must consider this fact when replenishing their fluids (see Chapter 5 for additional information on hydration).

Risk factors for heat illness

Athletes who exercise at high intensity but who are not acclimatized to the conditions in which they are competing are more likely to suffer from exertional heat illness. Those who are less conditioned or less fit may also be more likely to suffer symptoms of heat illness. Athletes who are acclimatized to exercising in conditions of high temperature extremes but not high humidity are also at considerable risk. As mentioned, evaporation is the major mechanism by which sweating effects heat loss. High ambient humidity reduces the rate of sweat evaporation and therefore impairs the athlete's heat loss capacity. This situation has occurred in beach volleyball athletes who train year round on warm coastal beaches,

then travel to compete in summer tournaments held in locales where the humidity may exceed 90%. Without the benefit of effective evaporation, the athlete's body core temperature can rise quickly, resulting in heat illness. All outdoor volleyball players should therefore be closely monitored for signs of heat illness. It is particularly important to identify and watch those athletes who have suffered from heat illness in the past, as they are more likely to be affected again. Medical personnel caring for outdoor volleyball athletes should monitor the environmental conditions and be willing (and authorized) to limit or postpone practice or competition should the wet bulb globe temperature (WBGT) exceed predetermined, agreed upon safety levels.

Certain types of medication may also put individuals at risk for heat illness. Diuretics ("water pills") may result in relative dehydration. Both caffeine and alcohol have diuretic properties. Athletes on these medications should be cautioned about the increased risk of dehydration and heat-related illness. Decongestant medications result in vasoconstriction, which impairs heat loss at the skin surface. Anticholinergic medications, such as some antidepressants, block parasympathetic tone—thereby inhibiting sweat production. Beta-blockers (a popular class of high blood pressure medication) may also decrease skin blood flow. Phenothiazides and other antipsychotic medicines such as haloperidol may result in decreased thirst, even in the face of significant dehydration.

Heat stress

Heat stress may precipitate three different types of heat illness in athletes: heat cramps, heat exhaustion, and heat stroke. While there are unique identifying characteristics for each of these conditions, more typically there is some overlap between them clinically. Certainly athletes can experience two of these conditions at the same time, such as concurrent heat cramps and heat exhaustion. Often, serious problems can be avoided if the affected athlete is identified early on, prior to the onset of severe symptoms. Players who feel dizzy or restless or who exhibit even minimal mental status changes (i.e. confusion) should (in the appropriate setting) be suspected of having heat stress. Vital signs will demonstrate an elevated core temperature, an increased heart rate, and reduced blood pressure. Cooling the athlete in a shaded area and giving cool fluids by mouth may prevent the onset of more serious, life-threatening symptoms.

Heat cramps

Heat cramps are tetanic contractions or spasms of exercising muscles. The athlete's core body temperature may be elevated or normal. Heat cramps may even occur hours after exercise. The mechanism by which heat cramps occur has not been fully elucidated. Almost certainly, dehydration plays a major role. The role of electrolytes in the etiology of heat cramps has been investigated, and it appears that sodium deficiency may be a contributing factor. There have been anecdotal reports of magnesium deficiency contributing to symptoms in some individuals.

In volleyball players, the muscles most frequently involved are the muscles of the lower limb such as the gastrocnemius and hamstrings. Forearm and hand muscles may cramp in hand setters. However, severely affected individuals may experience tetanic contractions of several different muscle groups simultaneously, including the rectus abdominus and the shoulder girdle musculature. Acute treatment includes stretching the involved muscle as quickly and completely as possible. Stretching is often more easily performed passively, by an athletic trainer or physical therapist who may be attending to the athlete. Application of ice is often beneficial as well. Oral rehydration should be attempted, preferably with a beverage containing replacement electrolytes (such as a sports drink). Some individuals may respond better to an infusion of intravenous saline (0.9 normal saline or lactated Ringer's solution are the iv fluids of choice).

Prevention of heat cramps involves acclimatization to exercise in conditions of high heat and humidity. It may take 10–14 days of training in such conditions before the athlete adapts physiologically. For some, a training regimen of longer duration and greater intensity may help to prevent symptoms in the future. All outdoor volleyball athletes should be counseled regarding "prehydration." It is recommended that outdoor athletes consume approxi-

mately 500 mL of fluid roughly 1.5 h before training or competition. Prehydration is essential to maintaining fluid balance during exercise. Athletes should not rely on thirst as a trigger for fluid replacement, as significant fluid losses can occur before they become thirsty. Athletes who have suffered from heat cramps in the past should probably be advised to liberally salt their food. Predisposed individuals may benefit from regular dietary salt supplementation, although little well-designed research on this topic exists in the literature.

Heat exhaustion

Heat exhaustion is characterized by symptoms of irritability, light-headedness, nausea with or without vomiting, and generalized weakness. Findings on examination may include a rapid heart rate (pulse), low blood pressure, "goose bumps," profuse sweating, and reduced urinary output. The core temperature is elevated, but is less than 41.8°C (105°F). Heat exhaustion is felt to occur because of dehydration and hypovolemia (reduced intravascular fluid volume). Electrolyte loss, particularly sodium, may also be a contributing factor.

The acute treatment for heat exhaustion is to rapidly cool the affected athlete, reducing their core temperature to 38.9°C (102°F) or less. The athlete should be placed in a cool environment and sprayed with cool or lukewarm water to facilitate evaporation and conductive heat loss. Placing the athlete in front of a fan helps to maximize convective heat loss. Oral rehydration is the preferred method of fluid replacement. Athletes who are suffering from severe nausea or experiencing emesis may need IV rehydration. In this situation, 0.9 normal saline or lactated Ringer's solution are again the intravenous fluids of choice.

Heat stroke

The definition of exertional heat stroke varies depending on the source, but the clinical hallmark is an elevated core temperature of 40.6°C (105°F) or greater. Heat stroke results from a global decompensation of the body's mechanisms for heat loss. Volume depletion and peripheral vasoconstriction impair the ability to transfer heat to the environment. Signs and symptoms of exertional heat stroke include hypotension (very low blood pressure), tachycardia (technically defined as a heart rate exceeding 100 beats·min^{-1}—although in well-trained athletes, a pulse of 90 beats·min^{-1} may represent a significant elevation of heart rate), reduced urine output, vomiting, and diarrhea. The athlete may go into hypovolemic shock, possibly resulting in kidney failure. Mental status changes, including disorientation and delirium, are common. There may even be bleeding into the brain, and seizure activity and coma have been reported to occur. The liver may be damaged, resulting in increased liver enzymes that can be monitored by serial blood tests. Other organ systems can fail as well, including the hematologic system (resulting in disseminated intravascular coagulation), and the muscles themselves may break down, resulting in rhabdomyolysis. Finally, cardiorespiratory overload can result in lung failure and/or myocardial infarction. Heat stroke must be regarded as a medical emergency and as a potentially fatal condition.

The most important goal in the treatment of exertional heat stroke is to cool the body to below 38.9°C (102°F) as quickly as possible. The most effective cooling method is to immerse the body in ice water, since heat is lost from the skin much more quickly by conduction to cold water than it is to the air. Athletes with exertional heat stroke are quite sick, so total body immersion should probably be done only if there are emergency medical personnel present capable of intubating the patient to protect the airway and maintain respiration. Obviously, most medical areas at volleyball competitions or tournaments are not equipped with this level of acute care personnel or facilities. Therefore, it is vitally important that athletes with heat stroke are transported to an emergency medical center as quickly as possible. However, cooling should not be delayed. Packing the entire body in towels that have been immersed in ice water is often effective in rapidly lowering the core temperature. Remember that the skin is the organ responsible for heat loss. The more skin in contact with cold water, the more effectively heat will be lost. It was once felt that placing ice packs over the large vessels in the groin and axilla was an effective way to cool heat stroke patients. However, this intervention may actually result in a reflex peripheral vasoconstriction, so the practice should probably be avoided. Spraying cool water on the skin (to maximize heat loss via conduction and evaporation) and fanning air over the athlete (to maximize convection) are also beneficial.

Prevention of heat illness

Heat illness is preventable. Note, however, that although the American College of Sports Medicine has established guidelines for prevention of thermal injury during running, no volleyball-specific guidelines for the prevention of heat illness have been developed. Nevertheless, based upon our scientific understanding of heat illness, prevention strategies should emphasize athlete education and physiological adaptation (Fig. 9.1). It is therefore important to discuss heat illness with all athletes—particularly those who have been affected by it in the past. Acclimatization to exercise in the environment in which the athlete will be competing is probably the most important consideration. As discussed, the process of acclimatization should begin at least 10–14 days prior to the first day of competition. Advise athletes that they will probably begin sweating earlier and at a greater rate as they adapt physiologically. Athletes should keep in mind that muscle is about 80% water and that they can lose up to 1.5 L of water before they demonstrate significant thirst.

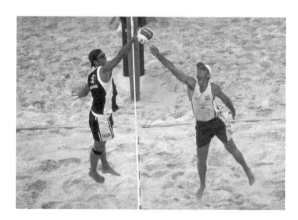

Fig. 9.1 Beach volleyball athletes are at risk for heat illness when competing in hot, humid conditions. Appropriate precautions include adequate hydration and acclimatization. Protection from the harmful effects of exposure to the sun's ultraviolet radiation is also recommended. (© Allsport/ Shaun Botterill.)

The loss of 2% of body weight due to dehydration can noticeably impair athletic performance. Outdoor volleyball athletes should therefore be urged to prehydrate themselves to help prevent dehydration and to permit ongoing high-level activity. Reasonable fluid intake guidelines include:

1 Drink 500 mL of water or fluid replacement beverage 90 min before competition.

2 Drink 250 mL every 20 min while competing. If the duration of a competition is less than 1 h, then water is probably the ideal fluid replacement beverage. If the competition lasts more than 1 h, then a carbohydrate/electrolyte solution (containing 4–8% carbohydrate) may be more beneficial.

3 After exercise, drink 1 L of fluid replacement beverage per kilogram of body weight lost during exercise.

Heat illness and the medical team

The medical team covering tournament play should be prepared to measure core body temperature accurately should the need arise. The only reliable means of measuring core temperature is rectally, and thus the tournament medical bag should include a rectal thermometer measuring up to 45°C (113°F). Aural, oral, and axillary thermometers all have significant shortcomings in the evaluation of heat illness. Normal saline or lactated Ringer's solution should be available in quantities sufficient for an entire tournament. A shaded area (or tent) with adequate air circulation should be available with cots or tables on which athletes may lie down. A mechanism for rapid cooling of athletes with heat exhaustion and heat stroke should be immediately available. A plan for rapidly transporting an athlete with heat stroke to a nearby emergency medical or intensive care facility should also be agreed upon in advance.

Sun exposure

One of the attractions of beach volleyball is that it is played outdoors during the summer months. As a result, participants typically wear swimming attire or other clothing that exposes their skin to the sun. Unfortunately, excessive exposure to ultraviolet (UV) radiation is damaging to the skin. A single episode of prolonged UV-B exposure can cause sunburn, a thermal injury which may vary in severity based on the duration of exposure, the intensity of the light source, and the amount of pigment in the individual's skin. UV-B radiation is not filtered by cloud cover and is reflected off both sand and water—further increasing the athlete's UV exposure. Sunburn can be quite painful, and if severe can cause blistering, fluid loss, and temperature dysregulation. Prevention of sunburn is considered the best treatment, as no intervention is uniformly effective for sunburn once it occurs.

The cumulative effects of long-term exposure to UV light include weathered, wrinkled skin that appears prematurely aged. Significant sunburn acquired as a youth increases one's risk of developing malignant melanoma, a particularly dangerous form of skin cancer, in later life. Furthermore, UV exposure increases an individual's risk of developing basal cell and squamous cell carcinomas of the skin. Outdoor volleyball athletes should therefore take appropriate precautions to protect themselves from excessive sun exposure. Recommendations include:

1 Avoid direct sun exposure when possible. Stay in the shade when not playing. If possible, avoid playing during midday (when the sun is at its highest point in the sky), since this is when the amount of UV radiation penetrating the atmosphere is highest.

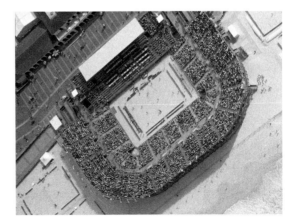

Fig. 9.2 Beach volleyball is the only Olympic sport to be contested on sand. The Bondi Beach venue at the Sydney 2000 Summer Olympics was a popular destination for fans of beach volleyball. (© Allsport/ Mike Powell.)

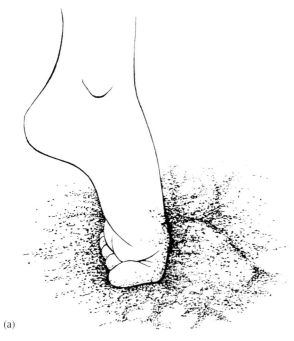

(a)

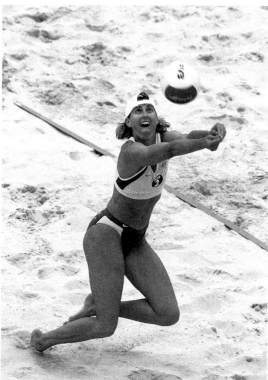

(b)

2 Wear loose fitting clothing and head coverings. This will permit sweat to evaporate while providing direct protection from the sun.

3 Use topical sunscreen preparations on uncovered skin to minimize UV-A and UV-B exposure. A sun protection factor (SPF) of 15 or greater is recommended. It may be necessary to reapply the sunscreen throughout the day, particularly if the athlete has been sweating heavily.

4 Wear sunglasses to protect the eyes from damaging UV radiation.

Injuries unique to competition on the sand

Beach volleyball is one of very few sports contested on the sand, and it is the only Olympic sport played on sand (Fig. 9.2). This puts beach volleyball athletes at risk for some unique injuries; "sand toe," for example, is an injury to the great toe that occurs when a beach volleyball player lands from a jump or other movement of the lower limb with their great toe plantar flexed in the sand (Frey *et al*. 1996). The subsequent forced plantar flexion of the great toe underneath the foot results in a sprain of the dorsal aspect of the first metatarsophalangeal (MTP) joint (Fig. 9.3). Severe cases of sand toe may result in open dislocation of the first MTP joint. Obviously, such an injury would require significant irrigation and antibiotic treatment. Fortunately, most cases of sand toe are not severe and can be managed with taping to support the first MTP joint. The injury typically results in significant pain and may impair jumping ability. With rest, these capsular sprains can be expected to heal over a period of approximately 8 weeks. The extent to which the incidence of sand toe is related to sand quality and the degree of compact-

Fig. 9.3 Sand toe results from forced plantar flexion of the metatarsophalangeal joint of the great toe. This occurs when the athlete lands on or transfers a significant load onto a neutral or plantarflexed toe (a), as Kerri Pottharst appears to do during this defensive play on day 10 of the Sydney 2000 Olympic Games (b). (© Allsport/ Scott Barbour.)

ness is unknown. There is anecdotal evidence, however, that suggests that knee injuries occur more frequently when beach volleyball is played on hard, compact sand. The FIVB has established guidelines to insure a minimum standard of sand quality on the courts used by the Beach Volleyball World Tour athletes.

Since beach volleyball is contested in bare feet on an uneven surface that may occasionally conceal unknown foreign objects, the tournament medical director must also be prepared for other foot and lower limb injuries, including nail avulsions, puncture wounds, lacerations, and other toe sprains/dislocations. At large tournaments, facilities and personnel for suturing lacerations should be available, if possible. Tetanus booster shots should also be available and administered when the athlete's immunization history is unknown or out of date. Athletes may continue competing even after a foot laceration has been sutured, if an occlusive dressing is worn. However, even the most adhesive of tapes or bandages are often not equal to the stresses placed on them by beach volleyball players, and as a result the dressings may come off during competition, leaving the wound exposed and vulnerable to infection. In such circumstances, a synthetic, fine-woven, nylon sock worn over the dressing will allow the athlete to continue to compete.

Reference

Frey, C., Andersen, G.D. & Feder, K.S. (1996) Platarflexion injury to the metatarsophalangeal joint ("sand toe"). *Foot and Ankle International* **17** (9), 576–581.

Recommended reading

Armstrong, L.E., Epstein, Y., Greenleaf, J.E. *et al.* (1996) Heat and cold illness during distance running: position stand of the American College of Sports Medicine. *Medicine and Science in Sports and Exercise* **28** (12), i–x.

Convertino, V.A., Armstrong, L.E., Coyle, E.F. *et al.* (1996) Exercise and fluid replacement: position stand of the American College of Sports Medicine. *Medicine and Science in Sports and Exercise* **28** (1), i–vii.

International Olympic Committee Medical Commission (2000) *Sport Medicine Manual*. International Olympic Committee, Lausanne, Switzerland.

Chapter 10
Injury prevention

Roald Bahr

Injury patterns in volleyball

The risk of injury in volleyball is lower than that documented for other team sports such as basketball, soccer, or ice hockey (Bahr & Bahr 1997; Bahr *et al.* 2002). Presumably, this difference can be attributed to the non-contact nature of the game of volleyball, since players from opposing teams are separated by the net. As is the case for all other sports, the injury pattern seen in volleyball is unique, and medical personnel who care for volleyball athletes should be familiar with the type of injuries to which volleyball players are prone. The sports medicine professional's responsibility does not stop at treating injuries, however; they also have an obligation to try to *prevent* injuries. To accomplish this goal, the volleyball medical professional must have a thorough understanding of volleyball injury patterns, injury mechanisms, and risk factors.

Ankle sprains account for approximately half of all acute time-loss injuries in volleyball (Bahr & Bahr 1997). The rate of ankle sprains is about one sprain per 1,000 player-hours of exposure (Bahr *et al.* 1994; Bahr & Bahr 1997). Most injuries are mild to moderate, but the injury rate is close to that observed in soccer and basketball—sports where the athletes are not separated by a net. In other words, ankle sprains are a significant source of disability in volleyball.

The most important overuse injury in volleyball is jumper's knee (patellar tendinopathy). Cross-sectional studies among high-level volleyball players have shown that the prevalence of patellar tendinopathy is 40–50% (Ferretti *et al.* 1984; Ferretti 1986; Lian *et al.* 1996b). However, the true proportion of affected players may be even greater, since none of the aforementioned studies included players with disabling problems.

Risk factors for sport-related injuries may be generally classified as either "intrinsic" or "extrinsic." Intrinsic risk factors are those qualities or features that are inherent to the athlete and which may predispose them to certain types of injury. Intrinsic risk factors might include the athlete's age, morphotype, a history of prior injury, degree of strength and conditioning, and psychological make-up. Extrinsic factors are inherent to the sport and the athlete's participation therein, and include the volume of training, playing surface, equipment used, position(s) played, environmental conditions, and the rules of the game. From these few examples, it is also evident that certain risk factors are "modifiable," while others are "unmodifiable." Clearly, only interventions targeting modifiable risk factors are likely to be successful in reducing the incidence of injuries. For example, athletes who are well conditioned and physically fit are generally more resistant to overuse injuries than are those athletes who may be less well conditioned (possibly as the result of attempting to return to competition too soon after an injury, for example). This chapter describes the injury mechanisms, risk factors, and prevention strategies for some of the most common injuries in volleyball, focusing on ankle sprains as the most common acute injury, and on patellar tendinopathy as the most common overuse injury. The chapter also briefly covers other common injuries, including acute knee and finger injuries, and overuse conditions including low back pain and shoulder pain.

Preventing ankle sprains

Injury mechanisms

Ankle sprains typically occur at the net when the athlete lands on the foot of an opponent or of a teammate after blocking or attacking (Fig. 10.1) (Hell & Schönle 1985; Schafle *et al.* 1990; Bahr *et al.* 1994). About half of all ankle sprains occur when a blocker lands on the opposing attacker's foot, while about one-quarter result from a player landing on

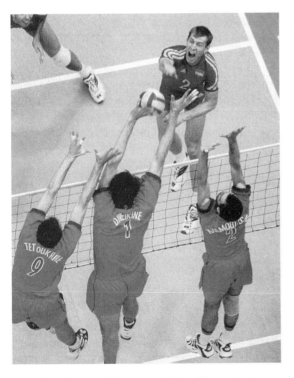

Fig. 10.1 The main "danger zone" for ankle sprains in volleyball: injuries mainly occur in the area around the centerline when landing after blocking or attacking. This happens when the attacking player lands on or across the centerline, or when one of the blockers lands on his teammate's foot.

their teammate's foot following a two- or three-person block (Bahr *et al.* 1994).

One common high-risk situation occurs when the volleyball is set too "tight," i.e. too low, too quick, and too close to the net. In trying to reach the ball in this situation, many attackers try to *outjump* the ball, thereby risking a landing on or across the centerline (Fig. 10.2). This in turn puts the opposing blocker at risk for landing on the attacker's foot. Of the injuries caused by landing on an opponent, about one-half take place in the legal "conflict zone" under the net without violating the current centerline penetration rule. The remaining 50% result from a centerline violation (the attacker is almost always at fault). It is important to understand that the present centerline violation rule allows a player to step across the centerline, as long as a part of their foot remains on or above the centerline.

In summary, the most common mechanism for acute ankle injury occurs when a blocker lands on the opposing attacker's foot, which may or may not have penetrated the centerline in violation of the current rule. In addition, it appears that most of the ankle sprains in volleyball result from what could be termed technical errors, including an inadequate approach or flawed take-off or landing technique when blocking or attacking.

Risk factors

The most important risk factor that has been identified for ankle sprains is a previous ankle injury. In fact, research has shown that among senior players, four out of five ankle sprains occur in previously injured ankles (an observation made in other sports as well) (Ekstrand & Tropp 1990; Milgrom *et al.* 1991). Compared to an ankle with no prior injury, the risk of injury is fourfold greater for an ankle that has been sprained one or more times (Bahr & Bahr 1997). Furthermore, the more recent the injury, the higher the risk. The injury rate during the first 6–12 months after an ankle sprain is nearly 10-fold higher than for an ankle without previous injury.

Possible preventive strategies

Several intervention strategies have been proposed based on the typical injury mechanisms and risk

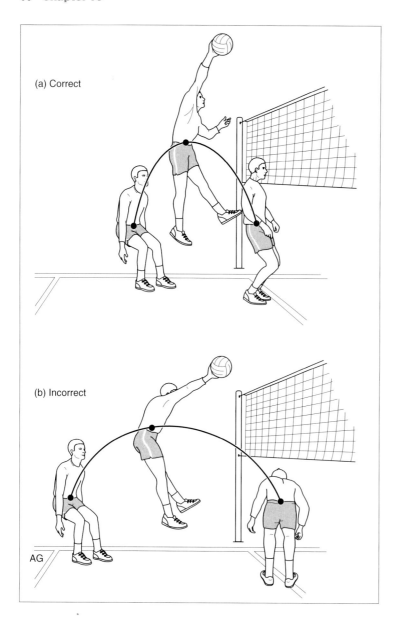

(a) Correct

(b) Incorrect

AG

Fig. 10.2 The main injury mechanism for an ankle sprain in volleyball. Injuries result from the attacker trying to "out jump" a set that is faster, lower, or closer to the net than anticipated, causing him to land on or across the centerline (b) and thereby putting the opposing blocker at risk for landing on his foot. This situation could be avoided if the attacker attempts to reach the ball with a final long approach step (a), instead of trying to reach the ball by jumping.

factors for ankle sprains (Bahr *et al.* 1994; Bahr & Bahr 1997): (i) change the centerline rule to reduce the "conflict zone" under the net; (ii) provide athletes with specific training on take-off and landing techniques during attack and multiperson blocks; (iii) use tape or ankle braces as external ankle protection; and (iv) adequately rehabilitate sprained ankles.

Rule change

A more restrictive centerline violation rule has been suggested as a simple measure, since it would deter players from landing on the opponent's side of the court and thereby reduce the number of conflicts between opposing players when landing. It is possible, and perhaps even likely, that changing the centerline violation rule would significantly reduce the incidence of ankle sprains. However, a previous attempt at reducing injury risk by making any penetration of the centerline a fault resulted in an unacceptable number of game interruptions, and the proposed rule change was therefore abandoned (Bahr 1996). However, it is also important to note that research has demonstrated that the majority of centerline violations occur in "low injury risk" situations, e.g. setters approaching the net to set the ball, or blockers and attackers turning away from the net *after* landing. It may be, therefore, that a rule which discriminates between centerline contact/penetration based on the injury risk inherent in the situation (e.g. centerline contact within the conflict zone = fault vs penetration occurring away from the area in which the volleyball is being played = no fault) would be able to reduce the risk of ankle sprain injury while minimizing the stoppages of play, which players and spectators alike find disruptive to the game.

Technical training

A second prevention strategy is to teach proper movement, take-off, and landing techniques. Technical training and information have previously been shown to reduce the injury rate in soccer (Ekstrand *et al.* 1983). A training program for volleyball should include drills specifically designed to teach players how to reach tight sets without stepping on the centerline (Fig. 10.2), as well as blocking drills (Fig. 10.3). The ability to block effectively, including the ability to mount a two- or three-person block to gain a tactical advantage over the opposing attacker, requires the ability to move quickly sideways along the net and time both the movement pattern and the take off between the players involved. Every

practice session should include block movement drills performed in pairs as part of the warm-up routine to improve footwork, balance, and timing.

Tape/brace

The protective effects of taping and bracing have been persuasively shown in intervention studies in soccer and basketball, but only for players with a history of prior ankle injury (Tropp *et al.* 1985; Sitler *et al.* 1994; Surve *et al.* 1994). Although there is no direct evidence from volleyball-specific studies, there is strong evidence from studies focusing on other sports that the use of taping or bracing should be recommended for a period of up to 12 months after an ankle sprain, when risk of injury is increased several fold. The mechanism by which such ankle orthoses are thought to work is not known with certainty, but may involve simply enhancing the athlete's proprioceptive awareness of the ankle joint. This view is corroborated by the fact that the preventative effect of braces is limited to players with previous injury, where proprioceptive function is reduced (Tropp *et al.* 1985; Konradsen & Ravn 1991; Karlsson *et al.* 1992). In addition, orthoses do not seem to restrict ankle inversion in a substantial enough way to explain their prophylactic effect on ankle sprain incidence. If the protective effect were mechanical, one would expect an effect in healthy, previously uninjured ankles as well.

Many different ankle supports are commercially available. Ankle taping has also been shown to be beneficial in restricting inversion motion, although it appears that ankle supports are superior to ankle taping since ankle supports do not lose their ability to restrict inversion, while tape does "loosen up" after several repeated cycles of vertical jumping. Unlike semirigid orthoses, the effectiveness of ankle

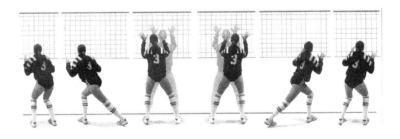

Fig. 10.3 Movement skills in blocking are important, and drills should be included in the training program with players performing in pairs.

taping has not been tested in randomized controlled
trials, but if the effect is mainly through enhancement of proprioception, there is no reason to expect
taping to be less effective than orthoses. Other factors, such as cost and skin care obviously should also
be considered in the choice between tape and orthoses. Furthermore, there is no evidence that wearing an ankle orthosis increases the incidence of knee
injuries, and most studies suggest that semirigid
orthoses do not significantly impair athletic
performance.

Adequate rehabilitation, including "proprioceptive" training

Tropp *et al.* (1985) and others (Konradsen & Ravn
1991; Karlsson *et al.* 1992) have shown that proprioceptive function is reduced in athletes who
complain of a feeling of persistent instability following an ankle sprain. Proprioceptive control of
the affected ankle joint is impaired in the immediate
recovery period following an acute sprain (Konradsen *et al.* 1998), but studies have shown that this
function can be restored through a balance board
training program (Gauffin *et al.* 1988; Holme *et al.*
1999; Wester *et al.* 1996). In these studies, proprioceptive function was quantified by measuring the reaction time to a sudden inversion strain, or the
degree of postural sway during a one-legged balance
test. It should be noted that the use of the term proprioceptive function, which is defined as the function of the *afferent* components only, may be
inappropriate in this context. The ability to react to a
sudden inversion stimulus or balance on one
leg clearly depends on both sensory and motor
function, and should perhaps therefore be termed
sensorimotor control.

A balance board training program has been shown
to reduce the risk of reinjury in functionally unstable
ankles in soccer players (Tropp *et al.* 1985). The effect
of balance training alone in preventing ankle sprains
has not been tested in volleyball players, but balance
board training has been included as part of a comprehensive volleyball injury prevention program
(see below). The available data suggest that intensive
balance board training is effective in previously injured players. The program is performed as balance
exercises on one leg on a disk (Fig. 10.4). Based on the

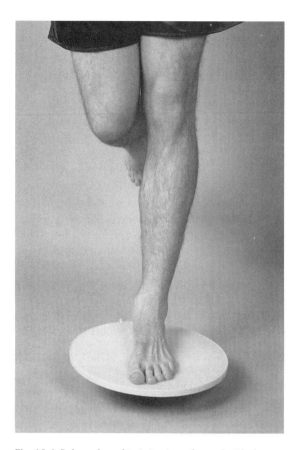

Fig. 10.4 Balance board training is performed with the
player standing on one leg on a balance board. The
objective is to control balance without using the hands,
hips, or knees to adjust body position, but to correct
balance using the ankle only. Thus, arms are held across
the chest and the opposite leg is held still in 90° knee
flexion.

available literature, it appears reasonable to recommend a program of 10 min of balance board training
five times a week over 6–10 weeks for all players with
a history of ankle sprain.

Effect of a prevention program

An intervention program consisting of injury awareness information, specific technical training, and a
program of proprioceptive training for players with
a history of ankle sprains, demonstrated a 47%
reduction in the incidence of ankle sprains in the
course of a single season (the rate of ankle sprain

injury fell from 0.9 to 0.5 per 1,000 player-hours) (Bahr *et al.* 1997). However, it should be noted that direct contact with each team participating in the study was (for practical reasons) limited to one visit. No information regarding how the coaches and players complied with the advice and information offered to them was collected. Although the athletes appeared well motivated, it is likely that the effectiveness of the prevention program could have been even better if it was reinforced on a regular basis. The results of this study should encourage medical personnel working with volleyball teams to institute a program of ankle injury prevention, as positive results can be expected if coaches and medical staff cooperate in establishing and promoting an injury-prevention program.

Preventing patellar tendinopathy

Injury mechanisms

Patellar tendinopathy or "jumper's knee" is the most common overuse injury in volleyball. Athletes with jumper's knee are usually unable to recall one specific traumatic event that precipitated their symptoms. It is therefore assumed that in most cases the injury results from repetitive overloading of the tendon fibers. Histological findings of degeneration and fibrotic scarring in the tendon itself, as well as in the bone–tendinous junction, suggest that the injury consists of an unhealed partial tendon tear. This view is supported by the demonstration of abnormalities in the tendinous tissue using ultrasonography, computerized tomography, and magnetic resonance imaging (King *et al.* 2000).

Risk factors

The prevalence of jumper's knee increases with the frequency of jump training, and is higher among players who train or compete on hard, unforgiving surfaces (Ferretti *et al.* 1984). The tactics of the game require middle blockers to jump more than other front row players, and not surprisingly they demonstrate a higher prevalence of jumper's knee. Thus, there is ample evidence that the prevalence of

jumper's knee in volleyball players is closely related to the volume of jumping.

However, it is not known why some players have problems whereas others do well despite an equally high training volume. Biomechanical evidence is limited, but there is no convincing evidence in support of suggestions that injury may be associated with malalignment of the extensor mechanism of the knee, the patella alta, abnormal patella laxity, or other structural abnormalities (Kujala *et al.* 1986, 1987; Lian *et al.* 1996b). Interestingly, one study revealed that volleyball players with jumper's knee actually performed better than asymptomatic athletes in a standardized jump test emphasizing eccentric force generation (Lian *et al.* 1996a). This suggests that those athletes who jump well might be better able to eccentrically activate their knee extensor muscles, thereby placing increasing load on the patellar tendon–bone junction. The same study also showed that the right knee was affected significantly more often than the left knee among volleyball players. One reason for this may be the right–left take-off technique normally used by right-handed spikers. This results in a deeper flexion angle and a state of functional valgus rotation malalignment during the eccentric phase of take off in the right knee, which is likely to cause higher tendon tension on the right side. Similarly, players who develop the deepest knee flexion angle during landing from a spike jump have been shown to be more likely to suffer from jumper's knee (Richards *et al.* 1996).

Preventive measures

No evidence-based methods for the prevention of patellar tendinopathy have been published. However, epidemiological and biomechanical studies suggest that the cause of the syndrome is simply too much jumping, particularly in talented, "natural" jumpers. A typical scenario may be the following: a young, promising player is recruited to play on a higher level (e.g. secondary school to university), and among the primary selection criteria are jumping ability and agility. This transfer from a "safe" training environment (2–3 days of training per week, no weight lifting) to a higher level with a sudden increase in strength, muscle mass, and jumping ability may result in progressive overload of the extensor apparatus.

Based on this scenario, coach and player education (with special emphasis on the pathophysiology) would seem to be an important component of a jumper's knee prevention program. In particular, training loads must be increased gradually. Weight training and plyometric training lead to increases in strength and jumping ability within weeks, especially in adolescents; whereas tendons may need months to adapt to the new level of physiological demand placed on them. Therefore, the athlete's response to training—especially weight and plyometric training—must be closely monitored. It is clearly important to take the athlete's first pain episode seriously, and to take appropriate action at once to avoid developing a chronic pain condition.

Secondary prevention of patellar tendinopathy must also be considered. Comparing the forces used in rehabilitation with the forces and rates of force development in eccentric–concentric contractions incurred during training and games, it is not surprising that treatment programs emphasizing immobilization, rest from athletic activity, or isometric exercises frequently fail to provide significant therapeutic benefit. Strength training must be specific to the proposed task of the tendon, and preliminary studies using specific eccentric training programs have shown promising results, even in athletes with recalcitrant tendinopathy (Stanish *et al.* 1986; Fyfe & Stanish 1992; Alfredson *et al.* 1998). However, further studies are necessary to understand the forces involved in jumping in order to design proper rehabilitation training programs for injured high-performance athletes and thereby avoid reinjury.

Preventing finger injuries

Injury mechanisms

Although they rarely result in time loss, finger injuries occur frequently in volleyball. These injuries mainly result from blocking, when a player tries to stop or deflect a spike from the opponent by reaching across the net with one or both hands (with fingers extended). Defensive plays, such as diving or

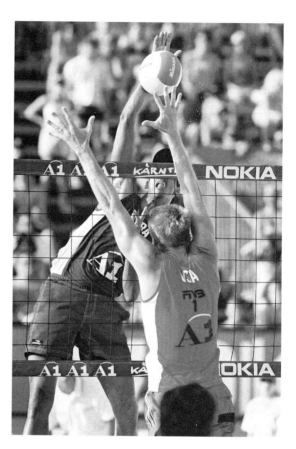

Fig. 10.5 Fingers are exposed when blocking, especially the thumb and little finger. (Courtesy of Mike Ranz, FIVB Official Photographer.)

rolling to retrieve the ball, may result in injury to the digits. The thumb and little finger are the most vulnerable phalanges. That these two digits are injured more frequently than others is easy to understand, considering their vulnerable position when blocking and playing defence (Fig. 10.5). The metacarpophalangeal joint of the thumb is the most frequent location of ligamentous injury, but unlike some other sports (such as skiing) it is the radial, not the ulnar, collateral ligament that is typically injured.

Risk factors

As with ankle injuries, a history of previous injury is the most significant risk factor for finger injuries. The skill level of the player may also be expected to play a role, both when blocking and playing defence. Proper finger position and timing is essential to be able to withstand the considerable forces involved when the spiked ball impacts on the extended fingers. While the forces are higher at the elite level, unexperienced players often injure their fingers because of inadequate hand/finger positioning and timing when blocking or playing defence.

Preventive measures

The most important preventative measure is to teach players proper hand and finger positioning when blocking. Timing is also important, since being too early or too late on the block means that the player may not be prepared for ball contact at the proper time. Players with previous injury and instability problems should tape their fingers. "Buddy taping" the affected digit to an adjacent digit is an effective way to protect the injured finger from further injury. Finally, players should not wear jewelry while playing volleyball, since rings may get entangled in the net and result in traumatic amputation.

Preventing acute knee injuries

Injury mechanisms

The rate of volleyball-related acute knee injuries, including anterior cruciate ligament (ACL) injuries, is considerably lower than in other team sports (Arendt & Dick 1995). ACL injuries in other team sports are for the most part non-contact injuries, and result from landing or plant-and-cut maneuvers with the knee in a vulnerable position, usually in valgus. This seems to be the case in volleyball too, and most of the injuries occur during landing after attacking or blocking (Ferretti *et al.* 1992). Since jumping and cutting characterize the movement pattern in volleyball, it might be expected that ligamentous knee injuries would be as common in volleyball as in basketball or soccer. Curiously, this does not seem to be the case. One possible explanation for the lower incidence of ACL injuries in volleyball may be that landing and cutting skills can be performed in a more predictable manner than in basketball and soccer. In both of these other sports, it is not uncommon for an opponent to suddenly block the way, forcing the player to perform the skill in a different way than anticipated.

Unlike ACL injuries, meniscus injuries occur predominantly during the defensive phase of play, when players perform rapid twisting movements with the knee in the typical defensive position of near 90° of flexion. In this position, the meniscus is subjected to considerable compression and torsion stress, and the athlete is therefore at increased risk of menisceal injury.

Risk factors

Knee injuries, and ACL injuries in particular, occur more frequently among female volleyball players than among male volleyball players. This gender disparity has been observed in most other sports as well. Several explanations for this phenomenon have been proposed. A disproportionate number of knee injuries also seem to occur during games compared with training, probably reflecting the maximum effort expended and the greater risks taken in a competitive situation.

Preventive measures

A balance board training program has been shown to reduce the risk of ACL injury in healthy soccer players and there is reason to believe that balance training alone may be an effective means of preventing not only ankle injuries, but also ACL injuries. The program is carried out in a similar way as the ankle program, but particular attention must be paid to knee positioning during training (have the athlete keep the knee above the toe). Strength training and plyometric training may also have a protective effect against acute knee injuries, particularly in adolescent athletes.

Preventing low back pain

Injury mechanisms

Low back pain is a common complaint among volleyball players. Data collected by the National Collegiate Athletic Association (NCAA, Indianapolis, IN USA) on women's collegiate volleyball suggest that back pain is the fourth leading cause of time lost due to injury. Common diagnoses include discogenic low back pain, acute spondylolysis (stress reaction of the pars interarticularis, which may progress to stress fracture), and lumbar strain (acute muscular overload) or sprain (acute ligamentous overload). Often the exact cause or anatomical basis of the athlete's low back pain cannot be accurately diagnosed. "Mechanical low back pain" is a non-specific term used to describe a syndrome of low back pain that worsens with activity. Volleyball athletes are at considerable risk for low back disorders, in view of the movement patterns involving trunk rotation and lumbar flexion and extension that are common to volleyball skills—particularly spiking and jump serving.

Risk factors

Risk factors for low back pain and injury that have been identified include repetitive lumbar extension and trunk rotation, and cigarette smoking. Athletes who are particularly tall may be at increased risk by virtue of the longer lever arm of the spine when compared with shorter individuals. Athletes with spondylolysis are frequently found to have a flattening of the normal lumbar lordosis and relative inflexibility of the hamstrings. However, it is not clear whether these findings represent an intrinsic risk factor for the condition or a compensatory adaptation by the body in an effort to minimize the degree of lumbar extension to which the spine is subjected in these athletes.

Preventive measures

To minimize the risk of low back pain, volleyball athletes should follow a program of generalized strength and conditioning, in addition to maintaining flexibility through the low back, hips, and lower limbs through regular stretching. Exercises designed to specifically improve the athlete's "core" stability and the endurance of the muscles that dynamically stabilize the lumbar spine should (theoretically) enhance the athlete's ability to withstand repetitive overload of the spine, which is inherent to the skill set of the sport, particularly at the elite level.

Preventing shoulder pain

Injury mechanisms

Shoulder injuries account for 8–20% of all volleyball injuries. Shoulder injuries occur largely as the result of chronic overuse, and only rarely result from acute trauma. Although the incidence of time-loss injuries is low, the prevalence of shoulder pain and dysfunction may be much higher (Kugler *et al.* 1996). The mechanism of injury is complex, but most likely is the result of repeated spiking and serving. The kinematics of these skills are similar to those of other overhead throwing or racquet sports, such as baseball and tennis. The high angular velocities generated at the often extreme range of motion observed at the end of the cocking phase of the arm swing places the shoulder under great stress (Fig. 10.6). When considering the multiple repetitions involved—an elite attacker spikes about 40,000 times a year—this can lead to overload of the structures at risk.

When these stresses are applied at a rate exceeding that of tissue repair, progressive damage to both the static and dynamic stabilizing structures of the shoulder can occur. In keeping with the complex mechanism of injury, volleyball players with shoulder problems often present with vague complaints. In addition to, or instead of, pain they may report fatigue, discomfort, apprehension, paresthesia, or numbness as their principle symptom(s), and only rarely do they describe any feeling of instability. Apprehension is a term specifically used to describe the fear exhibited by patients with unstable shoulders that their shoulder will sublux or dislocate. In these cases, the athlete experiences a sharp pain on extreme external rotation. This may lead to transient loss of muscular control over the extremity ("dead arm" syndrome). The severe pain usually subsides quickly, but soreness and weakness may persist for a period of time.

Risk factors

The main risk factor for shoulder pain is the volume of training performed. Elite volleyball athletes are at particular risk for overuse syndromes of the shoulder girdle. Older athletes are also at increased risk of developing shoulder pain, although problems may occur in younger athletes after a sudden increase in training intensity. Talented spikers—who are able to hit the ball with superior speed—may also be at higher risk; in their case, the ability to develop extreme velocities and torques in the spiking arm puts the passive and active stabilizers of the glenohumeral joint at greater risk of fatigue and dysfunction.

It is felt that a combination of lax tissues on the anterior side of the glenohumeral joint and contracted tissues on the posterior side of the joint may contribute to instability by "pushing" the humeral head forward. Consequently, players with restricted range of motion and muscle weakness/imbalance are at risk for compromised glenohumeral joint

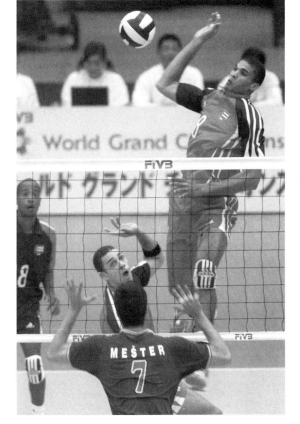

Fig. 10.6 Cocking phase during spiking. Note the maximal external rotation and abduction of the shoulder, which leads to large stresses on the anterior stabilizers of the shoulder joint. (Courtesy of Mauro de Sanctis, FIVB Official Photographer.)

function. Volleyball players typically develop reduced shoulder internal rotation and increased shoulder external rotation of the dominant (spiking) limb, which can be interpreted as indirect evidence of anterior capsular laxity. At the same time, there is often reduced rotator cuff function and impaired scapular control, which can result in lateralization or even in winging of the scapula.

Preventive measures

The prevention of shoulder pain and injury begins with a preseason conditioning program and continues thoughout the season. The program should focus on stretching and strengthening exercises.

Stretching exercises should focus on the posterior structures (Fig. 10.7). Exercises should be performed as repeated slow, sustained stretches, holding the stretch at the point of slight discomfort for at least 45 s. However, it is important to note that too much flexibility can become a liability. In someone who already possesses a lax glenohumeral joint capsule, further stretching may predispose to increased laxity and even joint instability. Thus, a stretching program must be individually designed for each athlete, stressing development of flexibility where it is lacking.

Strengthening exercises should focus on the main stabilizers of the glenohumeral joint—the rotator cuff muscles—and the scapular stabilizers (Fig. 10.8). It should be noted that the shoulder exercises traditionally used in the weight-training program for

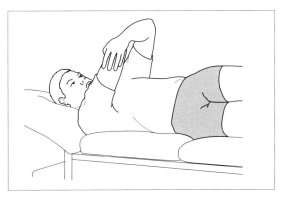

Fig. 10.7 Shoulder-stretching exercises should focus on the posterior structures of the shoulder.

volleyball players—bench press, pull down, and pull over—actually are more likely to increase rather than reduce the risk of shoulder injury if used in isolation. This can be explained by the fact that isolated strengthening of the deltoid, pectoralis major, and latissimus dorsi is likely to increase arm speed and torque, and therefore put additional strain on the glenohumeral stablilizers. These exercises must therefore be combined with a program aimed at improving rotator cuff strength and scapular control.

Finally, warming up prior to repetitive overhead use of the shoulder is critical to prevent shoulder injury. The warm-up program should include exercises designed to increase core temperature first, followed by stretching. Warm up then finishes with exercises incorporating the ball, hitting first at low intensity and then progressing to full-intensity spiking.

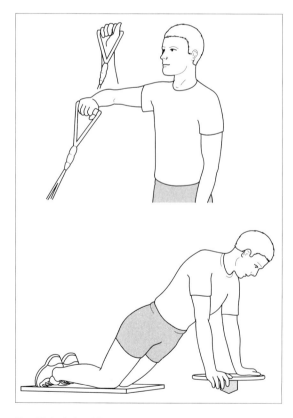

Fig. 10.8 A shoulder-strengthening exercise program should include a number of drills to strengthen to rotator cuff, as well as the ability to stabilize the scapula.

Role of the medical staff

The traditional role of the sports medicine staff has been to diagnose and treat injury and illness. However, there is a need to redefine the role of the team physician and physical therapist. As stated in the introduction to this chapter, their responsibility does not stop at treating injuries—there is also an obligation to prevent injuries. This requires a thorough understanding of injury patterns, injury mechanisms, and risk factors, in addition to close cooperation between the coaching and medical staff. Both groups must simultaneously acknowledge each other's expertise while assuming an active partnership role in the other's area. The coaching staff needs to involve the medical team when planning the training program, and medical personnel

Table 10.1 A comprehensive injury prevention program.

General
Warm up and stretching
Preseason medical screening to assess status of previous injuries
Have adequate first aid equipment (at least ice and elastic wrapping) available at all times

Ankle
Include drills to improve take-off and landing techniques for attackers and blockers in warm-up routine
Introduce a restrictive centerline during practice and scrimmage games
Include a 10-week balance board training program for players with previous ankle sprains
Use taping and bracing for previously injured players that have not undergone an adequate balance training program

Knee
Gradual increase in training load
Introduce weight training and plymometrics gradually into training program
Prompt and adequate rehabilitation of new episodes of patellar tendon pain

Fingers
Teach proper finger positioning and timing when blocking
Taping of injured fingers
Do not wear rings

Shoulder
Gradual increase in training load, particularly spiking and serving
Shoulder strengthening and stretching, with particular attention to rotator cuff and scapula-stabilizing exercises

need to involve the coaching staff in the rehabilitation of injured players. The value of medical staff involvement has previously been shown conclusively in soccer. In cooperation, the medical and coaching staff can introduce a comprehensive injury prevention program taking the skill level, practice and game schedule, injury status of the team, and other factors into consideration (Table 10.1).

Although the cost:benefit ratio of the preparticipation medical examination in mass participation sports may be questioned, for the team physician the preseason exam is an essential part of the injury prevention process. It is important to conduct the preseason exam as early as possible before the actual start of the competitive season, so as to allow sufficient time to implement special conditioning programs before the start of the season. For the same reason, it may even prove beneficial to perform a postseason exam to survey injury status in preparation for the next season. The purpose of the medical examination, which ideally should be a joint effort between the team physician and physical therapist, is to get to know the player, and to identify risk factors for injury. The main risk factors for injury are previous injury and minor present injuries that might progress. The examination should therefore include an evaluation of all previous injuries, with special attention to passive and active stability of the knee, ankle, and shoulder joint.

References

Alfredson, H., Pietilä, T., Jonsson, P. & Lorcutzon, R. (1998) Heavy load eccentric calf muscle training for the treatment of Achilles tendinosis. *American Journal of Sports Medicine* **26**, 360–366.

Arendt, E. & Dick, R. (1995) Knee injury patterns among men and women in collegiate basketball and soccer. NCAA data and review of literature. *American Journal of Sports Medicine* **23**, 694–701.

Bahr, R. (1996) The effect of a new center line violation rule on the quality and flow of volleyball games. *International Volleytech* **2**, 14–19.

Bahr, R. & Bahr, I.A. (1997) Incidence of acute volleyball injuries: a prospective cohort study of injury mechanisms and risk factors. *Scandinavian Journal of Medicine and Science in Sports* **7**, 166–171.

Bahr, R., Bahr, I.A. & Lian, Ø. (1997) A twofold reduction in the incidence of acute ankle sprains in volleyball after the introduction of an injury prevention program—a prospective cohort study. *Scandinavian Journal of Medicine and Science in Sports* **7**, 172–177.

Bahr, R., Lian, Ø., Karlsen, R. & Øvrebø, R.V. (1994) Incidence and mechanisms of acute ankle inversion injuries in volleyball—a retrospective cohort study. *American Journal of Sports Medicine* **22**, 601–604.

Ekstrand, J., Gillquist, J. & Liljedahl, S.O. (1983) Prevention of soccer injuries. Supervision by doctor and physiotherapist. *American Journal of Sports Medicine* **11**, 116–120.

Ekstrand, J. & Tropp, H. (1990) The incidence of ankle sprains in soccer. *Foot and Ankle* **11**, 41–44.

Ferretti, A. (1986) Epidemiology of jumper's knee. *Sports Medicine* **3**, 289–295.

Ferretti, A., Papandrea, P., Conteduca, F. & Mariani, P.P. (1992) Knee ligament injuries in volleyball players. *American Journal of Sports Medicine* **20**, 203–207.

Ferretti, A., Puddu, G., Mariani, P.P. & Neri, M. (1984) Jumper's knee: an epidemiological study of volleyball players. *Physician and Sportsmedicine* **12**, 97–103.

Fyfe, I. & Stanish, W.D. (1992) The use of eccentric training and stretching in the treatment and prevention of tendon injuries. *Clinics in Sports Medicine* **11**, 601–624.

Gauffin, H., Tropp, H. & Odenrick, P. (1988) Effect of ankle disk training on postural control in patients with functional instability of the ankle joint. *International Journal of Sports Medicine* **9**, 141–144.

Hell, H. & Schönle, C. (1985) Ursachen und Prophylaxe typischer Volleyballverletzungen. *Zeitschrift fuer Orthopaedische* **123**, 72–75.

Holme, E., Magnusson, S.P., Becher, K., Bieler, T., Aagaard, P. & Kjaer, M. (1999) The effect of supervised rehabilitation on strength, postural sway, position sense and re-injury risk after acute ankle ligament sprain. *Scandinavian Journal of Medicine and Science in Sports* **9**, 104–109.

Karlsson, J., Peterson, L., Andreasson, G. & Högfors, C. (1992) The unstable ankle: a combined EMG and biomechanical modeling study. *International Journal of Sports Biomechanics* **8**, 129–144

King, J.B., Cook, J.L., Khan, K.M. & Maffulli, N. (2000) Patellar tendinopathy. *Sports Medicine and Arthroscopy Review* **8**, 86–95.

Konradsen, L. & Ravn, J.B. (1991) Prolonged peroneal reaction time in ankle instability. *International Journal of Sports Medicine* **12**, 290–292.

Konradsen, L., Olesen, S. & Hansen, H.M. (1998) Ankle sensorimotor control and eversion strength after acute ankle inversion injuries. *American Journal of Sports Medicine* **26**, 72–77.

Kugler, A., Krüger-Franke, M., Reininger, S., Trouillier, H.H. & Rosemeyer, B. (1996) Muscular imbalance and shoulder pain in volleyball attackers. *British Journal of Sports Medicine* **30**, 256–259.

Kujala, U.M., Friberg, O., Aalto, T., Kvist, M. & Österman, K. (1987) Lower limb asymmetry and patellofemoral joint incongruence in the etiology of knee exertion injuries in athletes. *International Journal of Sports Medicine* **8**, 214–220.

Kujala, U.M., Österman, K., Kvist, M., Aalto, T. & Friberg, O. (1986) Factors predisposing to patellar chondropathy and patellar apicitis in athletes. *International Orthopaedics* **10**, 195–200.

Lian, Ø., Engebretsen, L., Ovrebo, R.V. & Bahr, R. (1996a) Characteristics of leg extensors in male volleyball players with jumper's knee. *American Journal of Sports Medicine* **24**, 380–385.

Lian, Ø., Holen, K.J., Eugebretseu, L. & Bahr, R. (1996b) Relationship between symptoms of jumper's knee and the ultrasound characteristics of the patellar tendon among high level male volleyball players. *Scandinavian Journal of Sports Medicine* **6**, 291–296.

Milgrom, C., Shlamkovitch, N., Finestone, A. *et al.* (1991) Risk factors for lateral ankle sprain: a prospective study among military recruits. *Foot and Ankle* **12**, 26–30.

Richards, D.P., Ajemian, S.V., Wiley, J.P. & Zernicke, R.F. (1996) Knee joint dynamics predict patellar tendinitis in elite volleyball players. *American Journal of Sports Medicine* **24**, 676–683.

Schafle, M.D., Requa, R.K., Patton, W.L. & Garrick, J.G. (1990) Injuries in the 1987 National Amateur Volleyball Tournament. *American Journal of Sports Medicine* **18**, 624–631.

Sitler, M., Ryan, J., Wheeler, B. *et al.* (1994) The efficacy of a semirigid ankle stabilizer to reduce acute ankle injuries in basketball. A randomized clinical study at West Point. *American Journal of Sports Medicine* **22**, 454–461.

Stanish, W.D., Rubinovich, R.M. & Curwin, S. (1986) Eccentric exercise in chronic tendinitis. *Clinical Orthopaedics and Related Research* **208**, 65–68.

Surve, I., Schwellnus, M.P., Noakes, T. & Lombard, C. (1994) A fivefold reduction in the incidence of recurrent ankle sprains in soccer players using the sport-stirrup orthosis. *American Journal of Sports Medicine* **22**, 601–606.

Tropp, H., Askling, C. & Gillquist, J. (1985) Prevention of ankle sprains. *American Journal of Sports Medicine* **13**, 259–262.

Wester, J.U., Jespersen, S.M., Nielsen, K.D. & Neumann, L. (1996) Wobble board training after partial sprains of the lateral ligaments of the ankle: a prospective randomized study. *Journal of Orthopaedic and Sports Physical Therapy* **23**, 332–336.

Recommended reading

Bahr, R., van Mechelen, W. & Kannus, P. (2002) Prevention of sports injuries. In: Kjaer, M. (ed.). *Scandinavian Textbook of Sports Medicine*. Munksgaard, Copenhagen.

Renstrom, P.A.F.H. (ed.) (1993) *Sports Injuries: Basic Principles of Prevention and Care*. Blackwell Science. Oxford.

Chapter 11
Principles of volleyball injury rehabilitation

Jonathan C. Reeser

Introduction

Injuries are an unfortunate and seemingly unavoidable consequence of sports participation. As has been discussed in previous chapters, volleyball athletes are primarily at risk for acute ankle sprains, in addition to chronic overuse injuries of the shoulder, knees and low back. The injured player generally experiences a decrement in performance, and pain associated with the injury may prevent athletic participation altogether. Consequently, athletes are typically well motivated to seek treatment to relieve the symptoms related to their injury, and to rehabilitate the affected body part to permit ongoing sports training and competition.

The goal of injury treatment and rehabilitation is the restoration of optimal function. Ideally, this goal can be attained by identifying the mechanism of injury, making an accurate diagnosis, and then formulating a treatment plan that will enable the athlete to return to competition and training while minimizing the risk of reinjury. First and foremost the sports medicine physician or physiotherapist needs to make an accurate and complete diagnosis. In some cases a precise pathoanatomical diagnosis is not possible based on the clinical presentation alone, and if detailed knowledge of the anatomy in question will influence the athlete's treatment plan then diagnostic imaging should be obtained as appropriate. A comprehensive treatment plan for any sport-related injury should include not only an understanding of the symptomatic, anatomical, and functional consequences of the specific injury, but should also identify the athlete's modifiable intrinsic and extrinsic risk factors for injury.

The tissue injury cycle

The injured athlete may present with a variety of complaints, including pain (either with activity or at rest), swelling, erythema, bruising, stiffness, or simply an inability to perform at their usual level. Collectively, these observations may be referred to as the injured athlete's "clinical symptom complex." Symptoms are generally reflective of some sort of underlying tissue alteration or damage that has occurred due to the mechanism of injury; this damage may be termed the "tissue injury complex." Based on the athlete's history, mechanism of injury, and symptom complex, the nature of the injury can be conveniently categorized as either an acute injury, a chronic injury, or as an acute exacerbation of a chronic injury. As a direct result of the injury, or as a consequence of the abnormal movement patterns that result from the injury, other tissues and structures may be placed under increased physiological demand and/or anatomical stress; the affected structures may be collectively referred to as the "tissue overload complex." Structural deficits may subsequently lead to deficits of function and biomechanics (i.e. technique), which have been referred to as the "functional biomechanical deficit complex." In an effort to prevent recurrence of their

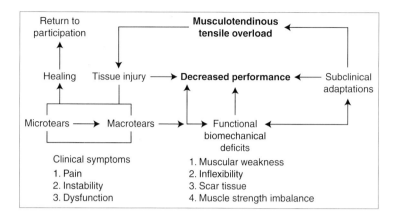

Fig. 11.1 The tissue injury cycle. Deficits in one area "feed forward" to perpetuate the injury cycle in a self-reinforcing manner. (From Kibler *et al*. 1992.)

symptoms while performing provocative skills, or in an attempt to compensate for any decrement in performance, the athlete is likely to substitute new or altered movement patterns (often subconsciously). This "subclinical adaptation complex" can in turn lead to additional tissue overload, injury, symptoms, biomechanical deficits, and further (mal)adaptations. In this way a feed-forward injury cycle is established (Fig. 11.1). This conceptual "vicious" injury cycle—originally introduced by Kibler—is particularly applicable to chronic overuse injuries, but also provides a useful framework for understanding and predicting the possible sequelae of acute musculoskeletal injuries if left untreated (Kibler *et al*. 1998).

It is important to note that only in the case of an acute injury is the athlete likely to be symptomatic at the time of initial tissue injury. For example, the athlete who suffers a lateral ankle inversion sprain is immediately distressed. Conversely, the athlete who develops a chronic overuse injury has likely been accumulating subclinical microdamage (at a rate exceeding the tissue's intrinsic ability to repair itself) for some time. Unless the athlete or an observant coach identifies a drop off in performance or an alteration in technique, the process and consequences of chronic overload may go unrecognized until the cumulative trauma exceeds the athlete's individual threshold for pain perception or tolerance. For example, a newly disabled volleyball athlete may attempt to resume training without making conscious technical accommodation for their physical impairment. Consequently, the increased physiological and biomechanical demand on the involved structures precipitates an overuse injury. A similar sce-

nario could be envisioned for the acutely injured athlete who attempts to return to play too quickly, thereby placing the healing body part at increased risk of reinjury or provoking a secondary overload injury of associated soft tissues. Unless interrupted by a comprehensive treatment and rehabilitation program emphasizing strength, endurance, flexibility, neuromuscular control (proprioception), and proper technique, this vicious injury cycle can result in prolonged and often incomplete recovery from both acute and chronic injuries. Incomplete rehabilitation therefore places the injured athlete in jeopardy of recurrent symptoms with long-term functional consequences (Kibler *et al*. 1998).

Phases of treatment

It follows from the above discussion that the treatment plan may differ based on the type of injury suffered. For example, an acute contusion or sprain injury should not be treated in the same way as a chronic overuse injury is treated. Although the exact treatment protocol for different types of injuries varies, the process of treating any injury, regardless of type, can nevertheless be divided into three successive phases: the acute phase, the recovery phase, and the functional phase. Different portions of the "injury cycle" are addressed as the athlete progresses through each phase of treatment (Kibler 1990; Kibler *et al*. 1998).

In the acute phase, after a diagnosis is made, the athlete's clinical symptoms are addressed. The initial treatment of most injuries focuses on pain relief, management of swelling, restoration of range of motion, and prevention of secondary complications. Common interventions include analgesic medications, thermal modalities (ice and, in appropriate circumstances, heat), and protection and relative rest of the injured body part. Relative rest permits the injured tissues to begin healing while minimizing the deleterious effects of inactivity on the athlete as a whole (potentially including deconditioning, disuse atrophy, and inflexibility).

During the recovery phase of care, the emphasis of treatment shifts to providing appropriate stimulation to initiate and facilitate gradual functional restoration of the affected body part and associated structures. Typically this involves a program of progressive strengthening and conditioning, emphasizing flexibility and proprioceptive training throughout the kinetic chain. Biomechanical alterations and subsequent tissue overload should be identified and similarly treated. At the conclusion of the recovery phase the athlete is ready to progress to volleyball-specific functional exercises, culminating in their return to participation.

Toward the end of the final "functional" phase of rehabilitation, the emphasis of treatment shifts towards prevention of reinjury, or "prehabilitation." For this reason, some clinicians refer to this final phase as the "maintenance" phase of care. When approached from within this framework, it is clear that the injured athlete should always be rehabilitated beyond the mere absence of symptoms. Although it is often possible to quickly relieve the athlete's pain through a number of different interventions, long-term goals such as the restoration of optimal function and a reduced risk of injury recurrence are only achievable through a comprehensive treatment program (Herring 1990; Kibler *et al.* 1998). For example, an athlete who complains of shoulder pain with spiking may feel considerably improved following administration of a corticosteroid injection, but unless the underlying basis for their symptom complex has been identified and addressed their symptoms will without doubt recur.

This structured approach to the injury rehabilitation process facilitates goal setting on the part of both the athlete and the volleyball medical professional. Setting realistic goals requires that the athlete understand the phases inherent to the recovery process, and helps keep the injured athlete motivated during what can be a physically and psychologically challenging period. Clearly defined goals can also help the athlete's coaches and teammates appreciate what is required before the athlete is permitted to return to play.

Therapeutic interventions

Most injury treatment and rehabilitation programs are multifaceted, involving both passive and active therapeutic interventions. Passive modalities are by definition those which require little to no active participation on the part of the injured athlete. Commonly employed passive techniques include compression, application of heat or cold, massage, and electrical stimulation. Active interventions require the injured athlete's participation, and commonly include exercise programs involv-ing resistance training or stretching/flexibility training.

Massage therapy, thought to accelerate tissue recovery and minimize postexercise soreness, is a popular technique and has become incorporated into the training regimens of most elite volleyball athletes. Thermal modalities are also widely used. Recreational and elite players alike depend on the topical application of ice to reduce pain and swelling after an acute musculoligamentous injury. This practice is so universally accepted that ice is part of the PRICE acronym for the treatment of acute sports injuries (protection, rest, ice, compression, and elevation) (Fig. 11.2). Heat is also a useful therapeutic agent, as it is an effective analgesic and is helpful in relaxing/mobilizing tight or contracted soft tissues characteristic of chronic overuse injuries. Deep heat is also thought to promote blood flow into an area and thereby accelerate healing. Therapeutic ultrasound penetrates and heats soft tissues more deeply than do hot packs, which have a more superficial effect (Fig. 11.3). Electrotherapy can provide a variety of beneficial effects, depending on the current intensity, waveform, duty cycle, and the placement of electrodes. Transcutaneous electrical nerve stimulation (TENS) may provide local analgesia after trauma; functional electrical stimulation can assist in muscle re-education and maintenance of tone during recovery; while interferential current may be useful in minimizing soft tissue edema as well as

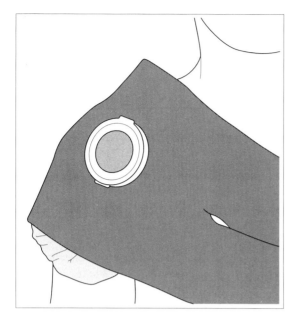

Fig. 11.2 Ice, applied superficially for up to 20 min several times a day, can limit pain and swelling in the affected area.

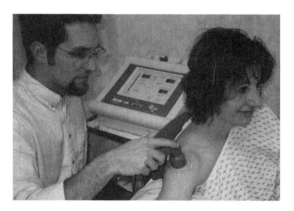

Fig. 11.3 Therapeutic ultrasound can provide analgesia and enhance joint range of motion, and is often a useful adjunctive therapy.

pain. Electrical current can also be used to drive anti-inflammatory medication into the subcutaneous tissue through a process known as iontophoresis.

Therapeutic exercise is the cornerstone of most rehabilitation programs. Exercise programs can be designed around a specific joint or muscle group that is injured (tissue injury complex) or otherwise affected (tissue overload complex), and can also be designed to produce or maintain whole-body cardiorespira-tory fitness. Joint-specific exercise programs generally include components of both resistance training (building strength and endurance) and flexibility training. During the acute phase of injury rehabilitation, greatest emphasis is placed on restoration of pain-free active range of motion. Isometric exercises may be useful during this phase to maintain—or in some cases retrain—muscles that work together to provide dynamic joint stability. During the recovery and maintenance phases of rehabilitation, the recovering athlete should be guided through a progressively more challenging program of functional restoration. Strength training in the later periods of the rehabilitation plan should emphasize eccentric muscular activity (Kibler *et al.* 1998).

Eccentric muscular activation is defined as a voluntary lengthening of force-generating muscle. Generating more force per cross-sectional area than concentric muscular activity, eccentric activation produces considerable tensile strain on muscle and the actomyosin cross-bridges. The myofibrillar damage that results from such intense "negative work" may result in a syndrome of delayed-onset muscular soreness in an untrained athlete. Eccentric muscular activity is critical to the sport-specific function of several essential muscle groups. For example, the muscles of the rotator cuff act eccentrically to decelerate the upper limb during follow-through after a spike or serve, and the quadriceps of the thigh act eccentrically to limit knee flexion upon landing from a jump. Performed repetitively, these eccentric actions place considerable mechanical load upon the involved muscles, rendering them at increased risk of acute strain injury. Furthermore, as muscles fatigue from repetitive work, the joint(s) about which they act may be at increased risk of ligamentous sprain injury (Mair *et al.* 1996).

Fortunately, muscles (and other tissues) adapt in direct response to the specific demands placed on them. It is therefore important for the athlete to progress through the rehabilitation program to increasingly functional and (eventually) sport-specific exercises in order to restore the affected body part to a level of strength, endurance, and integrated neuro-muscular function that will enable it to withstand the demands of sporting activity. Thus, in the acute stage of treatment the injured athlete might be instructed in isometric, closed kinetic chain exercises designed to enhance proprioceptive awareness and produce minimal shear across the affected joint. In the recovery phase, the athlete will graduate to more advanced isotonic or isokinetic eccentric exercises through a functional range of motion before finally progressing to a supervised program of sport-specific skills emphasizing proper technique in the functional (maintenance) phase of rehabilitation (Fig. 11.4). Once the recovering athlete can perform volleyball-specific skills involving the affected body part without pain, they can return to training and competition.

Effectively and comprehensively treating and rehabilitating volleyball injuries is a complex process. The ability to rehabilitate the athlete beyond the absence of symptoms requires a sound understanding of the structure and function of the affected body part in a volleyball-specific context. In order to pro-

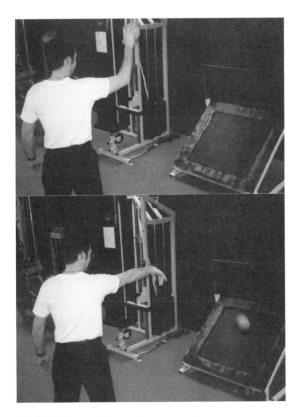

Fig. 11.4 Plyometric exercises, such as the one demonstrated here, allow the athlete to exercise the affected limb in a more functional manner than is possible with traditional resistance training.

vide some practical examples of these principles, the chapter will conclude with a structured clinical overview of, and general treatment recommendations for, three of the most common volleyball-related injuries: rotator cuff tendinopathy, jumper's knee, and lateral ankle sprains.

Rotator cuff tendinopathy

Rotator cuff injuries are typically overuse injuries. Of the four muscles comprising the rotator cuff, the supraspinatus is the most frequently injured. The explanation for this observation is principally anatomical—the supraspinatus tendon travels in the space beneath the acromion and the coracoacromial ligament to insert on the humeral head and can become injured/inflamed as it is cyclically compressed with repetitive overhead motion. The mechanism by which the tissue injury occurs can be a primary phenomenon, wherein the rotator cuff simply deteriorates with time, age, and overuse. In athletes, however, tissue injury is typically a secondary phenomenon due to scapular dysfunction and the resultant dynamic instability of the glenohumeral joint (Meister 2000a, 2000b). By the time the athlete complains of symptoms, the supraspinatus tendon shows little histological evidence of inflammation and thus it is probably more appropriate to diagnose the athlete with tendinosis or tendinopathy rather than tendinitis *per se*.

If, through repetitive overload or acute trauma, the shoulder's well-coordinated system of static and dynamic glenohumeral stabilization is compromised (tissue injury complex), the athlete will begin to substitute altered movement patterns in an effort to minimize symptoms and maintain performance (subclinical adaptation complex). This may in turn lead to imbalances in flexibility (functional biomechanical deficit complex). One nearly universal sign of disturbed shoulder girdle mechanics is scapular dysfunction. Clinically, this is manifest by anterolateral displacement of the involved scapula on the thoracic cage (referred to as the "lateral scapular slide"), and by restricted internal rotation when actively (or passively) assessing shoulder girdle range of motion. As a result of this scapular dysfunction, glenohumeral control is typically impaired. Increased anterior translation of the humeral head in the glenoid fossa creates, in effect, a "functionally unstable" shoulder and places the athlete at risk for impingment of the supraspinatus tendon and attrition of the glenoid labrum (Levine & Flatow 2000). Given its crucial role in shoulder function, therefore, the scapula should not be overlooked when evaluating the volleyball athlete who complains of anterior shoulder pain with overhead activity. Indeed, early rehabilitation of rotator cuff injuries should emphasize scapular motion and strengthening in order to provide a sound, stable "base" for upper limb function.

Acute phase management of rotator cuff tendinopathy also focuses on relieving the athlete's pain (through medication and the judicious use of thermal modalities, such as ice, ultrasound, electrical stimulation, and/or iontophoresis). The goal is to

provide an environment that permits tissue healing, while minimizing the deleterious effects of rest and time off from competition. Once the athlete has minimal pain through a full range of motion, they can progress on to the recovery phase of rehabilitation. This stage emphasizes strengthening, range of motion, and progressive scapular control (Fig. 11.5). Spiking and serving are reintroduced in the functional phase of rehabilitation. During this third and final stage the physician or physiotherapist should seek to identify and correct any underlying biomechanical deficits and subclinical adaptations elsewhere within the kinetic chain that might have precipitated the rotator cuff injury. Indeed, the shoulder girdle musculature does not generate tremendous upper limb torque: roughly, the legs and back generate 85% of the energy required to spike or serve a volleyball. However, when a proximal segment of the kinetic chain is injured, the more

Table 11.1 A rehabilitation plan for rotator cuff tendinopathy (modified from Kibler *et al.* 1998).

Mechanism of injury	Chronic overload/overuse of the shoulder, resulting in repetitive microtrauma and gradual symptom onset
Clinical symptom complex	Anterior shoulder pain, worse with flexion/elevation above shoulder girdle height and abduction/internal rotation, mild weakness of abduction and internal rotation, pain which worsens at night
Tissue injury complex	Tendinosis of the supraspinatus at the musculotendinous junction, perhaps with some concomitant attritional labral wear and tear and subacromial bursitis
Tissue overload complex	Muscles of the rotator cuff, anterior laxity and posterior tightness of the shoulder capsule, scapular dysfunction
Functional biomechanical deficit complex	Limited shoulder internal rotation, weak shoulder abduction and external rotation, scapular slide, possibly with concomitant trunk inflexibilities
Subclinical adaptation complex	Altered spiking and serving mechanics, decreased abduction, increased elbow and wrist action to maintain velocity
REHABILITATION PROTOCOL	
Acute phase	
Goals:	Minimize pain and restore pain-free active range of motion, begin program of scapular control, maintain cardiorespiratory fitness/generalized conditioning
Interventions:	Thermal modalities, including ultrasound, active range of motion/stretching exercises, isometric exercises, closed kinetic chain exercises emphasizing scapular control and glenohumeral proprioception, relative rest
Recovery phase	
Goals	Increase shoulder girdle strength and endurance, improve range of motion, improve scapular control, correct flexibility imbalances
Interventions	Active range of motion/stretching exercises, concentric and eccentric isotonic exercises isolating the rotator cuff and progressing to sport-specific movement patterns
Functional phase	
Goals	Increase power, increase endurance, restore sport-specific function (spiking and serving), return to play, establish program of prehabilitation
Interventions	Exercises to strengthen the entire kinetic chain, upper limb plyometrics emphasizing skill-specific movement patterns, analysis of technique

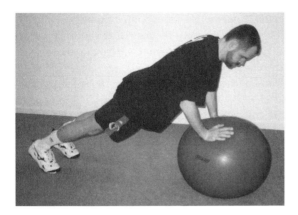

Fig. 11.5 Incorporating a Swiss ball into an exercise program makes routine exercises more challenging and helps to develop dynamic neuromuscular control along the kinetic chain.

distal segments often attempt to "catch up" the deficit so as to maintain performance—thereby placing these structures at higher risk of overload injury. Thus, an athlete with low back pain may attempt to compensate for a drop off in spike velocity by altering their spiking mechanics—which in turn may overload the shoulder girdle and precipitate an episode of shoulder pain. Because of the fine coordination needed throughout the entire kinetic chain to perform volleyball-related overhead sports skills, optimum shoulder function is dependent on maintaining balanced strength and flexibility—not only in the shoulder girdle but in the hips and trunk as well. Once the athlete can perform sport-specific skills through a pain-free range of motion, they can return to play. Table 11.1 summarizes a comprehensive rehabilitation program for rotator cuff tendinopathy.

Jumper's knee (patellar tendinopathy)

Jumper's knee is probably the most common overuse injury suffered by volleyball athletes—by some estimates, approximately 40% of volleyball players experience symptoms of jumper's knee. The knee joint must withstand high forces during jumping that render it vulnerable to overload and injury. The patella plays a critical role in the biomechanics of the knee and in jumping ability. By lengthening

the moment arm on which the quadriceps acts, the patella increases knee extensor torque and enhances the mechanical advantage of the quadriceps muscle group, increasing extensor force production by approximately 50%. Komi has estimated that the knee extensors contribute in excess of 50% of the force required to produce a forceful jump (Luhtanen & Komi 1978). Thus, jumping ability would appear to be highly dependent on the patella's role in amplifying the force-producing capacity of the quadriceps. Some of the force generated during activation of the quadriceps is directed through the patella toward the knee joint's center of rotation. The patellofemoral joint reaction force is a measure of the compression of the patella against the femur, and is dependent on the angle of knee flexion and the load applied. In general, with increasing knee flexion there is greater contact between the patella and femur, serving to distribute the increasing force—which with a deep knee bend can approach eight times the body weight. Maximal patellofemoral joint reaction force occurs at 60–90° of knee flexion. Not surprisingly, research has shown that there is a correlation between knee joint kinematics and jumper's knee: in one study, those volleyball athletes with the deepest knee flexion angle during landing from a spike jump were more likely to experience symptoms of jumper's knee (Richards *et al.* 1996).

Epidemiological studies have shown that patellar tendinopathy is related to repetitive loading of the knee extensor mechanism: the prevalence of jumper's knee increases with the frequency of jump training, and is higher among players who train or compete on hard, unforgiving surfaces. Research has also shown that athletes with superior jumping ability may be at increased risk of developing patellar tendinopathy (Lian *et al.* 1996). As the study attempted to control for the volume of jump training, it seems unlikely that this association is simply due to a training effect. Rather, there may be intrinsic structural and biomechanical properties of the lower limbs that are unique to athletes who jump well, particularly in regard to the athlete's ability to eccentrically activate the knee extensors. It is also important to note that weakness of the hip external rotators may be seen in athletes with jumper's knee, as can tightness of the hip flexors, tensor fascia lata and iliotibial band, hamstrings, and gastrocnemius

–soleus complex. Again, it is not clear whether these inflexibilities should be considered causal or secondary in relation to the pathomechanics of patellar tendinopathy. Inspection of the entire kinetic chain may reveal evidence of prior lower limb injury, or other predisposing factors, including a rigid, cavus foot. Insufficiency of the medial quadriceps can predispose the athlete to abnormal patellar tracking, as can excessive pronation or a large Q angle (the angle formed by the femur and tibia at the knee). More re-

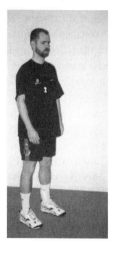 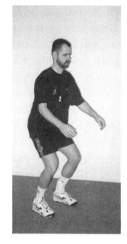 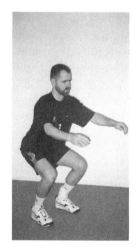

Fig. 11.6 Drop squats eccentrically exercise the knee extensors and are often employed in the treatment of jumper's knee.

Table 11.2 A rehabilitation plan for jumper's knee (modified from Kibler *et al.* 1998).

Mechanism of injury	Overuse through excessive jump training
Clinical symptom complex	Anterior infrapatellar knee pain—worse with activity and resolved with rest, tenderness over the patellar tendon, reduced knee extensor torque
Tissue injury complex	Patellar tendon (microtearing at the bone–tendon junction)
Tissue overload complex	Patellofemoral joint, quadriceps, hamstrings, hip girdle
Functional biomechanical deficit complex	Inflexibility of the hip, thigh, and leg musculature, including the hamstrings and gastrocnemius–soleus complex, pain inhibition of the knee flexors/extensors
Subclinical adaptation complex	Altered gait and jumping mechanics, including reduced stride length and avoidance of knee extension/eccentric quadriceps activation on the involved side
REHABILITATION PROTOCOL	
Acute phase	
Goals	Reduce pain, restore pain-free range of motion, maintain general cardiorespiratory fitness
Interventions	Passive thermal and electrotherapy modalities, active range of motion/stretching exercises, isometric quadriceps exercises, closed kinetic chain (CKC) exercises—limiting CKC knee flexion to 50°, relative rest
Recovery phase	
Goals	Improve lower limb and trunk flexibility, screen for and address lower limb and core imbalances of strength and flexibility, improve proprioception/neuromuscular control of the knee
Interventions	Active range of motion/stretching exercises, eccentric quadriceps exercises (including drop squats), closed kinetic chain exercises through a functional range of motion
Functional phase	
Goals	Regain sport-specific function (countermovement and squat jumping), return to play, begin prehabilitation
Interventions	Therapeutic/prophylactic taping/bracing as needed, sport-specific functional progression including plyometrics, analysis of jumping technique

cently, attention has focused on the role of the pelvis and the athlete's "core" strength and dynamic stability as intrinsic risk factors for knee injuries, an idea proposed in the literature by Sommer (1988). Rehabilitation should therefore focus on correcting strength and flexibility imbalances throughout the trunk and entire lower limbs. Strengthening exercises should initially be performed at knee flexion angles that minimize patellar loading, beginning with isometric exercises and progressing through a functional continuum emphasizing eccentric strength training (Fig. 11.6). Attempting to correct abnormal patellar tracking through bracing or taping can be a useful therapeutic adjunct to control symptoms while rehabilitating the knee. Table 11.2 summarizes the principles of rehabilitation for jumper's knee.

Lateral ankle sprains

The lateral ankle sprain is the most common acute volleyball-related injury. The true ankle joint consists of the tibiofibular talar joint, but in a practical sense the "ankle" also includes the subtalar joint. The typical volleyball-related ankle sprain mechanism of injury involves net play—most often a blocker landing on a teammate's foot or on the foot of the opposing spiker who has crossed over the centerline. As the blocker lands, their feet are typically plantar flexed in anticipation of accepting and dissipating the ground reaction force associated with landing. This is an anatomically disadvantageous position for the ankle, since when the foot is plantar flexed there is inherently greater laxity in the true ankle joint. When landing on an uneven surface, unless the dynamic (muscular) ankle stabilizers can maintain the joint in a stable alignment, the ligaments that passively stabilize the ankle are suddenly overloaded. As the foot inverts and the subtalar joint oversupinates, a predictable pattern of ligamentous loading occurs which can lead to failure of one or more of the lateral ankle ligaments. The anterior talofibular ligament (ATFL) fails initially, followed by the calcaneofibular ligament, and then the posterior talofibular ligament. In mild (grade 1) sprains, the ATFL may be simply stretched. In more

serious (grade 2) injuries, one or more ligaments may be partially disrupted, while a grade 3 injury indicates complete diastasis of one or more lateral ankle ligaments.

The athlete who has suffered an inversion ankle injury usually recalls a definite mechanism of injury with immediate functional disability proportional to the severity of the injury. The athlete may have felt or even heard a distinct "pop." On early examination, the amount of swelling typically correlates with the severity of the injury. The athlete will be tender over the ligaments involved. Palpatory examination should include the entire leg and foot to rule out associated proximal fibular (maisonneuve) fractures or avulsion injuries of the peroneal tendons off their insertion onto the lateral aspect of the fifth metatarsal. Grade 1 and 2 injuries are more common than grade 3 injuries, and can be treated non-operatively with aggressive early weight bearing and

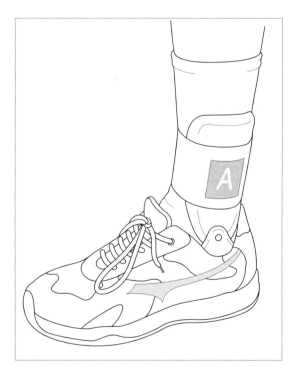

Fig. 11.7 Semi-rigid ankle orthoses are thought to enhance proprioceptive awareness about the ankle, and have been shown to help reduce the risk of recurrent ankle sprain injury.

range of motion, progressing on to strengthening and proprioceptive retraining exercises prior to return to play. Studies have demonstrated that proprioceptive training not only reduces the risk of reinjury, but also the incidence of acute lateral ankle sprains if used prophylactically (Bahr *et al.* 1997). Furthermore, there is evidence that chronic ankle instability might place volleyball athletes at a higher risk of eventually developing arthritic changes in the ankle (Gross & Marti 1999). Thus, a comprehensive rehabilitation program should include proprioceptive retraining. Use of an ankle-stabilizing orthosis can provide protection during early ambulation, and in some cases may actually reduce the risk of reinjury, particularly within the first 12 months following an ankle sprain injury (Thacker *et al.* 1999) (Fig. 11.7). Table 11.3 summarizes the rehabilitation plan for an acute lateral ankle sprain injury.

Prevention of reinjury

Although appropriate treatment and rehabilitation of injuries permit the athlete to return to play as quickly as possible, the ideal situation would be to prevent injuries entirely. The above discussion suggests that one way to prevent overuse injuries is to attend to the strengthening and conditioning of muscle groups routinely overloaded by the sport. Such an approach has been termed "prehabilitation." Flexibility is also a key factor in optimizing muscle function and joint motion. Endurance is a critical component of athletic fitness: there are several studies that suggest that fatigue results in abnormal muscular activation patterns, thereby placing the joint(s) acted upon by those muscles (and the muscles themselves) at increased risk of injury. Thus,

Table 11.3 A rehabilitation plan for an acute grade 1 lateral ankle sprain (modified from Kibler *et al.* 1998).

Mechanism of injury	Inversion sprain after landing on the opposing attacker's foot, which had penetrated the centerline
Clinical symptom complex	Local swelling and acute ecchymosis, tender to palpation over the anterior talofibular ligament, antalgic gait
Tissue injury complex	Sprain injury of the ATFL
Tissue overload complex	Peroneal muscles may be slightly strained from inversion stress and eccentric activation while attempting to stabilize the ankle
Functional biomechanical deficit complex	Swelling and pain may limit ankle range of motion and motor function. Some degree of ankle instability will persist unless fully rehabilitated
Subclinical adaptation complex	Reduced stride length, altered cadence, limited weight bearing
REHABILITATION PROTOCOL	
Acute phase	
Goals	Reduce oedema, minimize pain, improve active range of motion
Interventions	PRICE, anti-inflammatory medications, electrotherapy, and thermal modalities, support (tape or orthosis), weight bearing as tolerated, active range of motion/stretching exercises, isometric exercises, open kinetic chain exercises
Recovery phase	
Goals	Increase strength and endurance of dynamic ankle stabilizers, improve proprioception at the ankle
Interventions	Generalized lower limb conditioning, advanced weight bearing, active range of motion/stretching exercises, isotonic exercises, closed kinetic chain exercises, proprioceptive retraining.
Functional phase	
Goals	Restore normal neuromuscular control of the ankle joint and regain sport-specific function (explosive jumping, landing, cutting), return to play, begin prehabilitation
Interventions	Advanced proprioceptive exercises, sport-specific functional progressions, including resistance training of muscles acting about the knee and hip, agility drills, and plyometrics

in order to achieve maximum performance and reduce the risk of injury, the volleyball athlete should participate in a structured, volleyball-specific training program, periodized to minimize the risk of overtraining, with appropriate attention to nutrition and rest.

References

Bahr, R., Lian, Ø. & Bahr, I.A. (1997) A twofold reduction in the incidence of acute ankle sprains in volleyball after the introduction of an injury prevention program: a prospective cohort study. *Scandinavian Journal of Medicine and Science in Sports* **7**, 172–177.

Gross, P. & Marti, B. (1999) Risk of degenerative ankle joint disease in volleyball players: study of former elite athletes. *International Journal of Sports Medicine* **20**, 58–63.

Herring, S.A. (1990) Rehabilitation of muscle injuries. *Medicine and Science in Sports and Exercise* **22** (4), 453–456.

Kibler, W.B. (1990) Clinical aspects of muscle injury. *Medicine and Science in Sports and Exercise* **22** (4), 450–452.

Kibler, W.B., Chandler, T.J. & Pace, B.K. (1992) Principles of rehabilitation after chronic tendon injuries. *Clinics in Sports Medicine* **11** (3), 663–671.

Kibler, W.B., Herring, S.A. & Press, J.M. (1998) *Functional Rehabilitation of Sports and Musculoskeletal Injuries.* Aspen Publishers, Gaithersburg, MD.

Levine, W.N. & Flatow, E.L. (2000) The pathophysiology of shoulder instability. *American Journal of Sports Medicine* **28** (6), 910–917.

Lian, Ø., Engebretsen, L., Ovrebo, R.V. & Bahr, R. (1996) Characteristics of the leg extensors in male volleyball players with jumper's knee. *American Journal of Sports Medicine* **24** (3), 380–385.

Luhtanen, P. & Komi, R.V. (1978) Segmental contribution to forces in vertical jump. *European Journal of Applied Physiology and Occupational Physiology* **38** (3), 181–188.

Mair, S.D., Seaber, A.V., Glisson, R.R. & Garrett, W.E. (1996) The role of fatigue in susceptibility to acute muscle strain injury. *American Journal of Sports Medicine* **24** (2), 137–143.

Meister, K. (2000a) Injuries to the shoulder in the throwing athlete. Part 1: biomechanics/pathophysiology/classification of injury. *American Journal of Sports Medicine* **28** (2), 265–275.

Meister, K. (2000b) Injuries to the shoulder in the throwing athlete. Part 2: evaluation/treatment. *American Journal of Sports Medicine* **28** (4), 587–601.

Richards, D.P., Ajemian, S.V., Wiley, J.P. & Zernicke, R.F. (1996) Knee joint dynamics predict patellar tendinitis in elite volleyball players. *American Journal of Sports Medicine* **24** (5), 676–683.

Sommer, H.M. (1988) Patellar chondropathy and apicitis, and muscle imbalances of the lower extremities in competitive sports. *Sports Medicine* **5**, 386–394.

Thacker, S.B., Stroup, D.F., Branche, C.M., Gilchrist, J., Goodman, R.A. & Weitman, E.A. (1999) The prevention of ankle sprains. *American Journal of Sports Medicine* **27** (6), 753–760.

Recommended reading

Burkhart, S.S., Morgan, C.D. & Kibler, W.B. (2000) Shoulder injuries in overhead athletes. *Clinics in Sports Medicine* **19** (1), 125–158.

Hecox, B., Mehreteab, T.A. & Weisberg, J. (1994) *Physical Agents.* Appleton & Lange, Norwalk, CT.

Whiting, W.C. & Zernicke, R.F. (1998) *Biomechanics of Musculoskeletal Injury.* Human Kinetics, Champaign, IL.

Chapter 12
Shoulder injuries in volleyball

Andrea Ferretti and Angelo DeCarli

Introduction

Shoulder injuries are among the most common volleyball-related overuse injuries. Shoulder injuries also frequently occur in other "overhead" sports such as baseball, tennis, and swimming, i.e. sports whose skills require repetitive arm elevation to 90° (shoulder level) or above. The shoulder joint is designed for mobility rather than stability, and is therefore susceptible to injury when subjected to the athletic demands of these sports. Volleyball skills such as spiking and serving place a tremendous load on the shoulder girdle. These forces must be absorbed and dissipated by the stabilizing mechanism of the shoulder, which consists of both static stabilizers (including the glenohumeral joint, the glenoid labrum, and the ligamentous shoulder capsule) and dynamic stabilizers (the four muscles of the rotator cuff: the supraspinatus, infraspinatus, teres minor, and subscapularis).

Although differences clearly exist, the kinematics of volleyball spiking and serving resembles those of throwing a baseball. Both skills subject the dominant shoulder girdle to repetitive stresses. If these stresses are applied at a rate exceeding the rate of tissue repair, such overload can result over time in cumulative damage to the shoulder. Therefore, to better understand the mechanism of overuse shoulder injuries in volleyball athletes, the volleyball medical professional should have a basic familiarity with the kinematics of the volleyball spike and serve. Like the baseball throwing motion, the mechanics of

these skills can be divided into three phases (first described by Tullos and King 1973): cocking, acceleration, and deceleration/follow-through.

The cocking phase may be defined as the period between the preparation for movement and the moment at which the shoulder begins the explosive phase of acceleration. This phase has been further described as "cocking the hammer." Initially the athlete abducts and externally rotates the hitting limb at the shoulder, keeping the elbow flexed. At the conclusion of this phase, the shoulder is maximally externally rotated and extended, with the upper limb abducted 90° or more (Fig. 12.1a). Spikers and jump servers typically combine this movement pattern with trunk rotation and lumbar extension, while "float" servers tend to maintain a more neutral trunk position. The acceleration phase actually begins with lumbar flexion and trunk derotation. The momentum thereby generated is funneled up though the scapula to the shoulder girdle and on to the wrist and hand (the most distal links in the kinetic chain). The "cocked" upper limb moves forward, and begins to accelerate through a combination of flexion, adduction, and internal rotation. At the moment of contact with the volleyball (Fig. 12.1b), the upper limb is typically abducted to 150–180° (i.e. nearly vertical), slightly flexed (so as to contact the ball out in front of the body), and extended at the elbow (to permit contact with the ball at the highest point possible). This position also maximizes the moment arm of the upper limb, resulting in a faster arm swing and a more powerful spike. After the ball is contacted, the deceleration

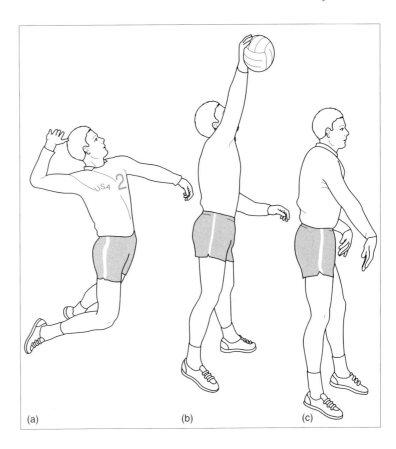

Fig. 12.1 Phases of the arm swing: (a) cocking, (b) acceleration, (c) follow-through.

phase begins. The primary purpose of the deceleration/follow-through phase is to dissipate the energy accumulated during acceleration, while trying to minimize stresses about the shoulder. Follow-through occurs via a combination of upper limb adduction and shoulder internal rotation (Fig. 12.1c), and is mediated by the eccentric action of the rotator cuff. Indeed, if not for the dynamic stabilizing action of this group of four muscles, the shoulder joint would dislocate anteriorly after every spike or jump serve!

Thus, the spiking or overhead serving motion takes the shoulder through a wide active range of motion at high speed. Significant forces are generated in the upper limb, placing the structures of the shoulder girdle at great risk of injury. Furthermore, it has been estimated that the elite volleyball athlete will perform 40,000 spikes in one season of competition. Given this volume and load, it should not be too surprising to learn that the most common

volleyball-related shoulder injuries are overuse in character, and include: the syndrome of glenohumeral instability, impingement syndrome (rotator cuff tendinopathy), and suprascapular neuropathy.

Shoulder instability

Clinical scenario

An elite volleyball player presents to the sports medicine clinic with complaints of acute anterior superior shoulder pain on his dominant (hitting) side. He had attempted to make a diving save with his upper limb fully forward flexed (Fig. 12.2), and experienced the immediate onset of severe pain that prevented him from competing further. Since the onset of symptoms, he has experienced persistent pain

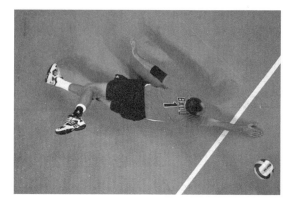

Fig. 12.2 A fall onto an outstretched arm is a common mechanism by which trauma to the glenoid labrum may be sustained. (Photo courtesy of Olympic Museum, Lausanne.)

with spiking and blocking. Often this pain is so intense that it virtually "paralyses" him. He also reports a frequent "clunking" sensation in the shoulder with upper limb abduction.

Pathophysiology

The glenohumeral joint is the most mobile joint in the human body. While this available range of motion permits volleyball athletes to serve and spike and block, the intrinsic instability of the shoulder predisposes the volleyball athlete to joint-related injury. There are several factors influencing glenohumeral stability, which results from a hierarchy of both "active" (dynamic) and "passive" (static) mechanisms. The passive mechanism, or static stabilizers of the shoulder, consists of the glenoid labrum (a rim of fibrocartilage that serves to deepen the glenoid fossa) and the joint capsule, which is in turn reinforced by the superior, middle, and inferior glenohumeral ligaments. Dynamic stability is an active process mediated by the rotator cuff (principally the subscapularis muscle–tendon unit), in concert with the tendon of the long head of biceps brachii. Dysfunction of one or more of these components can result in a functionally unstable shoulder.

The syndrome of glenohumeral instability is characterized by abnormal mobility of the humeral head in relation to the glenoid fossa. Glenohumeral insta-

bility may be classified according to the degree of instability (dislocation vs subluxation), the etiology of instability (traumatic vs atraumatic), and the position of the translated humeral head in relation to the glenoid fossa (anterior vs inferior vs posterior vs multidirectional instability). Dislocation of the humeral head may be defined as the complete separation of the articular surfaces of the humeral head and the glenoid fossa. Immediate relocation (reduction) of a dislocated shoulder does not typically occur spontaneously. Subluxation of the glenohumeral joint, on the other hand, can be defined as a momentary translation of the humeral head along the glenoid fossa, but without complete separation of the articular surfaces. Subluxations by definition are transient, and reduction is virtually instantaneous.

The etiology of glenohumeral joint instability can be either traumatic or atraumatic. For example, a previously normal shoulder may become unstable as a result of trauma (most commonly a fall on an outstretched upper limb). As the humerus translates forward during anterior dislocation, the glenoid labrum may be avulsed from its attachment, and capsule and periosteum stripped off the scapular neck. After reduction, the labrum and capsule often do not reattach to the glenoid and scapular neck, respectively, thereby producing a persistently weak area that may predispose the athlete to recurrent anterior dislocations. Atraumatic instability can develop in athletes with constitutionally lax ligaments with little to no history of overt injury. More commonly, however, atraumatic shoulder instability is the consequence of chronic overload with resultant attrition of the static and dynamic stabilizers.

The humeral head can dislocate or sublux anteriorly (anterior instability is the most frequent type of shoulder instability among overhead athletes), posteriorly, inferiorly, or in all directions. This latter condition, usually associated with laxity of the capsuloligamentous restraints, is referred to as multidirectional instability. In volleyball, pure traumatic dislocation of the shoulder is quite rare; however, if a certain degree of ligamentous laxity predisposes the shoulder, dislocation may occur during a defensive action resulting in a fall on an outstretched arm, particularly if the limb is abducted and externally rotated. There have also been case reports of elite volleyball athletes dislocating anteriorly following a spike.

In volleyball, as in other sports requiring repetitive upper extremity activities, recurrent glenohumeral subluxation can occur even in the absence of discrete trauma. Presumably, the repetitive abduction and external rotation of the upper limb during serving and spiking results in gradual stretching of the anterior capsular structures. This secondary capsular laxity permits the humeral head to sublux anteriorly. Players with transient anterior subluxation, or "dead arm" syndrome, may complain of "paralysing pain" that causes the arm to go "lame" or "dead" when attempting a hard spike, service, or other overhead skill.

Diagnostic and therapeutic considerations

If possible, the direction of the instability should be determined in order to permit proper treatment, which may be conservative (physical therapy based) or surgical. The diagnosis of anterior glenohumeral instability is straightforward in the case of recurrent shoulder dislocation. However, the diagnosis of glenohumeral instability can be considerably more difficult in athletes without a history of shoulder dislocation or precipitating trauma. In addition to a careful history, the volleyball medical professional should therefore confirm the suspected diagnosis by performing a careful physical examination and by obtaining other diagnostic (imaging) tests as indicated.

The apprehension sign (Fig. 12.3) is a reliable indicator of anterior shoulder instability. The test is performed as part of a comprehensive physical examination by passively externally rotating the shoulder with the upper limb abducted to 90° and the elbow flexed to 90°. The sensitivity of the test may be increased if the examiner places anteriorly directed pressure on the proximal humerus to further stress anterior structures. As external rotation progresses, the athlete with an unstable shoulder will become apprehensive, fearing that the shoulder is about to dislocate. Similarly, a posteriorly directed force on the proximal humerus should eliminate the athlete's apprehension and sense of impending

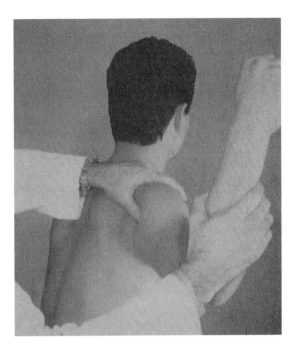

Fig. 12.3 Apprehension test for shoulder instability. (Photo courtesy of Nuova Cesi.)

dislocation (this has been termed the "relocation sign"). Radiographic examination of the suspected unstable shoulder should be obtained to detect any bone abnormalities stemming from prior dislocation (Fig. 12.4). Contrast-enhanced cross-sectional imaging modalities (e.g. magnetic resonance imaging (MRI) or computerized tomography (CT) arthrography) provide the best views of the relevant anatomy—particularly of the glenoid labrum.

The treatment of anterior glenohumeral instability can be conservative or surgical. Conservative treatment is indicated in the early stages of anterior instability in the overhead athlete, after the initial episode or two of traumatic dislocation, and as a preliminary approach to atraumatic multidirectional instability. The principal goals of the rehabilitation program are to strengthen the dynamic stabilizers of the glenohumeral joint, particularly the subscapularis, and to correct any imbalances of strength or flexibility. Isotonic strength in internal (and external) shoulder rotation equal to 20% of the athlete's body weight has been suggested as an objective test of readiness for return to competition in overhead

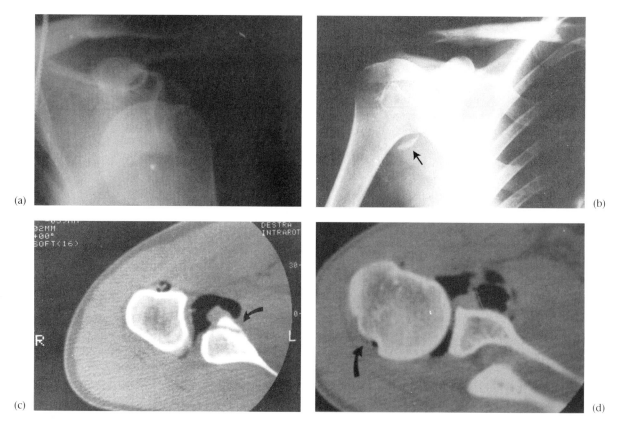

(a)

(b)

(c)

(d)

Fig. 12.4 Radiographic findings in shoulder dislocation: (a) radiographic/acute (unreduced) appearance of an anterior shoulder dislocation on plain film imaging, (b) plain film appearance of a Bankart lesion (arrow), defined as a fracture of the inferior glenoid rim, typically with associated labral pathology, (c) CT appearance of a glenoid fracture (arrow) in an athlete with recurrent anterior dislocation, and (d) CT appearance of a Hill-Sachs defect (arrow), defined as a depression fracture of the posterior aspect of the humeral head due to impact against the glenoid rim. (Photo courtesy of Nuova Cesi.)

athletes. The athlete should be taken through a functional progression of upper limb strengthening exercises, beginning with isometric exercises and advancing to isotonic exercises and then to eccentric training. In cases of recurrent dislocation, in selected cases of initial dislocation, and in functionally disabling anterior instability, surgical intervention may be the treatment of choice (Ferretti *et al.* 1998a). The nature of the surgical procedure is, of course, dependent upon the clinical scenario. Postoperative dislocation recurrence rates are relatively low, ranging from 2 to 11%. Elite volleyball athletes requiring shoulder surgery for the treatment of instability may not be able to return to their preinjury level of performance. Return to competition following surgical repair may take 6 months or longer and players may

experience a slight to moderate loss or restriction of external shoulder rotation.

Impingement syndrome

Clinical scenario

An Olympic volleyball player presents to the polyclinic with complaints of anterior shoulder girdle pain of insidious onset. She denies a history of specific recent or past trauma, but reports that her aching discomfort worsens with repetitive overhead activity. She has played on the international level as an outside hitter for 8 years.

Pathophysiology

Impingement syndrome describes a condition of anterior shoulder pain that is quite common in volleyball players and other overhead athletes. Classically, impingement syndrome has been thought to result from chronic irritation of the tendons of the rotator cuff muscles as they pass beneath the coracoacromial ligament and the anterior part of the acromion—rotator cuff tendinopathy (Neer 1983). The two tendons most commonly involved are those of the supraspinatus and the infraspinatus muscles. The supraspinatus acts principally to abduct the upper limb at the shoulder, while the infraspinatus serves as an external rotator; thus, both muscles are vital to overhead upper limb function and sporting skills. In some cases the tendon of the long head of the biceps brachii may be involved as well. Recently, a variant of the impingement syndrome has been described in which the posterior shoulder capsule may be pinched by the humeral head as the shoulder is abducted and externally rotated. For further information on this so-called "posterior impingement syndrome," the interested reader is referred to articles by Meister (2000a, 2000b).

Overlying the tendons of the rotator cuff at their

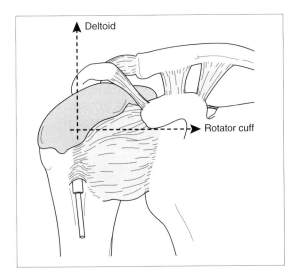

Fig. 12.5 Weakness of rotator cuff permits anterosuperior translation of the humeral head during overhead reaching (due to the unbalanced action of the deltoid), resulting in impingement syndrome.

attachment to the greater tuberosity of the humerus is the subacromial bursa. Normally this bursa is a thin sheet of tissue that reduces friction and allows the rotator cuff to glide beneath the coracoacromial arch and the anterior aspect of the acromion. In some volleyball athletes, repetitive serving and spiking results in a progressive impingement of the rotator cuff tendons against the coracoacromial ligament. As a result the intervening bursa is often irritated as well, producing a simultaneous inflammatory bursitis.

Impingement usually occurs when the arm is abducted and/or forward flexed at the shoulder to between 85 and 120°—particularly if the upper limb is internally rotated. As discussed, spiking or serving demand this kind of motion on a repetitive basis, which can result in chronic irritation of the rotator cuff tendons and the subacromial bursa. As the supraspinatus tendon becomes increasingly irritated and painful, it may become weaker and dysfunctional. Consequently, the supraspinatus and the other rotator cuff muscles may become less effective and coordinated, and the cuff as a whole may become less efficient at maintaining the humeral head within the glenoid fossa. Thereafter, with upper limb abduction the humeral head may tend to "ride up" as the dysfunctional rotator cuff fails to adequately depress the humeral head in the glenoid cavity (Fig. 12.5). This, in turn, further compounds the impingement of the rotator cuff tendons, producing increasing pain and limiting overhead activities. Over time and with repetitive use, the process of degeneration may lead to small attritional tears and eventually to large tears of the rotator cuff tendons. Thus, impingement and subsequent muscle hypotrophy can—over time—lead to a functionally unstable shoulder with recurrent symptomatic subluxation. Rotator cuff tears are especially common at the distal-most portion of the involved tendon near its insertion into the humeral head. Although complete rotator cuff tears are most likely to occur in athletes over 35 years of age, small, incomplete tears of the supraspinatus tendon have been documented in young players. This suggests that precautions should be taken to prevent young volleyball athletes from overspecializing and that skills should be taught to youth using a lighter weight ball to minimize the load on the developing shoulder.

Diagnostic and therapeutic considerations

Classification systems have been developed that describe three or four stages of rotator cuff involvement due to suprahumeral impingement. Most athletes are first treated with symptoms during stage I. The chief complaint during stage I is an aching discomfort in the anterior aspect of the hitting shoulder following overhead sporting activity. At this stage, performance is not significantly compromised. There is tenderness on palpatory examination, and the athlete will typically demonstrate a positive impingement sign (Fig. 12.6). Additional findings include a painful arc of motion during abduction from between 70 and 120°. This finding

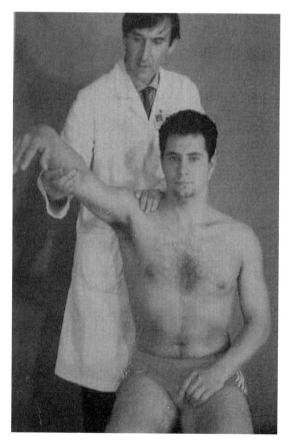

Fig. 12.6 Neer test: forced forward flexion causes pain and impingement of the greater tuberosity against the anterior acromion. (Photo courtesy of Nuova Cesi.)

is particularly common when the subacromial bursa is involved. Stage I lesions are considered to be reversible and generally respond well to conservative management consisting of relative rest, anti-inflammatory medications, ice, ultrasound/phonophoresis, and gradual initiation of a symptom-limited exercise program. Injection of corticosteroids for the treatment of tendinopathy is somewhat controversial. Although there is evidence that the process of chronic tendon injury is not inflammatory in character, many physicians nevertheless advocate the use of corticosteroids. If used, they may be employed as a first-line treatment or may be reserved pending the outcome of a short course of conservative therapy, depending on physician preference. Careful observation of the athlete while spiking or serving may reveal errors in technique. Such changes in technique are frequently precursors to impingement and therefore should be identified as a potential problem by the coaching staff or the athletic trainers. There may also be fatigue-related mechanical changes that can affect technique. Fatigue of the external rotators during the course of a workout or match may significantly alter the mechanics of the deceleration/follow-through phase, dramatically increasing impingement stress. In such situations, the faulty technique must be addressed and eliminated in order to manage the athlete's shoulder pain on a long-term basis. No lasting success will be achieved if the athlete is treated symptomatically and thereafter cleared to return to play without addressing the underlying mechanism of injury.

The athlete with stage II shoulder impingement may complain of pain both during and after activity but is able to compete without compromise. On examination, there may be some limitation in shoulder movement, although no true motor deficit is associated with this level of involvement. Supraspinatus and/or bicipital pain and pain-inhibited motor function are common, as are a positive impingement sign and a painful arc of motion during abduction. Pathologically, stage II lesions may demonstrate greater involvement of the subacromial bursa, along with thickening and fibrosis of the rotator cuff, which may lead to greater impingement stress as the available space under the coracoacromial arch is further restricted.

Conservative management as previously described is recommended in this phase.

Stage III impingement is characterized by pain both during and after sport activity and by an inability to compete at normal levels. The athlete with this level of involvement is typically older and has a long history of shoulder problems. There may be permanent degeneration of the rotator cuff tendons and thickening of the subacromial bursa with scar tissue formation. Frank tears of the rotator cuff of up to 1 cm in length are common. Radiographic evaluation may reveal subacromial or subclavicular spurring, calcific changes in the tendons or bursa, and possibly irregularities at the insertion of the supraspinatus (Fig. 12.7). CT and MRI can be helpful diagnostic tools, revealing degenerative changes of the rotator cuff and shoulder girdle. Ultrasound (sonography) is an inexpensive and reliable method useful for investigating the rotator cuff, although it is less sensitive than MRI in detecting partial tears of the rotator cuff. Physical examination findings are comparable between athletes with stage II and stage III impingement. The athlete may still achieve symptomatic improvement with conservative management (Fig. 12.8), although full return to competition without limitations is doubtful. Surgical intervention may be indicated if the athlete fails to respond to a therapy program.

The athlete with stage IV impingement may complain of disabling shoulder pain affecting normal daily activities. The athlete may be weak and have pain during shoulder abduction and external rotation, suggesting the possibility of a full-thickness rotator cuff tear. All previous impingement examination findings are exaggerated. Surgical management is almost certainly indicated at this stage. A variety of surgical procedures may prove therapeutic, depending on the clinical and anatomical findings. Although damage to the shoulder structures is significant at this point, athletes who have surgery can expect to be able to return to recreational athletics with minimal problems. However, return to high-level volleyball should not generally be expected.

Suprascapular neuropathy (volleyball shoulder)

Clinical scenario

During a routine preseason physical examination, the team physician for a university volleyball team notices unilateral atrophy in the infraspinatus fossa on the athlete's dominant side. The athlete denies significant pain or functional limitation, and their coach has not detected a noticeable decrease in performance. On examination, the physician documents weakness of the ipsilateral shoulder external rotators but there is no evidence of shoulder impingement. The athlete is tender to palpation over the spinoglenoid notch, and crossed-arm adduction provokes some mild discomfort ipsilaterally.

Pathophysiology

Volleyball shoulder is defined as a condition of frequently painless atrophy of the infraspinatus muscle caused by suprascapular neuropathy. This syndrome, which has not been systematically identified in other throwing athletes, is relatively common among high-level volleyball players. Studies have demonstrated that the prevalence of suprascapular neuropathy among elite volleyball players ranges from between 12.5 and 45%, although the actual prevalence may be higher due to underreporting. In

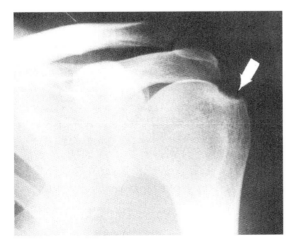

Fig. 12.7 Radiographic changes indicating insertional tendinopathy of the supraspinatus tendon (arrow). (Photo courtesy of Nuova Cesi.)

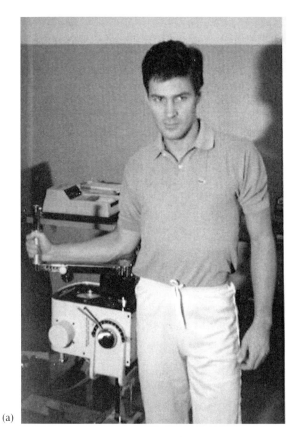

(a)

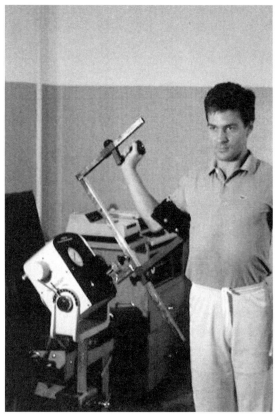

(b)

Fig. 12.8 Conservative treatment of impingement syndrome: isokinetic rehabilitation of rotator cuff (internal–external rotation): (a) arm adducted, (b) arm slightly abducted (modified neutral position). (Photo courtesy of Nuova Cesi.)

1985, during the European Volleyball Championships, 96 athletes from various national teams were examined. Twelve athletes (12.5%) demonstrated paresis of the infraspinatus on the dominant side (Ferretti *et al*. 1987) (Fig. 12.9). However, in another study, infraspinatus atrophy was detected in 64% of the athletes examined during the 1989 FIVB World Gala held in Singapore (Ferretti *et al*. 1998b). It is apparent, then, that suprascapular neuropathy is often overlooked as a cause of shoulder pain on the dominant side in overhead athletes—probably because the condition often presents with symptoms suggestive of rotator cuff tendinopathy.

There are two potential anatomical sites where the sûprascapular nerve may become compromised: the suprascapular notch and the spinoglenoid notch

(Fig. 12.10). Entrapment at the suprascapular notch results in palsy of the common trunk of the nerve with marked atrophy of both the supraspinatus and infraspinatus muscles, poorly localized pain, and loss of strength of the arm in abduction and external rotation. More distal involvement at the spinoglenoid notch is more common among volleyball players, and results in a more focal palsy of the terminal branch of the nerve, with isolated infraspinatus atrophy, loss of strength in external rotation, and inconstant pain.

Athletes with volleyball shoulder typically present with complaints of vague posterior shoulder pain affecting their dominant side, although they may be completely asymptomatic. Volleyball shoulder appears to affect all volleyball players equally,

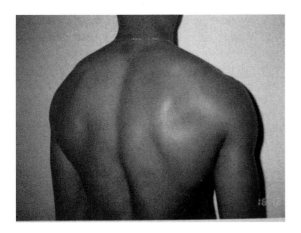

Fig. 12.9 Isolated atrophy of infraspinatus in a volleyball player. (Photo courtesy of Nuova Cesi.)

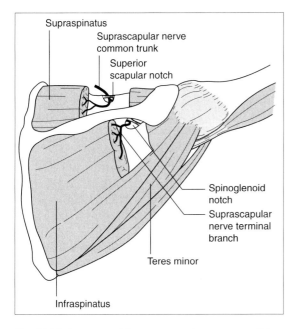

Fig. 12.10 Anatomy of the suprascapular nerve: possible sites of injury.

without regard for their position. Curiously, despite significant weakness of external rotation, these elite athletes often notice no deterioration in their sport performance. Although the dominant limb should generally be stronger than the non-dominant limb,

isokinetic testing has revealed that individuals with suprascapular neuropathy are on average 22% weaker in the affected arm during external rotation when compared with the unaffected limb.

The etiology of the paralysis of the terminal branch of the suprascapular nerve in volleyball players is still not definitively understood, and no consensus exists as to causation. Anatomical variations of the spinoglenoid ligament and the course of the nerve's terminal branch should be considered as potentially predisposing factors for suprascapular pathology. Rarely, ganglion cysts arising from the glenohumeral joint may be found to compress the nerve along its path. The observation that infraspinatus atrophy occurs almost exclusively on the dominant side suggests that repetitive spiking and serving might be causally related. Indeed, Sandow and Ilic (1998) have proposed that the suprascapular nerve is vulnerable to direct compression or impingement by the medial border of the supraspinatus and infraspinatus tendons within the spinoglenoid notch when the upper limb is abducted and externally rotated. However, since setters are equally affected when compared with players at other positions, spiking would seem to be mechanistically less important than serving.

The "float" serve is a skill that is clearly unique to volleyball. Unlike the jump serve, the server does not try for maximum speed, but rather tries to impart a "floating" trajectory to the volleyball that makes it's flight unpredictable and difficult to receive. A well-executed float serve may shift course by as much as 10 cm in the last 0.4 s before player contact. To "float," the ball must not rotate on its axis and its velocity should be approximately 13–14 $m \cdot s^{-1}$. The depth of the seams of the volleyball covering has been shown to affect the trajectory of the ball as well. The serve is dependent on technique: the server must contact the ball sharply at its dead center, then immediately arrest follow-through and retract the arm. This sequence of actions requires first eccentric and then concentric activation of the posterior muscles of the shoulder — particularly the infraspinatus and teres minor. This mechanism may result in impingement of the terminal branch of the suprascapular nerve at the spinoglenoid notch at the base of the spine of the scapula (Ferretti *et al.* 1995) (Fig. 12.11).

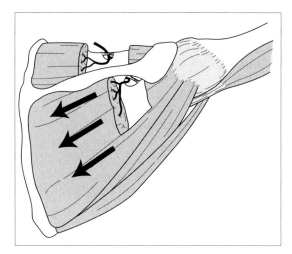

Fig. 12.11 Mechanism of stretching of the terminal branch of the suprascapular nerve during eccentric activation of the infraspinatus muscle, which occurs during the deceleration phase of the float serve.

Diagnostic and therapeutic considerations

The diagnosis of suprascapular neuropathy requires a high index of suspicion. On examination, there will be noticeable atrophy of the infraspinatus fossa (and possibly the supraspinatus fossa) on the dominant side, although the bulk of the overlying trapezius may obscure the muscle wasting if mild. The affected shoulder will be weaker in external rotation. The athlete may be tender to palpation at the site of impingement, and cross-body adduction of the upper limbs may be somewhat provocative of pain. Note that bilateral suprascapular neuropathy has been reported. The diagnosis may be confirmed by electromyography, which will demonstrate injury potentials in the affected muscle(s). MRI is warranted (particularly in elite athletes) to rule out compressive lesions such as ganglia, which, if present, might prompt consideration of early surgical intervention.

Treatment of volleyball shoulder consists most often of a rehabilitation program emphasizing strengthening of the shoulder external rotators (principally the teres minor, in addition to any residual infraspinatus activity). In fact, despite profound atrophy, the infraspinatus frequently is not com-

pletely denervated and therefore a daily strengthening program may be quite effective at restoring motor function. As indicated earlier, volleyball athletes rarely report negative effects on their performance, and thus volleyball shoulder should be considered to be a relatively benign entity in most cases. Although surgical treatment is rarely indicated in volleyball players with infraspinatus atrophy, several surgical procedures have been developed to release the nerve at the suprascapular notch or at the spinoglenoid notch. Athletes who continue to have pain despite conservative treatment may benefit from surgical release of the nerve at the site of entrapment. Despite clinical improvement in pain and strength, recovery of infraspinatus atrophy is seldom observed after surgery.

Thus, suprascapular neuropathy in top volleyball players usually represents a benign condition producing minimal disability in the short term. It should be noted, however, that the long-term consequences of suprascapular neuropathy are not entirely clear. The infraspinatus muscle also functions as a major depressor of the humeral head, acting in concert with the other muscles of the rotator cuff to dynamically stabilize the glenohumeral joint. Loss of infraspinatus function creates a potential imbalance in the force couple formed by the deltoid and rotator cuff. Such an imbalance might lead, over time, to a "secondary" impingement syndrome. For this reason, the volleyball medical professional should be careful to thoroughly assess complaints of shoulder pain by an athlete with known infraspinatus deficiency. While volleyball shoulder can on occasion prove painful, other coincident diagnoses including rotator cuff tendinopathy or functional shoulder instability should not be overlooked.

References

Ferretti, A., Cerullo, G. & Russo, G. (1987) Suprascapular neuropathy in volleyball players. *Journal of Bone Joint Surgery* **69A**, 260–2263.

Ferretti, A., De Carli, A. & Fontana, M. (1995) Entrapment of suprascapular nerve at spinoglenoid notch. In: M Vastamaki, M. & Jalovaara, P. (eds). *Surgery of the Shoulder,* pp. 385–392. Elsevier Science, Amsterdam.

Ferretti, A., De Carli, A., Calderaro, M. & Conteduca, F. (1998a) Open capsulorrhaphy with suture anchors for recurrent anterior dislocation of the shoulder. *American Journal of Sports Medicine* **26** (5), 625–629.

Ferretti, A., De Carli, A. & Fontana, M. (1998b) Injury of the suprascapular nerve at the spinoglenoid notch. The natural history of infraspinatus atrophy in volleyball players. *American Journal of Sports Medicine* **26** (6), 759–763.

Meister, K. (2000a) Injuries to the shoulder in the throwing athlete. Part 1: biomechanics, pathophysiology, classification of injury. *American Journal of Sports Medicine* **28** (2), 265–275.

Meister, K. (2000b) Injuries to the shoulder in the throwing athlete. Part 2: evaluation, treatment: *American Journal of Sports Medicine* **28** (4), 587–601.

Neer, C.S. (1983) Impingement lesions. *Clinical Orthopaedics* **173**, 70–77.

Sandow, M.J. & Ilic, J. (1998) Suprascapular nerve rotator cuff compression syndrome in volleyball players. *Journal of Shoulder and Elbow Surgery* **7**, 516–521.

Tullos, H.S. & King, J.W. (1973) Throwing mechanism in sports. *Orthopaedic Clinics of North America* **4** (3), 709–720.

Recommended reading

Burkhart, S.S., Morgan, C.D. & Kibler, W.B. (2000) Shoulder injuries in overhead athletes: the dead arm revisited. *Clinics in Sports Medicine* **19** (1), 125–158.

Levine, W.N. & Flatow, E.L. (2000) The pathophysiology of shoulder instability. *American Journal of Sports Medicine* **28** (6), 910–917.

Chapter 13
Knee and ankle injuries in volleyball

Karim Khan and Roald Bahr

Introduction

This chapter discusses two particularly troublesome lower limb conditions that cause volleyball athletes in general a great deal of inconvenience and discomfort, and which—on occasion—can cut short a player's career. The first of these is jumper's knee, a condition also known as patellar tendinopathy, patellar tendinosis, and, in the past, patellar tendonitis. The term "jumper's knee" is used here because it is well entrenched in volleyball circles and aptly describes the mechanism of injury. Note that clinicians generally use the term "patellar tendinopathy" to refer to this condition, as athletes who participate in sports that are not particularly jump intensive can also suffer from the condition (e.g. soccer players, sprinters, skiers) (Karlsson *et al.* 1991).

This chapter also considers ankle sprain—the single most common acute injury among volleyball players. The typical mechanisms of volleyball-related ankle sprain injuries are discussed in more detail in Chapter 10, but to summarize, these injuries result most commonly from landing on an opponent or teammate's foot. Ankle sprains have been shown to account for as much as half of all acute injuries in indoor volleyball with an incidence of about one sprain injury per 1,000h of activity (Bahr *et al.* 1994; Bahr & Bahr 1997).

Both ankle sprains and patellar tendinopathy are less common among beach volleyball athletes than among their indoor counterparts. The softness of

the sand reduces the load on the patellar tendon during jumping and landing, and the fact that there are only two players per team reduces the risk of contact-related ankle sprains. Nevertheless, ankle sprains and patellar tendinopathy account for a significant proportion of injuries in beach volleyball, as well (Bahr & Reeser, in press). Taken together, these observations should provide ample incentive for physicians and physiotherapists involved in the care of volleyball players to learn how to effectively diagnose and treat both jumper's knee and ankle sprain injuries.

Jumper's knee

Clinical scenario

An Olympic volleyball player reports to the team physician with complaints of infrapatellar pain that is aggravated by jumping. The athlete's pain tends to occur after particularly arduous on-court training, or after activities such as weight training or plyometric jump training. Symptoms improve with rest. The player has previously experienced similar problems, the first instance of which occurred when he was a youth. The player localizes their pain to the inferior pole of the patella.

Clinical approach to anterior knee pain

There are numerous possible causes of pain in the

scenario outlined. Table 13.1 lists the more common causes of anterior knee pain. In most instances, however, the volleyball medical professional must distinguish between jumper's knee and the patellofemoral syndrome, as these are by far the most frequent causes of anterior knee pain in this population. In general, distinguishing one from the other is not too difficult a task (Table 13.2). Even so, the clinical features of the two conditions can overlap, potentially creating some diagnostic confusion. Furthermore, jumper's knee and patellofemoral syndrome can in rare instances present simultaneously as a result of an underlying biomechanical abnormality or because of excessive jump training.

History

When a volleyball player presents to the doctor or physiotherapist with a complaint of atraumatic knee pain, the clinician must first establish an accurate diagnosis. Based on a knowledge of volleyball-specific injury patterns, jumper's knee should be high on the list of potential diagnoses. In addition, however, there are a number of important historical

details that facilitate the practitioner's ability to arrive at an accurate diagnosis, including the circumstances surrounding the initial onset of pain, the specific location of the pain, the nature of aggravating activities, and the presence of any associated clicking, giving way, or swelling.

If the athlete's pain is typically precipitated by activities that involve repetitive eccentric loading of the patellar tendon, such as repetitive spike or block training, the athlete is probably suffering from jumper's knee. If on the other hand the onset of pain is insidious and the athlete complains of a diffuse ache that is exacerbated by either activity or prolonged sitting ("movie-goer's knee"), the alternative diagnosis of patellofemoral pain syndrome must be considered. Pain that occurs with and which gradually worsens during running is more likely to be of patellofemoral origin, whereas pain that occurs at the start of activity, settles after warm-up, and returns after activity or the next morning is more likely to represent patellar tendinopathy.

The prevalence of jumper's knee is 40–50% among high-level volleyball players (Ferretti *et al.* 1984; Ferretti 1986; Lian *et al.* 1996b). Extrinsic risk factors identified to date for jumper's knee include total training load (including the amount of weight training) and the hardness of the playing surface. Information on intrinsic risk factors is sparse. Theoretically, clinically important intrinsic risk factors are likely to exist, since only one in two players develop symptoms of jumper's knee despite identical extrinsic risk factors. Studies on static biomechanical parameters of volleyball athletes generally have not yielded conclusive results (Ferretti 1986; Kujala

Table 13.1 Common causes of anterior knee pain.

Patellofemoral syndrome
Jumper's knee
Recurrent patellar subluxation
Osgood–Schlatter disease (younger athlete)
Fat pad impingement

Table 13.2 Comparison of the clinical features of two common causes of anterior knee pain. Note that these conditions may coexist.

Signs	Patellofemoral syndrome	Patellar tendinopathy
Onset	Running (especially downhill), steps/stairs, hills, any weight-bearing sport requiring repeated knee flexion/extension (e.g. distance running)	Activities involving jumping and landing (e.g. basketball, volleyball, high jump, netball, bounding, ballet)
Pain	Vague/non-specific, may be medial, lateral, or infrapatellar	Usually around inferior pole of patella, aggravated by jumping and mid to full squat
Tenderness	Usually medial or lateral facets of patella but may be tender in infrapatellar region. May have no pain on palpation due to areas of patella being inaccessible	Most commonly inferior pole of patellar tendon attachment. Occasionally in midtendon, rarely at distal attachment to tibial tuberosity

et al. 1986). However, studies of the dynamic performance of the leg extensor apparatus suggest that players with jumper's knee perform on average better than controls (Lian *et al.* 1996a). The right knee is affected more often than the left knee among volleyball players. One reason may be the dynamic biomechanical factors acting upon the leg extensor apparatus during a spike jump with a right–left take off, since this may be expected to cause higher eccentric–concentric loading of the right knee compared with the left (Fig. 13.1).

Diagnostic and therapeutic considerations

Reproducing the patient's anterior knee pain during the clinical assessment is critical to establishing an accurate diagnosis. A double- or single-leg squat will usually provoke the athlete's typical symptoms. This is important both for diagnostic purposes and to provide a baseline in order to determine the effectiveness of treatment. The clinician should palpate the anterior knee carefully to determine the site of maximal tenderness. If the athlete has jumper's knee, tenderness will be maximal at the junction of the patella and the patellar tendon, and this is most evident when the knee is slightly flexed (Fig. 13.2). Biomechanical examination is important in determining any predisposing factors.

Radiographic imaging is generally not required to confirm the suspected clinical diagnosis of jumper's knee. However, ultrasonography and magnetic resonance imaging (MRI) both display the patellar tendon anatomy well. The presence of hypo-

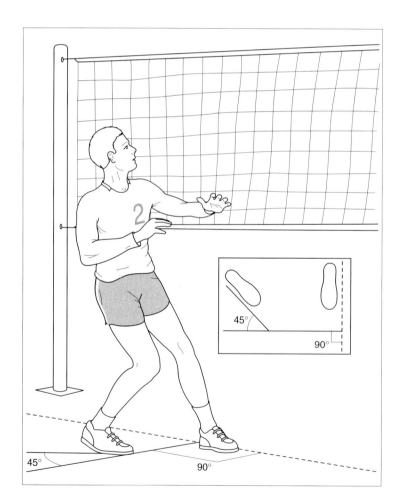

Fig. 13.1 Normal take-off position for a spike jump. Note how the right foot is externally rotated and that the flexion angle of the right knee is greater than the left. Presumably, this results in higher loads on the right knee during the eccentric phase of the take off.

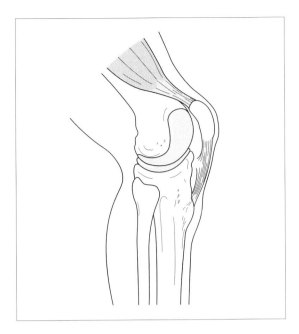

Fig. 13.2 Patellar tendinopathy—typical location of pathology.

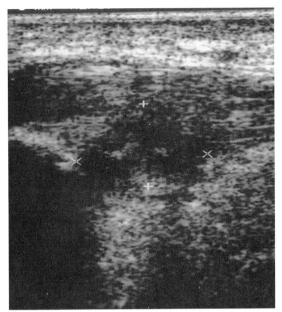

(a)

echogenicity on ultrasonography (Fig. 13.3a) or high signal abnormality on MRI (Fig. 13.3b) generally correlates with the symptoms characteristic of patellar tendinopathy. It should be noted, however, that asymptomatic athletes have been shown to have areas of abnormality on imaging of their patellar tendons. This observation reinforces the clinical nature of the diagnosis and the importance of a thorough history and physical examination (Lian *et al.* 1996b; Cook *et al.* 1998).

Once the diagnosis has been made, appropriate treatment can begin. Studies of the outcome of the treatment for jumper's knee indicate that some unfortunate players can suffer from prolonged symptoms. These athletes may require more than 6 months of treatment before they can return to sporting activities (Cook *et al.* 1997; Schiavone-Panni *et al.* 2000). To tackle this challenging problem, practitioners usually combine treatments that include self-care, medical management, and an exercise prescription. If this conservative approach fails, then surgical intervention is indicated.

Volleyball players must recognize that jumper's knee is potentially a very serious condition requiring

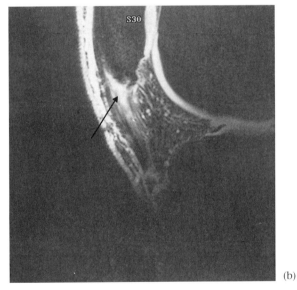

(b)

Fig. 13.3 Ultrasound evaluation of the athlete with symptoms of patellar tendinopathy may show the presence of hypoechogenicity (a), while MRI can reveal high signal abnormality (b).

a long period of rehabilitation. Thus, players should not defer seeking appropriate medical attention. Indeed, there is some evidence to suggest that early diagnosis and treatment of patellar tendinopathy helps to minimize the need for time off from volleyball.

Ice massage is one of the most effective therapies that a player can initiate. Ice should be applied over the affected tendon daily (or several times a day) for up to 15 min per session. The issue of whether or not a player should be treated with non-steroidal anti-inflammatory drugs (NSAIDs; available without prescription in many countries) is somewhat controversial.

Historically, the main pharmaceutical agents used to treat patellar tendinopathy have been NSAIDs and corticosteroids. Although jumper's knee was, at one time, considered to be an inflammatory disorder, it is now known to result from collagen disruption within the tendon—either due to degeneration or failed healing. Thus, the biological basis for using anti-inflammatory drugs is not obvious (Jozsa & Kannus 1997; Khan *et al.* 1999). Nevertheless, these drugs remain the most commonly used symptomatic therapy even though their efficacy in healing patellar tendinopathy remains unproven (Almekinders & Temple 1998). It would be reasonable to summarize current medical practice by saying that NSAIDs play a less-than-prominent role in the management of tendinopathy, particularly in chronic cases.

For the same reason that oral anti-inflammatory medication appears to be inappropriate in the treatment of tendinopathy, the role of corticosteroids also remains controversial (Shrier *et al.* 1996; Fredberg 1997). Jozsa and Kannus (1997) provide reasonable clinical guidelines for use of corticosteroid injections (Table 13.3). Note that after injection a tendon is at increased risk of rupture until appropriate strengthening has been undertaken.

A prescription of therapeutic exercise emphasizing eccentric strengthening of the knee extensors is the treatment of choice for patellar tendinopathy. Performing drop squats, among other eccentric exercises, theoretically stimulates tendon healing and effectively reduces the athlete's pain over time. The drop squat is performed in varying ways by different practitioners, but one description suggests beginning in a relaxed stance then suddenly dropping to a knee flexion angle of 100–120° (Fyfe & Stanish 1992; Cannell *et al.* 2001). Published studies recommend that patients perform three sets of 10 repeti-

Table 13.3 Guidelines for use of corticosteroid injections.

- Because corticosteroid injections are not without risk, attention must be paid to strict aseptic technique
- The number of injections to any one site should be restricted to a maximum of three, and successive injections should not be performed within 3–4 weeks
- It is important that the patient rest the area for 2–3 days after the injection and progress back to full activity gradually

tions once daily (Fyfe & Stanish 1992; Cannell *et al.* 2001). Studies are underway to determine whether slow eccentric squats with unloading in the concentric phase are even more effective.

Because volleyball players with patellar tendinopathy tend to "unload" the affected limb to avoid pain, the exercise program should progress to include single-leg exercises. In addition, squats performed on a 30° decline board appear to be more effective than those done on flat ground with the heels fixed, possibly by further loading the tendon (Cook *et al.* 2000). As the athlete progresses, the exercise prescription can be made more challenging by increasing the load and speed of the exercises. Endurance can subsequently be introduced once the athlete can perform these exercises well. Thereafter, combinations of load (weight), speed, and/or height (e.g. jumping exercises) can be added (Cook *et al.* 2000). These end-stage eccentric exercises can provoke tendon pain, and are recommended only if the athlete's sport demands intense loading (and then only after the athlete has completed a sufficiently long rehabilitation period). However, an eccentric training program, performed under close supervision and adjusted as needed, has been shown in clinical trials to be effective in improving or even eliminating symptoms associated with jumper's knee. For sports such as volleyball, jump training is also an essential component of a comprehensive rehabilitation program. Ice may be used to cool the tendon after eccentric training to minimize postexercise pain.

Of course, conservative treatment is not uniformly successful. There are numerous potential reasons why an eccentric strength training program might fail to produce the desired clinical outcome, including: excessively rapid progression through the rehabilitation program, inappropriate loading (e.g. insufficient strength or speed training, eccentric exercise started too early or too aggressively, insufficient single-leg training), excessive reliance on passive treatments (such as electrotherapeutic modalities), and inadequate monitoring of the patient's symptoms both during and after therapy.

Surgical intervention for jumper's knee is generally reserved for symptomatic volleyball players who have not improved after at least 6 months of conservative management. A variety of surgical techniques have been described but the outcome of surgery remains rather unpredictable. Success rates from between 46 and 100% have been reported, with a mean time for return to play ranging from 4 to more than 9 months. One long-term outcome study of patients who underwent open patellar tenotomy for patellar tendinosis revealed that only 54% were able to return to their previous level of sporting activity (Coleman *et al.* 2000).

Table 13.4 Diagnoses to consider after an acute ankle sprain.

Common	Less common	Do not miss
Lateral ligament injury	Fractures:	Syndesmosis injury
	lateral malleolus	Growth plate injury
	medial malleolus	
	base of the fifth	
	metatarsal	
	talus	
	calcaneus	
	Medial ligament injury	
	Dislocated ankle	
	Tendon rupture/dislocation:	
	tibialis posterior tendon	
	peroneal tendons	
	Achilles tendon	

Ankle injuries

Clinical scenario

A volleyball player reports to the team physician or therapist after suffering a sprained ankle. The sprain occurred when the athlete landed on the opposing attacker's foot after a block (note that it is also common for a player to land on a teammate's foot after a multiperson block). The athlete experienced immediate pain in the lateral aspect of the ankle, and noticed local swelling beginning only a few minutes later. Fortunately, the athlete had been given immediate first aid, including application of an ice bag and local compression to minimize swelling. At the time of the physician's visit, the player was limping noticeably, reluctant to bear full weight on the affected limb. This was the athlete's third lateral ankle sprain involving the same ankle.

Clinical approach to ankle sprain injuries

Although lateral ligament injury is by far the most common result of an ankle sprain, other possible sequelae have to be considered, as listed in Table 13.4. When a volleyball player presents to the physician

or physiotherapist after suffering an "ankle sprain," the practitioner must first determine which structures have been injured and to what extent. In most cases, a lateral ankle sprain injures one or more of the lateral ankle ligaments, but other structures may also be involved. Thus, the most important issue is to distinguish between ligament injuries and fractures. Fractures are rare among adolescents and young adults, but fractures of the lateral malleolus and fifth metatarsal occur more frequently among older recreational athletes. Since they may require early surgery, it is also important not to miss growth plate injuries in children or injuries to the syndesmosis. A careful history should be taken, since the mechanism of injury is an important clue to establishing an accurate diagnosis. A precise examination will reveal whether it is necessary to submit the patient to a radiographic examination to rule out fracture. If a fracture is suspected, X-rays should be obtained without delay. Surgery for an acute fracture—if necessary—should be performed within 6 h (before swelling is excessive).

Pathophysiology

The typical mechanism of ankle sprain injury is landing from a jump with the foot in an inverted position, i.e. plantar flexed, internally rotated, and supinated. With the foot in this position, the ankle joint is inherently unstable. The posterior talar plafond is narrower than the anterior portion, thereby reducing the bony stability of the ankle mortise when the foot is plantar flexed. Unless the dynamic musculotendinous ankle stabilizers can compensate for this reduced structural stability when the ankle joint is perturbed (such as when landing unexpectedly on an opponent's foot), the ligaments that statically stabilize the lateral ankle will be acutely overloaded. As the foot inverts and the subtalar joint oversupinates, the ligaments fail in a predictable pattern if the acute overload exceeds their tensile strength, rupturing sequentially in an anterior to posterior direction. The forces involved determine both the extent and degree of ligament injury. In about half the cases there is an isolated tear of the anterior talofibular ligament, while in about 25% there is a combined rupture of the anterior talofibular and calcaneofibular ligaments. Concomitant rupture of the posterior talofibular ligament is rare (1%). In the unusual event of an eversion injury (pronation and external rotation), a medial ligament injury must be suspected. In general, if the injury mechanism is atypical, the volleyball medical professional should maintain a heightened suspicion for injuries other than the typical lateral ligament tissue injury complex.

Diagnostic and therapeutic considerations

The goal of the initial physical examination is to decide whether the patient has a lateral ligament injury, and not a different injury requiring surgery or immobilization. According to the Ottawa ankle rules (Fig. 13.4), ankle X-rays are indicated only if there is bony tenderness to palpation or if the patient is unable to bear weight both immediately following the injury and at the time of the subsequent clinical assessment (Leddy *et al.* 1998). These guidelines, followed correctly, detect all clinically significant fractures (100% sensitivity).

Injury to the tibia–fibula syndesmosis can be diagnosed by a number of specific tests. The "squeeze test" is performed by compressing the fibula against the tibia about halfway between the knee and ankle. If the syndesmosis is injured, this maneuver will produce local pain. The "external rotation test," performed by externally rotating the foot with the ankle in 90° of flexion, is considered positive if the athlete

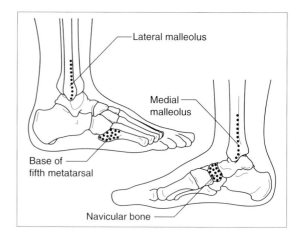

Fig. 13.4 According to the Ottawa rules the following four structures should be palpated to reveal bony tenderness: the midline, the lateral and medial malleoli, the base of the fifth metatarsal, and the navicular bone.

complains of pain in the region of the syndesmosis. These tests are reasonably specific, i.e. they usually do not cause significant pain if only the lateral ankle ligaments have been injured. A positive test necessitates radiographic evaluation to rule out injury to the syndesmosis.

Medical personnel may have learned that the anterior drawer and talar tilt tests can be used to clinically evaluate whether an ankle is mechanically unstable after a significant lateral ligament injury. From a theoretical anatomical and biomechanical perspective, the anterior drawer test should be positive if the anterior talofibular ligament is torn, while the talar tilt test should be positive if the calcaneofibular ligament is also ruptured. However, studies have shown that these tests have limited diagnostic value in the acute phase of injury, since they do not enable the clinician to distinguish between total and partial ligament ruptures, or between isolated or combined lateral ligament injuries. Furthermore, the treatment of ankle sprains is not dependent on the degree of ankle instability demonstrated on stress radiographic views. Therefore, the talar tilt and anterior drawer tests and stress X-rays have no clinical relevance in the evaluation of acute ankle sprain injuries.

If signs indicate that a fracture may be present according to the Ottawa ankle rules, a routine X-ray investigation is indicated (images obtained should include anteroposterior, lateral, and mortise views). Also, the same radiographic investigation is indicated if the physical examination has raised suspicion of a syndesmosis injury. Other imaging studies are usually not indicated in the acute phase.

Conservative management of lateral ligament injuries is recommended, even if there is evidence of a combined injury to the anterior talofibular and calcaneofibular ligaments. Non-operative, function-based treatments have been shown to result in outcomes rivaling the outcome of surgical repair and/or casting, regardless of degree of lateral ligament injury (Kannus & Jozsa 1991; Kaikkonen *et al.* 1996). Functional treatment provides the quickest recovery of full range of motion and return to physical activity, does not compromise mechanical stability any more than other treatments, and is safer and less expensive than surgical intervention. The goals of a functional treatment program are to minimize the initial injury, swelling and pain, to restore range of motion, muscle strength and proprioception, and then to graduate the athlete to a sport-specific exercise program prior to return to competition

The goal of the on-site treatment of acute ankle sprains is to minimize bleeding and swelling. This may be accomplished by providing immediate protection, rest, ice, compression and elevation (PRICE treatment, see Fig. 13.5). Of these early interventions, compression is probably the most important (so as to limit bleeding), while the main effect of cold therapy is to provide analgesia. If PRICE treatment is initiated immediately following the sprain injury and provided continuously for the first 24–48h thereafter, it is possible to significantly limit the amount of bleeding or swelling following a ligament injury.

Analgesics can be used to provide pain relief, but acetylsalicylic acid (aspirin) can prolong bleeding and should therefore be avoided. Non-aspirin pain relievers and over-the-counter NSAIDs are reasonable alternatives, and may also accelerate recovery by permitting earlier active range of motion and weight bearing.

After the initial bleeding phase is over, the goal of treatment is to regain normal, pain-free range of motion. Increased range of motion can be achieved through passive, active, or active-assisted stretching

exercises, and by submaximal exercise on a cycle ergometer. The exercise program should progress (according to the improvement in function and degree of symptoms) from progressive linear movements—e.g. toe raises, squats, jogging, jumping in place on two legs, then one, and skip-rope jumping—to cutting movements—e.g. running "figure of 8s", sideways jumping, and sideways hurdle jumps. The goal of these exercises is to gradually progress towards sport-specific exercises.

During the rehabilitation period, it is important to protect the ankle from new or recurrent injury by taping or bracing the ankle. Tape or a semirigid brace should be worn during both everyday and sporting activities where there is an increased risk of reinjury (e.g. walking over uneven terrain). The athlete should protect the injured ankle with an orthosis until a proprioceptive training program has been completed.

Re-establishing neuromuscular control of the injured ankle through a program of balance exercises is an important goal in the successful rehabilitation of an ankle sprain. Proprioceptive function is impaired in patients with residual functional instability after previous sprains (Konradsen & Ravn 1991), and can be improved by balance board exercises (Gauffin *et al.* 1988). Such programs can reduce the risk of reinjury to the level of a previously uninjured ankle (Tropp *et al.* 1985). A program of proprioceptive training is described in detail in Chapter 10. Proprioceptive training should be carried out for 6–10 weeks after an acute injury.

"Problem ankles"—persistent pain or instability

While most patients with a lateral ligament injury seem to do well following functional treatment, some athletes will develop residual symptoms and persistent complaints. The prevalence of chronic ankle problems following sprain injury has ranged between 18 and 78% in different studies (Karlsson & Lansinger 1993; Shrier 1995). It is therefore important to instruct athletes during the acute phase of rehabilitation to follow-up with their physician if they have persistent problems after completing a program of functional rehabilitation.

Do not bear weight on the ankle – no walking or testing. A quick examination to determine that there is lateral injury is all that is needed at this stage. Mix the contents of an ice bag by crushing the inner bag and shaking the bag carefully.	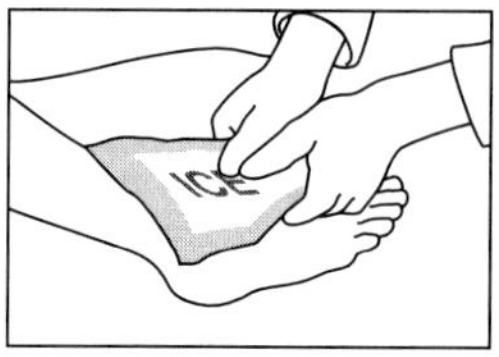
Place the ice bag with the center over the tip of the lateral malleolus. Fasten the proximal end of the ice bag with an elastic wrapping.	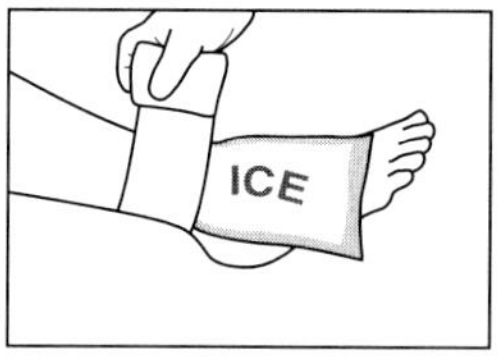
Fasten the distal end of the ice bag – continue fastening the ice bag with the elastic wrapping to apply firm compression using the ice bag as a compression tool.	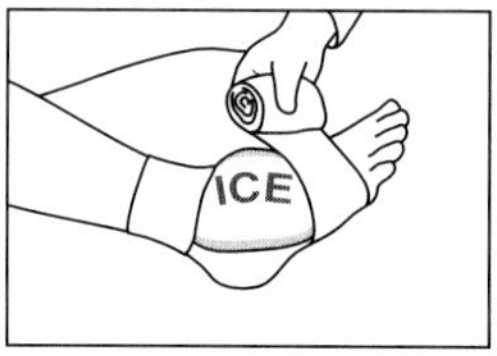
Place the patient with the ankle elevated as much as possible and the cold/compression bandage on for at least 30 minutes.	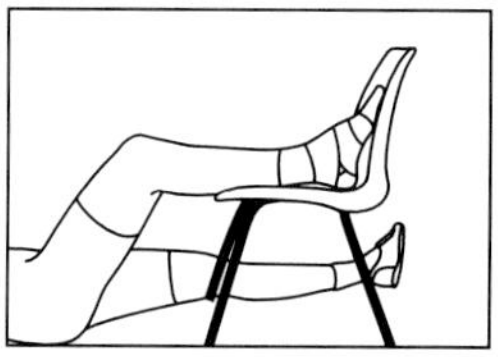
Avoid weight bearing when the patient needs to be moved – provide crutches if possible. Keep the cold/compression bandage on during transportation even after the cold effect has subsided.	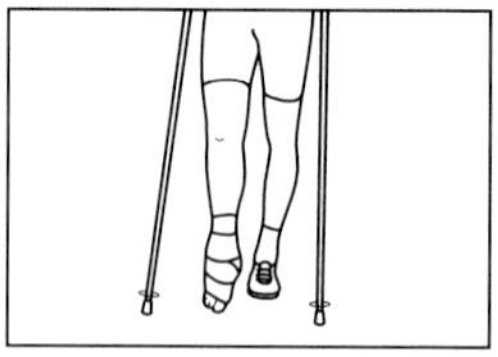
A more complete examination can be done after the initial 30-minute PRICE treatment has been completed. Continued compression bandage treatment is continued for the first 48 hours using an elastic wrapping with a felt or paper filling around the malleolus to provide maximum pressure on the injured ligaments.	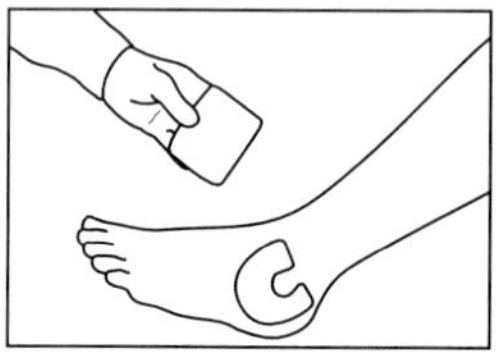
Cold treatment provides effective pain relief and intermittent cold treatment can be given for 20–30 minutes every 2–3 hours. Cold treatment can be given by simply using cold, running water or dedicated cold therapy equipment as shown here.	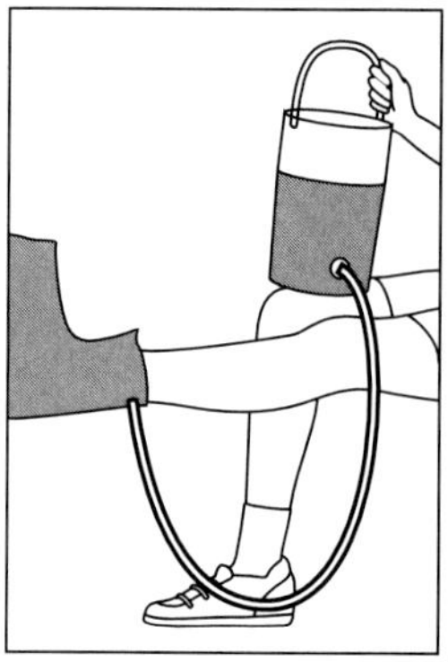

Fig. 13.5 Initial management of acute ankle sprains.

Patients with residual complaints can be broadly classified into two groups: those complaining of pain, stiffness, and swelling, and those with recurrent sprains and episodes of ankle instability. The cause of pain, stiffness, and residual swelling is often chondral or osteochondral injury of the ankle joint. Such lesions are more common after high-energy injuries, such as when landing after a maximal jump—and may therefore be expected to occur more often in volleyball players than in some other sports. Focal uptake on a bone scan may indicate that there is an osteochondral injury. A computerized tomography or MRI scan can be used to differentiate between subchondral fractures and chondral fractures with or without separation and/or displacement. Patients with persistent symptoms and chondral injuries should be referred to an orthopedic surgeon. Pain may also result from impingement of scar tissue, particularly in the anterolateral corner of the ankle joint.

Ankle instability may be described as either mechanical or functional in etiology. Mechanical instability can occur after complete ligament tears if the scar tissue is lengthened and provides inadequate mechanical support, while functional instability results from inadequate sensorimotor control of the ankle joint. Some patients can suffer from both mechanical instability and loss of sensorimotor control. Subtalar instability may also result from ankle sprains, and the sinus tarsi pain syndrome may occur as a sequela of a lateral ankle sprain injury.

The anterior drawer and talar tilt tests may be used to assess the mechanical stability of the ankle joint in such chronic cases, and stress X-rays are used by some clinicians to quantify and document the degree of instability. However, the large variability in talar tilt values in both injured and non-injured ankles precludes the routine use of these diagnostic tests. A simple functional balance test may be used to estimate sensorimotor control, although the predictive value of the test has not been properly documented. The patient is instructed to stand on one leg for 1 min with arms held across the chest, eyes fixed forward, and the opposite leg straight down. The test is said to be normal if the patient can complete 1 min on one leg and during at least 45 s of this time not have to adjust balance other than at the ankle (i.e. using the knees, hips, or shoulders to keep balance).

The test result is supranormal if the patient can complete an additional 15 s with their eyes closed.

Patients with persistent instability symptoms should complete at least 10 weeks of intensive proprioceptive training. The affected ankle should be taped or braced to prevent reinjury during this period. If instability episodes persist even after an adequate sensorimotor training program has been completed, the patient should be referred to an orthopedic surgeon for further evaluation and management.

References

Almekinders, L.C. & Temple, J.D. (1998) Etiology, diagnosis, and treatment of tendonitis: an analysis of the literature. *Medicine and Science in Sports and Exercise* **30**, 1183–1190.

Bahr, R. & Reeser, J.C. (2002) The FIVB beach volleyball injury study: injuries among professional beach volleyball players. *American Journal of Sports Medicine*, in press.

Bahr, R. & Bahr, I.A. (1997) Incidence of acute volleyball injuries: a prospective cohort study of injury mechanisms and risk factors. *Scandinavian Journal of Medicine and Science in Sports* **7**, 166–171.

Bahr, R., Lian, Ø., Karlsen, R. & Øvrebø, R.V. (1994) Incidence and mechanisms of acute ankle inversion injuries in volleyball—a retrospective cohort study. *American Journal of Sports Medicine* **22**, 601–604.

Cannell, L.J., Taunton, J.E., Clement, D.B., Smith, C. & Khan, K.M. (2001) A randomized clinical trial of the efficacy of drop squats or leg extension/leg curl exercises to treat clinically-diagnosed jumper's knee in athletes. *British Journal of Sports Medicine* **35**, 60–64.

Coleman, B.D., Khan, K.M., Kiss, Z.S., Bartlett, J., Young, D.A. & Wark, J.D. (2000) Outcomes of open and arthroscopic patellar tenotomy for chronic patellar tendinopathy: a retrospective study. *American Journal of Sports Medicine* **38**, 183–190.

Cook, J.L., Khan, K.M., Harcourt, P.R., Grant, M., Young, D.A. & Bonar, S.F. (1997) A cross sectional study of 100 athletes with jumper's knee managed conservatively and surgically. The Victorian Institute of Sport Tendon Study Group. *British Journal of Sports Medicine* **31**, 332–336.

Cook, J.L., Khan, K.M., Harcourt, P.R., Kiss, Z.S., Fehrmann, M.W. & Griffiths, L. (1998) Patellar tendon ultrasonography in asymptomatic active athletes reveals hypoechoic regions: a study of 320 tendons. *Clinical Journal of Sport Medicine* **8**, 73–77.

Cook, J.L., Khan, K.M., Maffulli, N. & Purdam, C. (2000) Overuse tendinosis, not tendonitis: Part 2. Applying the new approach to patellar tendinopathy. *Physician and Sports Medicine* **28** (6), 31–46.

Ferretti, A. (1986) Epidemiology of jumper's knee. *Sports Medicine* **3**, 289–295.

Ferretti, A., Puddu, G., Mariani, P.P. & Neri, M. (1984) Jumper's knee: an epidemiological study of volleyball players. *Physician and Sportsmedicine* **12**, 97–103.

Fredberg, U. (1997) Local corticosteroid injection in sport: a review of literature and guidelines for treatment. *Scandinavian Journal of Medicine and Science in Sports* **7**, 131–139.

Fyfe, I. & Stanish, W.D. (1992) The use of eccentric training and stretching in the treatment and prevention of tendon injuries. *Clinics in Sports Medicine* **11**, 601–624.

Gauffin, H., Tropp, H. & Odenrick, P. (1988) Effect of ankle disk training on postural control in patients with functional instability of the ankle joint. *International Journal of Sports Medicine* **9**, 141–144.

Jozsa, L. & Kannus, P. (1997) *Human Tendons. Anatomy, Physiology, and Pathology*. Human Kinetics, Champaign, IL.

Kaikkonen, A., Kannus, P. & Jarvinen, M. (1996) Surgery versus functional treatment in ankle ligament tears. A prospective study. *Clinical Orthopaedics* **326**, 194–202.

Kannus, P. & Jozsa, L. (1991) Histopathological changes preceding spontaneous rupture of a tendon. *Journal of Bone and Joint Surgery* **73**-A, 1507–1525.

Karlsson, J. & Lansinger, O. (1993) Chronic lateral instability of the ankle in athletes. *Sports Medicine* **16**, 355–365.

Karlsson, J., Lundins, D., Lossing, I.W. & Peterson, L. (1991) Partial rupture of the patellar ligament. Results after operative treatment. *American Journal of Sports Medicine* **19**, 403–408.

Khan, K.M., Cook, J.L., Bonar, F., Harcourt, P.R. & Astrom, M. (1999) Histopathology of common overuse tendon conditions: update and implications for clinical management. *Sports Medicine* **27**, 393–408.

Konradsen, L. & Ravn, J.B. (1991) Prolonged peroneal reaction time in ankle instability. *International Journal of Sports Medicine* **12**, 290–292.

Kujala, U.M., Österman, K., Kvist, M., Aalto, T. & Friberg, O. (1986) Factors predisposing to patellar chondropathy and patellar apicitis in athletes. *International Orthopaedics* **10**, 195–200.

Leddy, J.J., Smolinski, R.J., Lawrence, J., Snyder, J.L. & Priore, R.L. (1998) Prospective evaluation of the Ottawa Ankle Rules in a university sports medicine center. With a modification to increase specificity for identifying malleolar fractures. *American Journal of Sports Medicine* **26**, 158–165.

Lian, Ø., Engebretsen, L., Ovrebo, R.V. & Bahr, R. (1996a) Characteristics of leg extensors in male volleyball players with jumper's knee. *American Journal of Sports Medicine* **24**, 380–385.

Lian, Ø., Holen, K.J., Engebretsen, L. & Bahr, R. (1996b) Ultrasound characteristics of the patellar tendon and symptoms of jumper's knee among high-level male volleyball players. *Scandinavian Journal of Medicine and Science in Sports* **6**, 291–296.

Schiavone-Panni, A., Tartarone, M. & Maffulli, N. (2000) Patellar tendinopathy in athletes. Outcome of nonoperative and operative management. *American Journal of Sports Medicine* **28**, 392–397.

Shrier, I. (1995) Treatment of lateral collateral ligament sprains of the ankle: a critical appraisal of the literature. *Clinical Journal of Sport Medicine* **5**, 187–195.

Shrier, I., Matheson, G.O. & Kohl III, H.W. (1996) Achilles tendonitis: are corticosteroid injections useful or harmful? *Clinical Journal of Sport Medicine* **6**, 245–250.

Tropp, H., Askling, C. & Gillquist, J. (1985) Prevention of ankle sprains. *American Journal of Sports Medicine* **13**, 259–262.

Rcommended reading

El Hawary, R., Stanish, W. D. & Curwin, S. (1997) Rehabilitation of tendon injuries in sport. *Sports Medicine* **24**, 347–358.

Chapter 14
Other volleyball-related injuries

Jonathan C. Reeser

Introduction

In the preceding two chapters we have considered in some detail the diagnosis and treatment of the most common volleyball-related musculoskeletal injuries to the shoulder, knee, and ankle. Of course, volleyball athletes can and do suffer other forms of trauma, or injuries precipitated by overuse. According to data collected by the National Collegiate Athletic Association's Injury Surveillance System (NCAA, Indianapolis, IN USA), the fourth most common area to suffer a time-loss injury among women's collegiate volleyball players in the United States is the lower back. Trauma to the thumb and fingers is also quite common, as are contusion injuries or strains of the hip, pelvis, and thigh and the associated musculature. Elbow and foot injuries are frequently encountered. With regard to diagnostic considerations, the most common diagnoses recorded by the NCAA ISS (after sprain, strain, and tendinopathy) are stress fracture and contusion.

Stress fractures

Stress fractures are overuse injuries of bone, and—like most overuse injuries—are typically multifactorial in aetiology (Bennell 1999; Reeser 2001). Thus if a volleyball athlete has been diagnosed with a stress fracture (or if a stress injury is suspected), it is important to try to determine what factors precipi-

tated or contributed to the injury. Details of the athlete's training history should be noted, both in terms of volume and intensity. Intensive, prolonged muscular activity may itself result in bone strain and overload. Muscle fatigue, perhaps due to poor conditioning or as the result of overtraining, can attenuate the shock-absorbing capacity of the muscular system and thereby result in greater ground reactive forces transmitted to the tibia or femur (in the case of lower limb stress fracture). Structural malalignments (e.g. leg length discrepancies) or biomechanical inefficiencies (e.g. excessive subtalar pronation) can result in increased stress and strain on the tibiae. Concurrent injury may have resulted in subclinical biomechanical adaptations along the kinetic chain, thereby placing atypical loads on bone and precipitating a stress injury. Poor bone health, perhaps due to hormonal or dietary causes as seen in the female athlete triad, can weaken bone and make it more susceptible to injury. These and other intrinsic and extrinsic risk factors for the development of stress fractures are summarized in Table 14.1.

Stress fractures of the lower limb are among the most frequently encountered stress injuries among volleyball athletes (Ha *et al.* 1991). In addition, volleyball players appear to be at increased risk for developing stress fractures of the pars interarticularis of the vertebral bodies of the lower lumbar spine (Soler & Calderon 2000). This condition, referred to as spondylolysis, is common among athletes who participate in sports demanding repetitive lumbar hyperextension, truncal rotation, or axial loading,

Table 14.1 Risk factors for stress fracture.

Intrinsic risk factors	Extrinsic risk factors
Low bone mineral density	Excess volume or intensity of training
Lower limb malalignment	Change in training surface (density or topography)
Muscle fatigue or weakness	Worn out training shoes
Genetic predisposition	
Menstrual/hormonal irregularities	
Cigarette smoking	
Inadequate nutrition (calories or calcium)	

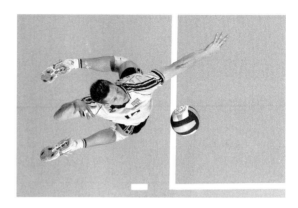

Fig. 14.1 The mechanical loading of repetitive jump serving and spiking places the volleyball athlete at risk for developing stress fractures of the lumbar spine, a condition known as spondylolysis. (© Dave Black, 2001.)

all of which perfectly describe the volleyball spiker or jump server (Fig. 14.1). Once considered to be a congenital variation, it is likely that (in most cases) spondylolysis is an acquired condition. However, genetic predisposition undoubtedly plays a role in the development of spondylolysis.

Studies suggest that the prevalence of spondylolysis among athletes who are at risk for developing the condition (including track and field athletes, gymnasts, and weight lifters) ranges anywhere from 1.5 to 8 times the 3–7% rate found among the general population (Soler & Calderon 2000). Spondylolysis most commonly affects a single level of the lumbar spine, typically the level of the fourth or fifth lumbar vertebral body (L5 > L4). Spondylolysis usually affects the pars bilaterally. Although the individual with spondylolysis can be asymptomatic, more often he or she complains of low back pain. Males and females appear to be equally affected, although females are more likely than males to have associated spondylolisthesis. The incidence of pars fractures among Caucasians is greater than that in African Americans, perhaps reflecting the generally higher bone density among African Americans (Bennell *et al.* 1999; Soler & Calderon 2000).

The most salient historical feature in the diagnosis of stress fracture is that of the insidious onset of activity-related pain. Early on, the pain is typically mild and occurs towards the end of the inciting activity. Subsequently, the pain may worsen and occur earlier during sporting activity, limiting participation. While rest may transiently relieve symptoms in the early stages, as the stress fracture progresses the athlete's pain may persist even after cessation of ac-

tivity. Night pain is a frequent complaint. Curiously, young children diagnosed with pars defects tend to be asymptomatic.

The symptomatic individual with a pars fracture will typically complain of localized axial low back pain. On physical examination, the individual will typically complain of pain upon palpation or percussion of the affected area. Inspection may reveal localized swelling, and possibly erythema. A thorough assessment of the athlete's flexibility, lower limb alignment (including leg lengths), foot structure (cavus vs flat feet), and motor function (evaluating for strength imbalances) should be performed. The pain associated with acute pars fracture may be provoked by lumbar extension, particularly while bearing weight on the ipsilateral lower limb. Hamstring inflexibility is a common finding among individuals with spondylolysis.

The clinical diagnosis of stress fracture may be confirmed radiographically. Plain films are often unrevealing, but if present the fracture line is best visualized on oblique views. Nascent or recently completed stress fractures of the pars may be detected on bone scan imaging (Anderson *et al.* 2000). Single photon emission computed tomographic (SPECT) views are considered the most sensitive and anatomically informative (Fig. 14.2a, b). Magnetic resonance imaging (MRI) is also a reasonable first-line imaging procedure (Bergman & Fredericson 1999), and allows concurrent evaluation of the lum-

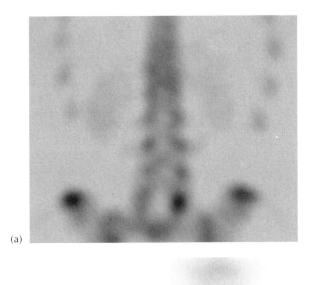

(a)

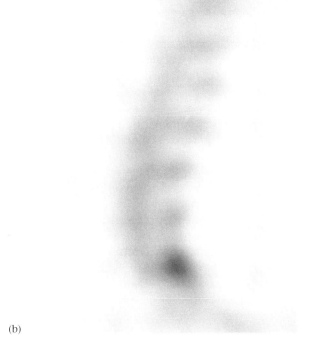

(b)

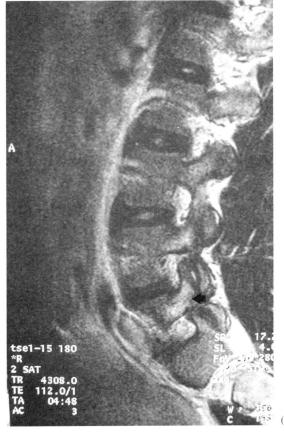

(c)

Fig. 14.2 Radiographic features of spondylolysis. (a, b) A three-phase bone scan with SPECT imaging is considered the "gold standard" in detecting areas of stress reaction. (c) However, MRI is increasingly useful in detecting areas of bone edema due to stress injury (arrow) in addition to demonstrating other anatomical details of the athlete's spine. These studies document a case of acute unilateral spondylolysis involving the pars interarticularis of the fifth lumbar vertebral body.

bar intervertebral discs as well as other potential pain generators in the spine (Fig. 14.2c).

The recommended treatment for acute spondylolysis has evolved considerably over the past decade and remains somewhat controversial. As with other stress fractures, the central tenet in such cases is relative rest with appropriate activity modification. Although some clinicians recommend bracing to minimize extension and resultant shear forces across the affected segment, the prevailing opinion appears to be that bracing is only necessary for those individuals who remain symptomatic despite limiting their activity, or who require a physical/tactile reminder to avoid provocative activities. Once the individual's symptoms permit, they should begin a rehabilitation program of flexibility training and dynamic lumbar spinal stabilization exercises. The program should emphasize pain-free functional progression, and once the athlete can perform sport-specific skills without symptoms they may return to training and competition. Radiographically documented pars interarticularis defects that are "cold" on bone scan probably represent remote injuries and have little chance of bony union. If symptomatic, these individuals can be treated with anti-inflammatories or other analgesics and should be instructed in a program of ongoing home exercises designed to strengthen the muscles that dynamically stabilize the lumbar spine.

Muscular injuries

Muscular injuries are among the most prevalent injuries in sports (Kibler 1990). Contusions, defined as blunt trauma to skin and the underlying soft tissues, are quite common among volleyball players. Defensive play in particular is associated with contusion injuries, as the defender may "dive" onto the playing surface in an effort to prevent the volleyball from contacting the flooring or ground (Fig. 14.3). Contusions that prevent the athlete from playing without pain should be treated acutely with relative rest and ice massage within the first 48 h. Thereafter, warm compresses may provide symptomatic relief and facilitate restoration of tissue flexibility and joint range of motion. In the immediate postinjury phase, compression and elevation may limit hemorrhage and bruising of the affected area. Early range of motion should be encouraged, and as soon as the athlete's pain is diminished he or she may begin (or resume) strengthening the affected muscle group(s) (Herring 1990). Deep bruises of muscles may precipitate heterotopic ossification, and this diagnosis should be considered if the athlete experiences a delayed increase in pain with associated warmth, swelling, and localized erythema over the contusion site.

Strain injuries are defined as stretch injuries of muscle. Strains typically result from forcible stretch-

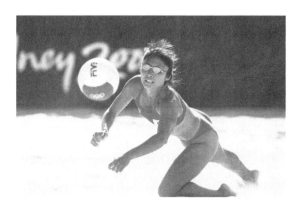

Fig. 14.3 Defensive play often results in soft tissue injuries, such as scrapes and contusions. (© Allsport/ Ezra Shaw.)

ing of eccentrically activated muscle. Long muscles with a parallel or fusiform architecture, and those that cross two joints (such as the hamstrings and rectus femoris), are most vulnerable to strain injury. Fatigued muscles are also less resistant to eccentric overload (Mair *et al.* 1996). Perhaps not surprisingly, muscles with a greater percentage of fast-twitch (type II) fibers are more susceptible to strain injury than are slow-twitch (type I) fiber-predominant muscles.

Following a strain injury, the affected muscle is weaker (and thus at increased risk of further injury) (Garrett 1996). Shortly after the injury, an inflammatory response occurs at the site of tissue damage, which occurs characteristically at the myotendinous junction. The inflammatory response subsides and the muscle regains the majority of its force-producing capacity within 7–10 days following injury. However, the muscle's tensile strength recovers more slowly, apparently in concert with the repair of muscular architecture. The initial treatment of strain injuries consists of protection, relative rest, ice, compression, and elevation. Acute phase interventions include early range of motion and isometric exercises, before rehabilitating the athlete through a functional continuum. An adequate warm-up period has been shown to reduce the incidence of strain injuries, possibly by enhancing muscular extensibility (Garrett 1996).

The role of anti-inflammatory medications in the treatment of contusions and strain injuries is somewhat controversial. Although these medications are used liberally by most health care professionals and indeed are generally available to patients for purchase without a physician's prescription, there is some evidence to suggest that their use may interfere with the inflammatory response that is essential to the normal tissue repair process (Almekinders 1999). The antiplatelet effect of many non-steroidal anti-inflammatory drugs (NSAIDs) may also increase the amount of bleeding associated with the injury, possibly increasing the risk of developing heterotopic ossification. Thus, a prudent approach would be to limit the use of NSAIDs following muscular injury, particularly during the first 48–72 h. Acetominophen (Tylenol) or other non-aspirin pain relievers may be used during the early stages of treatment to control pain and permit the athlete to better participate in range of motion and other therapeutic rehabilitative exercises.

Upper limb injuries

The distal upper limbs, consisting of the forearm, wrist, and hand, are vulnerable to injury in volleyball players (Bhairo *et al*. 1992). It has been estimated that the hand is moving at a speed of $20 \, \text{m} \cdot \text{s}^{-1}$ at the moment of contact with the volleyball when spiking. Furthermore, at the elite level, a spiked volleyball can travel at speeds approaching $150 \, \text{km} \cdot \text{h}^{-1}$. Trauma to digits of the upper extremity can occur while spiking, or more commonly while blocking (Fig. 14.4). Blocking is a skill generally performed with the digits spread and fully extended. This renders the digits—particularly digits 1 and 5—vulnerable to sprains or other ligamentous disruption involving the metacarpophalangeal and/or interphalangeal joints. Most injuries to the digits do not result in significant time lost from training or competition. Many elite volleyball players attempt to prevent acute ligamentous injury to the digits by reinforcing the proximal interphalangeal joints with adhesive tape. Tape performs the additional function of enhancing the athlete's coefficient of friction with the volleyball, permitting greater control and allowing more efficient transmission of force from hand to ball during spiking (Fig. 14.5). Fractures and dislocations of the phalanges can also occur, but

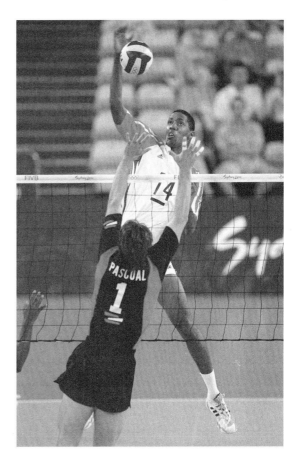

Fig. 14.4 Acute injury to the digits occurs frequently in volleyball, typically as the result of blocking. (© Allsport/ Darren McNamara.)

with less frequency. A defender who successfully "digs" or passes a hard-driven ball must absorb the impact either with the forearm or the hands. In the latter instance, the hands are typically extended and radially deviated at the wrist as the volleyball is received, and then quickly flexed and ulnarly deviated as the defender reflects the ball toward a teammate. The maneuver resembles a "set" but is referred to as an "open-handed dig" in this defensive situation. Performed repetitively, either in defence or when setting, this motion can lead to overload of the carpal bones, triangular fibrocartilage, and ligamentous structures of the wrist. Fatigue (stress) fractures of the carpal bones have been reported among volleyball players (Israeli *et al*. 1982), as have neurapraxic injuries of the ulnar nerve in the region of the hypothenar eminence. Appropriate orthope-

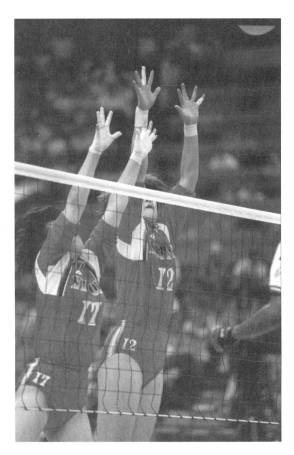

Fig. 14.5 Volleyball athletes frequently tape their digits — not only for therapeutic and preventive purposes, but also to enhance ball control. (Photo courtesy of Olympic Museum, Lausanne.)

dic intervention typically results in favorable clinical outcomes.

There is evidence in the literature to suggest that volleyball players are at risk for overuse-related circulatory disturbances of the upper limb. One study has documented higher vascular perfusion over the proximal interphalangeal joints of the hands in volleyball players when compared with healthy control subjects, although the clinical significance of this finding is unclear (McDougall *et al.* 1998). Non-invasive Doppler echographic screening of the forearm vasculature of professional volleyball players has also been performed, revealing evidence of predominantly asymptomatic aneurysms of the ulnar palmar arteries as well as lesions of the digital palmar arteries on the dominant side in approxi-

mately one-third of the athletes examined (Rosi *et al.* 1992). Furthermore, reports in the literature document at least six cases of volleyball athletes who complained of ischemic symptoms of the dominant distal upper limb who were subsequently diagnosed with traumatic aneurysmal dilatation of the posterior circumflex humeral artery (PCHA) resulting in secondary recurrent embolization to the arm and hand (Reekers *et al.* 1993). Mechanistically, it seems reasonable to hypothesize that the PCHA undergoes repetitive trauma within the quadrilateral space, although whether the artery is compressed or distracted in this region is not clear.

The quadrilateral space is defined by its borders, which include the teres minor, the teres major, the humerus, and the long head of the triceps (Fig. 14.6a). In addition to the PCHA, the axillary nerve also passes through this space, within which either the nerve or the artery may potentially be compressed when the volleyball athlete abducts and externally rotates the ipsilateral upper limb at the shoulder (Fig. 14.6b, c). Although two cases of axillary neuropathy in volleyball players have been reported in the literature (Paladini *et al.* 1996), this syndrome appears to be far less common among volleyball athletes than suprascapular neuropathy (Chapter 12). The athlete with axillary neuropathy may complain of vague shoulder girdle pain in addition to positional numbness over the deltoid muscle. The affected athlete may also demonstrate mild weakness of abduction of the upper limb at the shoulder (deltoid) and/or weakness of external rotation (teres minor). There is one case report in the literature of a volleyball player suffering a peripheral injury to the long thoracic nerve on the dominant side (Distefano 1989). This nerve supplies the serratus anterior muscle, one of the principal scapular stabilizers. Injury to the long thoracic nerve therefore may result in scapular dysfunction and predispose the athlete to impingement syndrome and shoulder pain.

Overtraining

There is compelling evidence to indicate that optimal strength and fitness are protective of both acute

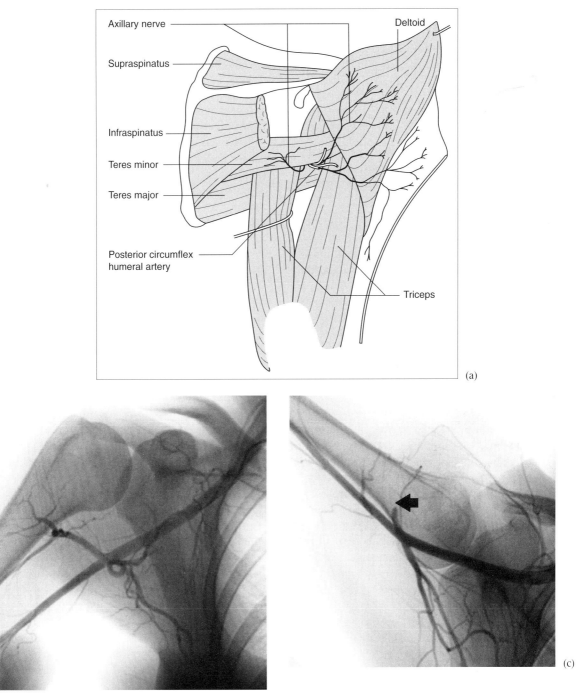

Fig. 14.6 (a) Anatomical line drawing of the quadrilateral space and its contents. (b, c) Angiographic appearance of the PCHA in a young volleyball player who reported shoulder pain when spiking or serving. With the arm at rest by the athlete's side, the vessel appears unremarkable (b). When the upper limb is abducted at the shoulder, however, the PCHA becomes occluded within the quadrilateral space (arrow) (c). The athlete underwent a surgical procedure to relieve the positional compression of the PCHA.

Table 14.2 Selected clinical features of the overtraining syndrome.

Deteriorating performance
Fatigue
Headaches
Impaired concentration
Lack of motivation; depressed mood
Loss of appetite
Menstrual dysfunction
Myalgias
Sleep disturbance
Susceptibility to colds and viral illnesses

and overuse injuries in sport. Strength and fitness also typically correlate positively with improved athletic performance. Consequently, strength training and conditioning programs have become essential to the development of elite athletes. However, training volumes below an optimal level do not generate sufficient stimulus to promote the desired physiological adaptation. Thus, coaches and the athletes themselves often push harder in an effort to run faster, jump higher, and become stronger.

Unfortunately, when athletes push (or are pushed) too hard, their risk of overuse injuries and acute overload injuries may increase. Training programs can therefore result in the desired positive effect of improved performance, but may also have potential negative effects. Over time, athletes who train excessively may develop sequelae of the overtraining syndrome (Table 14.2). This syndrome, which has been described in both endurance- and strength-trained athletes, is characterized by a constellation of symptoms and signs including deteriorating performance, loss of motivation, fatigue, myalgias, sleep and mood disturbance, and immunological deficits (Kentta & Hassmen 1998). Other terms used to describe overtraining include athlete "staleness" or "burn out", but overtraining *per se* should not be confused with the more transient effects of acute "overreaching." Generally, an athlete who fails to recover from a workout within 72 h should be considered to have overreached. If symptoms persist despite appropriate modifications in the training program, the athlete may have overtrained. Biochemical, hormonal, and physiological markers of the overtraining syndrome have been described, and the interested reader is referred to the excellent references noted at the end of the chapter for additional information.

What is clear is that the beneficial effects of training are maximized when the athlete is given sufficient time to recover. What is less clear, and often becomes apparent only in retrospect, is the appropriate balance between training and recovery for an individual athlete. Individual variation in exercise capacity, ability to recover, and tolerance for both physical as well as psychosocial stressors probably accounts for the varying degree of "staleness" experienced by athletes participating in identical training programs. Sports medicine professionals should maintain a reasonable degree of clinical suspicion for the overtraining syndrome, particularly in athletes who suffer multiple or recurrent injuries or who develop diffuse somatic complaints. Treating the overtraining syndrome effectively depends on accurate identification of the different physical and psychological stressors involved and intervening appropriately. Most often, the critical areas of intervention are nutrition and hydration, sleep, psychosocial status, and a sufficient quantity of low-volume/low-intensity activity ("active rest") to restore an appropriate athletic balance between training stress and recovery. Prevention of overtraining begins with individualized, structured (periodized) training programs which incorporate varied activities and which adjust training loads in anticipation of concurrent non-athletic stressors including travel or academic demands, which might push the athlete beyond their unique threshold for successful adaptation to stress.

Other problems

Although the emphasis of this chapter has been on musculoskeletal conditions affecting volleyball players, athletes are also at risk for other ailments. Viral upper respiratory illnesses occur commonly and may easily be transmitted among team members, particularly if the team members share living quarters. Gastrointestinal complaints are not uncommon, especially while traveling. Although competitive athletes at the collegiate and national team level are generally in good health, the older competitive athlete with underlying medical conditions may be at risk for exacerbating those conditions through intensive physical exertion. There is one case report in the literature of a recreational volleyball player who suffered a heart attack after being struck in the chest by a spike (Grossfeld *et al.* 1993). The authors speculate that the impact caused an acute thrombus to form at an atheromatous plaque in one of his coronary arteries, precipitating the myocardial infarction. Thus, medical personnel who care for volleyball athletes but are not themselves trained to provide general medical care should be prepared to triage non-musculoskeletal conditions to an appropriate health care provider who can help these individuals return to health and to sports participation.

References

Almekinders, L.C. (1999) Anti-inflammatory treatment of muscular injuries in sport. *Sports Medicine* **28** (6), 383–388.

Anderson, K., Sarwark, J.F., Conway, J.J., Logue, E.S. & Schafer, M.F. (2000) Quantitative assessment with SPECT imaging of stress injuries of the pars interarticularis and response to bracing. *Journal of Pediatric Orthopaedics* **20**, 28–33.

Bennell, K., Matheson, G., Meeuwisse, W. & Brukner, P. (1999) Risk factors for stress fractures. *Sports Medicine* **28** (2), 91–122.

Bergman, A.G. & Fredericson, M. (1999) MR imaging of stress reactions, muscle injuries, and other overuse injuries in runners. *MRI Clinics of North America* **7** (1), 151–174.

Bhairo, N.H., Nijsten, W.N., van Dalen, K.C. & ten Duis, H.-J. (1992) Hand injuries in volleyball. *International Journal of Sports Medicine* **13**, 351–354.

Distefano, S. (1989) Neuropathy due to entrapment of the long thoracic nerve. *Italian Journal of Orthopedics and Traumatology* **15** (2), 259–262.

Garrett, W.E. (1996) Muscle strain injuries. *American Journal of Sports Medicine* **24** (6), S2–S8.

Grossfeld, P.D., Friedman, D.B. & Levine, B.D. (1993) Traumatic myocardial infarction during competitive volleyball: a case report. *Medicine and Science in Sports and Exercise* **25** (8), 901–903.

Ha, K.I., Hahn, S.H., Chung, M., Yang, B.K. & Yi, S.R. (1991) A clinical study of stress fractures in sports activities. *Orthopedics* **14** (10), 1089–1095.

Herring, S.A. (1990) Rehabilitation of muscle injuries. *Medicine and Science in Sports and Exercise* **22** (4), 453–456.

Israeli, A., Engel, J. & Ganel, A. (1982) Possible fatigue fracture of the pisiform bone in volleyball players. *International Journal of Sports Medicine* **3**, 56–57.

Kentta, G. & Hassmen, P. (1998) Overtraining and recovery. *Sports Medicine* **26** (1), 1–16.

Kibler, W.B. (1990) Clinical aspects of muscle injury. *Medicine and Science in Sports and Exercise* **22** (4), 450–452.

Mair, S.D., Seaber, A.V., Glisson, R.R. & Garrett, W.E. (1996) The role of fatigue in susceptibility to acute muscle strain injury. *American Journal of Sports Medicine* **24** (2), 137–143.

McDougall, J.J., Ferrell, W.R., Bray, R.C., Wadley, V.M.R. & Frank, C.B. (1998) Repetitive activity alters perfusion of proximal interphalangeal joints of the human hand. *Clinical Journal of Sports Medicine* **8** (2), 106–110.

Paladini, D., Dellantonio, R., Cinti, A. & Angeleri, F. (1996) Axillary neuropathy in volleyball players: report of two cases and literature review. *Journal of Neurology, Neurosurgery and Psychiatry* **60**, 345–347.

Reekers, J.A., de Hartog, B.M.G., Kuyper, C.F., Kromhout, J.G. & Peeters, F.L.M. (1993) Traumatic aneurysm of the posterior circumflex humeral artery: a volleyball player's disease? *Journal of Vascular and Interventional Radiology* **4** (3), 405–408.

Reeser, J.C. (2001) Stress fractures. *Emedicine Journal* **2** (8). Available online @www.emedicine.com.

Rosi, G., Pichot, O., Bosson, J.L., Calabrese, G. & Carpentier, P. (1992) Echographic and doppler screening of the forearm arteries in professional volleyball players. *American Journal of Sports Medicine* **20** (5), 604–606.

Soler, T. & Calderon, C. (2000) The prevalence of spondylolysis in the Spanish elite athlete. *American Journal of Sports Medicine* **28** (1), 57–62.

Recommended reading

Brukner, P., Bennell, K. & Matheson, G. (1999) *Stress Fractures*. Blackwell Science Asia, Victoria, Australia.

Kreider, R.B., Fry, A.C. & O'Toole, M.L. (eds) (1998) *Overtraining in Sport*. Human Kinetics, Champaign, IL.

Watkins, R.G. (1996) *The Spine in Sports*. Mosby, St Louis, MO.

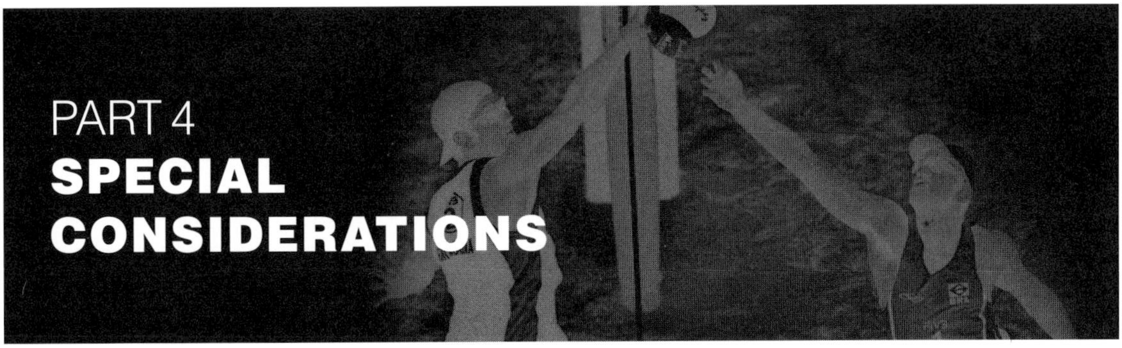

PART 4
SPECIAL CONSIDERATIONS

Chapter 15
The young volleyball athlete

Jonathan C. Reeser

Introduction

The rate of youth participation in organized sport in the United States and in many other countries around the world has increased exponentially over the past 50 years. Whereas youthful pastimes used to consist largely of unstructured free play, recently the trend has been for children to become involved in competitive sports programs as early as age 5. In the United Kingdom, nearly 80% of children aged 5–15 participate in organized sport. Perhaps more significantly, 11% of those took part in "intensive training" (Bruns & Maffulli 2000). In the United States, it has been estimated that up to half of boys and 25% of girls aged 8–16 participate in organized sport annually. Approximately 75% of male and 50% of female secondary school students in the USA compete in an organized sport.

Although there are many potential benefits from such a programmatic approach to youth sports, a number of potential drawbacks exist as well—not the least of which is the dramatic increase in the incidence of pediatric athletic injuries that has resulted from the increasing number of youth participants in sports. Nearly 40% of all injuries to children in the United States are thought to occur as the result of sports participation (Bijur *et al.* 1995). Interestingly this increase reflects more than a simple proportionate rise in the number of injuries. Rather, it appears likely that the inherent risk of injury increases with increasing rates of participation. For example, from 1983 to 1998, in Wales the actual rate

of sport-related injury to girls increased by a factor of 2.1, while the risk for boys increased 3.5-fold (Jones *et al.* 2001). Adolescents appear to be at higher risk for sport-related injuries than preadolescents and children.

The sport of volleyball has enjoyed explosive growth over the past half century. By some estimates, volleyball is now the most popular participation sport in the world. Nowhere has the growing popularity of volleyball been more evident than among the youth. Over the last two decades, the number of junior and youth athletes registered with USA Volleyball has increased 22-fold, from 4,833 in 1982 to 108,112 in 2001 ("junior" is defined by the FIVB as younger than age 21 for males and younger than age 20 for females, while "youth" is defined as younger than age 19 for males and younger than age 18 for females). Approximately 72% of the 149,216 registered members of USA Volleyball in 2001 were 20 years of age or younger. Most (nearly 94%) of these young athletes were female. Note that these figures do not reflect the numbers who participate in volleyball recreationally, or through school-based physical education curricula (for example, an estimated 426,814 secondary school age athletes in the United States participated in organized volleyball in 2000—more than 90% of whom were female). In response to the increasing popularity of volleyball among youth (and perhaps in turn contributing to its growth), many national volleyball federations sponsor youth and junior-level championship competitions for both genders, and the FIVB now holds biannual youth and junior World Championship

Table 15.1 Listing of FIVB Youth and Junior World Champions, since the inception of the respective competitions for both indoor and beach volleyball.

Date	Junior indoor		Youth indoor		Beach under 21		Beach under 18	
	Males	Females	Males	Females	Males	Females	Males	Females
1977	USSR	South Korea						
1981	USSR	South Korea						
1985	USSR	Cuba						
1987	South Korea	Brazil						
1989	USSR	Brazil	Brazil	USSR				
1991	Bulgaria	USSR	Brazil	South Korea				
1993	Brazil	Cuba	Brazil	Russia				
1995	Russia	China	Brazil	Japan				
1997	Poland	Russia	Italy	Brazil				
1999	Russia	Russia	Russia	Japan				
2001	Brazil	Brazil	Brazil	China	Brazil (Sigoli-Cunha)	Brazil (Maria Clara-Shaylyn)		
2002					Spain (Herrera-Mesa)	Brazil (Lima-Silva)	Brazil (Salgado-Borges)	Netherlands (Keizer-Stevens)

competitions for both males and females (Table 15.1).

Injuries in youth volleyball

Intuitively, it seems reasonable to speculate that, as youth participation in volleyball has increased, the incidence of volleyball-related injuries among this population must also have increased. Unfortunately, there is insufficient epidemiological data to permit a thorough analysis of the relative risk of injury among youth participating in volleyball compared with other sports. Similarly, based on the limited number of injury epidemiology studies reporting data for youth volleyball, it is not clear whether the injury pattern observed for adult volleyball players (discussed in Chapter 8) also applies to young volleyball athletes. *A priori*, one might assume that, as a non-contact sport, the risk of injury among young volleyball players would be low. In general, what few data are available suggest that volleyball is indeed relatively safe for youth when compared with other "major" sports.

Maffulli *et al.* (1996) published a retrospective study of injury patterns among children presenting to a sports injury clinic in Hong Kong over a 7-year period, and found that volleyball ranked fifth overall, behind track and field, basketball, cycling, and

soccer. Epidemiological data from Switzerland (de Loës 1995) revealed that volleyball accounted for only 1.2% of all sport-related injuries to youth from 1987 to 1989, but had the seventh highest incidence rate when corrected for exposure, with 3.0 injuries per 10,000 h (compared to ice hockey with 8.6 injuries per 10,000 h of exposure, and basketball with a rate of 3.5). Interestingly, volleyball was one of the few sports for which a gender difference was detected, with females having a slightly higher injury rate than males. Knee injuries in particular may have contributed to the observed gender difference in injury rates, as a subsequent study by the same author (de Loës *et al.* 2000) suggested that young females who participated in volleyball were 1.9 times more likely to suffer a serious knee injury than young males who played volleyball. Other investigators have documented similar gender differences in the incidence of anterior cruciate ligament injuries among university-level volleyball players (Arendt & Dick 1995) and among senior (adult) volleyball athletes (Ferretti *et al.* 1992).

Clearly, additional research in the area of injury epidemiology among both youth and junior, indoor and beach volleyball players is needed. Indeed, although the aforementioned studies suggest that volleyball is a relatively safe sport for children, a note of caution should be taken from an investigation by Backx *et al.* (1989). This study revealed that, among preteens participating in sport in the Netherlands, volleyball had the highest injury rate during practice, prompting the authors to conclude that "jump-intensive" sports (including volleyball) place young athletes at increased risk of lower limb injuries in particular. As discussed below, there are in fact several physiological reasons why children who participate in jump-intensive sports might be predisposed to lower limb injuries.

Pediatric physiology and the risk of injury

Perhaps the most important point to acknowledge from the outset of any consideration of pediatric sports medicine is that children are not simply miniature adults. By definition, a child is physiologically immature. As they grow and develop, anatomical and physiological changes occur which influence not only athletic potential and performance, but also the risk of injury. The musculoskeletal system of a young athlete is substantially different than that of an adult. In children, the "long" bones of the body (the humerus, radius, and ulna in the upper limb and the femur, tibia, and fibula in the lower limb) are still growing. The areas of longitudinal growth (termed the physeal plates) are located at the ends of the long bones and are quite vulnerable to injury—particularly fracture. As a result of these areas of relative skeletal weakness and immaturity, children (particularly preadoles-

cents) who suffer acute joint-related trauma are at increased risk of fracture compared with adults. Therefore, any child who suffers a sprained ankle should undergo radiographical evaluation to rule out a potentially serious fracture that might require casting or operative intervention. Salter and Harris developed a classification system (Fig. 15.1) to describe fractures involving the growth plate. This system has proven to be clinically useful in prognosticating the outcome of such fractures.

Areas of bony outgrowth at sites of musculotendinous insertion are termed apophyses, and these are potential sites of injury as well. Apophyses are vulnerable to traction injury, particularly when unequal rates of skeletal and muscular growth predispose the adolescent athlete to inflexibility. "Traction apophysitis" refers to a painful condition related to repetitive overload of the tendon inserting at the involved apophysis. Osgood–Schlatter disease, a common apophysitis involving the knee extensor mechanism at the tibial tubercle, is contrasted with another common overuse condition affecting the upper and lower limbs of young athletes in Table 15.2. Osteochondritis dissecans is a degenerative condition of the articular cartilage of a joint, typically affecting the knees and elbows. Young baseball pitchers who, through repetitive throwing, subject their dominant elbow to recurrent valgus stress are thought to be predisposed to osteochondritis dissecans of the elbow joint (also known as "Little League elbow") (Kocher et al. 2000). Research has demonstrated that young baseball players who limit

Table 15.2 Overuse conditions affecting young athletes.

Condition	Anatomic Location	Pathophysiology	Risk Factors	Treatment Options
Osgood Schlatter's Disease	Tibial Tubercle	Traction Apophysitis	Growth Spurt, Excess Jumping	Relative Rest
Sinding Larsen Johansson's Disease	Inferior Patellar Pole	Traction Apophysitis	Growth Spurt, Excess Jumping	Relative Rest
Sever's Disease	Calcaneus	Traction Apophysitis	Overpronation, Inflexibility	Rest, Orthoses, Stretching
Little League Elbow	Medial Elbow/Radiocapitellar Joint	Osteochondritis Dissecans	Excess Valgus Load on Elbow	Rest, Technique, Surgery
Little League Shoulder	Proximal Humeral Growth Plate	Stress Fracture	Overload, Excess Spiking	Rest, Technique, Surgery
Medial Tibial Stress Syndrome	Medial border of the Tibia/'Shins'	Soleus Enthesopathy	Excess Running, Overpronation	Relative Rest, Orthoses
Patellofemoral Pain Syndrome	Undersurface of the Patella	Chondromalacia	Excess Jumping, Malalignment	Quad Strengthening, Taping

Injuries to growth centres

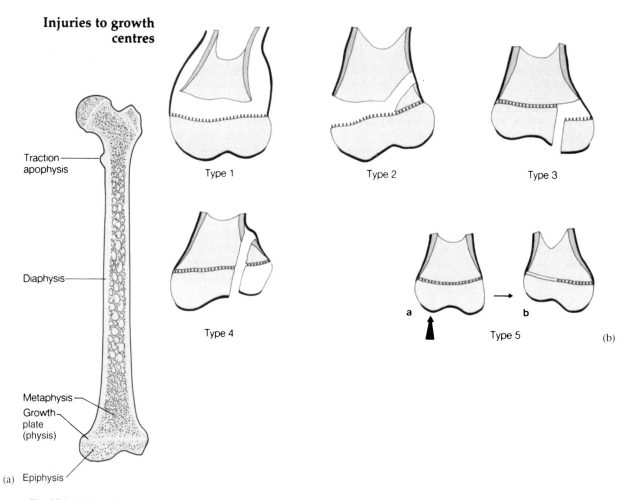

(a)

(b)

Fig. 15.1 (a) Long bones grow longitudinally from the physes, or growth plates, located at both the proximal and distal ends of the bone. (b) The Salter–Harris classification system for physeal injury describes five common injuries involving the growth plate and surrounding bone. Type 1 and type 2 injuries are considered horizontal injuries, and represent relatively benign fractures with typically good outcomes from treatment. Types 3–5 can be considered vertical injuries. These are less common than types 1–2, but are potentially more dangerous, with less favorable outcomes unless treated appropriately. Surgical fixation may be required to correct malalignment. If substantial injury to the cartilaginous growth plate occurs, future bone growth may be compromised. This is particularly problematic in type 5 injuries, which are difficult to detect acutely on radiographs since there is no accompanying fracture.

the number of maximal throws to fewer than 300·week^{-1} have a lower risk of developing elbow problems (Micheli *et al.* 2000). Although no studies have been performed investigating the optimal number of spikes for young volleyball players, it seems reasonable to limit the number of repetitions to avoid structural fatigue and overload. Children who are routinely given insufficient time to recover between training bouts are at risk for developing stress injury of weight-bearing bones. Stress fractures (such as

spondylolysis of the lumbar spine) are discussed in Chapter 14.

Treatment of overuse injuries

The general principle underlying treatment of these overuse conditions is to provide the young athlete with an appropriate amount of relative rest to permit healing, before beginning a program of therapeutic exercise emphasizing muscular endurance, joint flexibility, and neuromuscular control and coordination (proprioceptive awareness). Muscular development often lags behind skeletal growth in children, leading to periods of inflexibility and relative weakness of the soft tissues (muscles, tendons, and ligaments) surrounding the skeleton. Consequently, temporary structural malalignments are not infrequent in children and can render the pediatric athlete more susceptible to overload injuries. Regaining and maintaining balanced strength and flexibility is therefore an integral part of the rehabilitation of these injuries. It is equally important to assess the biomechanics of the athlete's sport-specific skills in an effort to identify and correct any flaws in technique which could be contributing to tissue overload (Hawkins & Metheny 2001). The importance of a thorough annual preparticipation examination by a well-trained sports medicine provider familiar with pediatric development and the demands of volleyball should not be overlooked either (Metzl 2000). The preparticipation examination is considered in detail in Chapter 6.

Other implications of developmental physiology

In addition to the musculoskeletal differences between children and adults, other physiological differences may contribute to the risk of injury among pediatric athletes. Specifically, children are mechanically less efficient than are adults, and as a result have a higher energy cost for athletic performance. Furthermore, although children produce more heat in response to activity than do adults, they are less efficient at dissipating the energy and thus are at increased risk of heat-related illness (American Academy of Pediatrics 2000a). Children sweat less than adults (limiting the amount of thermal energy that can be dissipated by evaporation) and they have a higher threshold for thirst, minimizing the amount of fluid replacement that they feel compelled to consume. Appropriate precautions should therefore be taken to safeguard young athletes when practicing or competing in hot and humid condi-

tions. Children also have reduced anaerobic capacities compared with adults, potentially making them even more susceptible to muscular fatigue and cramping. The aerobic capacities between children and adults do not differ significantly when corrected for weight. Finally, it is important to remember that neuromuscular coordination (and consequently skill acquisition) typically improves with age (and with practice). The motor control ability of a young athlete influences their risk of both acute traumatic and chronic overuse injuries. For example, bad timing when blocking may result in finger injuries, poor take-off technique when spiking may result in an increased risk of ankle sprain (to both the attacker and the opposing blocker), and faulty arm swing technique may excessively overload the shoulder and low back.

The nutritional needs of young athletes are not well understood, as limited research has been conducted in this area (Thompson 1998). It is evident, however, that adolescent athletes are in general poorly educated about the importance of sound nutrition. They may be susceptible to peer influence and misinformation. For example, studies have shown that as many as 11% of male and 2.5% of female pediatric athletes admit to taking anabolic steroids (American Academy of Pediatrics 1997). Use of "nutritional supplements" occurs on a similar scale and appears to be motivated by a desire for improved performance and concern over appearance. Like adults, young athletes should be encouraged to consume a varied and well-balanced diet. Coaches and parents should also be attentive to signs of disordered eating. Preoccupation with weight control and aesthetics among female athletes may begin as early as age 5–7 in some sports, and although volleyball is not typically included among the "aesthetic sports" there is a definite risk of developing maladaptive eating behaviors among young volleyball athletes with potentially dangerous consequences.

Pediatric injury prevention

Pediatric athlete injury prevention efforts should therefore include instruction in proper nutrition and hydration, in addition to attempting to match the demands of the sport to the physiological capacity of the growing athlete. There is, however, increasing support within the sports medicine community for introducing young athletes to strength and endurance training programs in an effort to prevent or minimize the risk of injury. Previously, there was considerable concern that pediatric athletes who participated in strength training programs were actually increasing their risk of injury, but research and experience have demonstrated the potential benefits of such programs.

The American College of Sports Medicine (1998) has recommended that athletes who are ready for participation in organized sports are in principle ready for some type of resistance training program so as to reduce the risk of injury. Indeed, it has been estimated that up to 50% of pediatric sport-related injuries may be preventable with a greater emphasis on generalized fitness. In addition to improved strength and endurance, other potential benefits from such training include reduced body fat, increased bone density, enhanced self-esteem, and improved performance.

Pediatric age programs are recommended to include flexibility, agility, and proprioceptive exercises in addition to strength and endurance training. Resistance training should be limited to one to three sets of 10–15 repetition maximum loads (10–15 RM) for six to eight different exercises, 2–3 days a week on non-consecutive days. Emphasis should be placed on proper technique and safety rather than the amount of weight lifted; additional load can be added as strength increases. Use of maximal weights is not recommended, due to concerns of overload of the vulnerable growth plates of the developing skeleton. However, submaximal training programs have not been found to affect linear growth. Furthermore, such programs have been shown to result in significant strength gains in preadolescents, exceeding by 30–40% the gains expected as the result of normal growth and development. Since preadolescents have minimal levels of circulating androgen anabolic hormones, it is thought the demonstrated strength gains result from improved neuromuscular coordination and motor unit recruitment rather than muscular hypertrophy (Faigenbaum 2000).

For young athletes who plan on participating in organized competitive sport, it may be therefore be advisable to initiate a program of fitness training 6–8 weeks before the competitive season begins rather than "playing their way into shape" as may have been done in the past. In order to avoid overtaxing involved structures, it is recommended that increases in training load (volume) be limited to less than 10% per week. Optimally, the program should incorporate adequate rest intervals to permit tissue recovery, and be sufficiently varied so that the youthful athlete (with a limited attention span) is not bored. Children have traditionally been advised against performing plyometric training. To be sure, advanced plyometrics such as those outlined in Chapter 4 are inappropriate for the young athlete. However, since exercises involving the muscular "stretch–shortening cycle" can help improve both speed and power of movement, it seems reasonable to incorporate simple plyometric exercises such as skipping, hopping, and rope jumping providing that the intensity and volume of training do not exceed the capacity of the athlete. Plyometric exercises involving the trunk (core) muscles may also be integrated in like fashion, and may theoretically help to reduce the risk of lumbar injuries (Fig. 15.2).

Goals of youth volleyball

As alluded to earlier, there are many potential benefits for enrolling youth in organized volleyball programs. Sport ideally promotes a healthy lifestyle, and fosters a sense of teamwork and fair play. Reasons that children participate in sport include "having fun," but in many instances this innocent motivation is cast aside by well-meaning but overzealous parents and coaches. Overly structured athletic programs may in many instances stifle long-term interest in fitness and athletics by children as they mature. Rather than focusing on skill development and enjoyable physical activity, many regimented youth athletic programs have over-emphasized winning, which has been postulated to account for the rather dramatic decline in athletic participation as children age. Consequently, the American Academy of Pediatrics has concluded that "reasonable goals for children and preadolescents participating in organized sports include acquisition of basic motor skills, increasing physical activity levels, learning social skills necessary to work as a

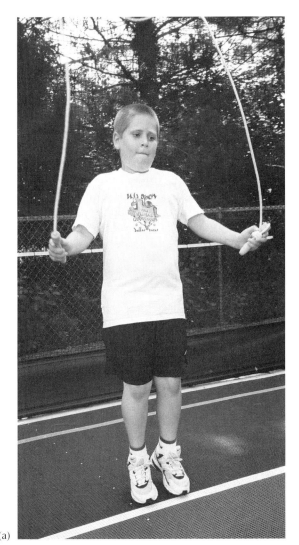

(a)

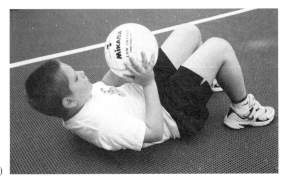

(b)

Fig. 15.2 Strength training and conditioning programs incorporating low-intensity plyometric exercises (a), and core strengthening and stabilization exercises (b) may help reduce the risk of injury for young athletes.

team, learning good sportsmanship, and having fun" (American Academy of Pediatrics 2001).

Increasing youth participation has helped to "grow the game" of volleyball worldwide. These youth feed the athlete developmental "pipeline" that produces talented volleyball athletes and which enable nations to sustain (or develop) "competitive excellence" in the sport. The youth of today may bring Olympic glory in the future and consequently there has been considerable interest in trying to identify the characteristics that contribute to volleyball proficiency and success. Anthropometric studies have been published which profile the body morphotype, height, jumping ability, and other physical and physiological traits of the elite volleyball athlete (Kioumourtzoglou *et al.* 2000; Gualdi-Russo & Zaccagni 2001). Not surprisingly, the elite adult volleyball athlete tends to be tall, lean (ecto- or mesomorphic/leptosomatic), and jumps well. However, no features have been identified which consistently and accurately predict future volleyball success at the international level.

Nature and nurture

So the question remains: are champions born or made? Certainly, features such as physical size and an athlete's physiological potential are genetically predetermined and contribute greatly to sports success. There is also undeniably a trainable component of sports talent. Increasingly, however, there is concern that starting sport-specific training at too young an age may prove detrimental in the long term. Intense physical training combined with premature sports specialization may jeopardize not only the developing athlete's health, but also detract from their advancement as a volleyball player. Research has demonstrated that there are potential adverse physiological consequences from intense physical training, including delayed menarche in females and an increased risk of overuse injuries to immature musculoskeletal systems (American Academy of Pediatrics 2000b). The International Federation of Sports Medicine (FIMS), in conjunction with the World Health Organization, examined the issue and concluded that "there is growing evidence that excessive and intensive training may increase the rate of overuse and catastrophic injuries" (FIMS 1997).

Furthermore, recent research on talent identification, profiling, and athlete development suggests that the best athletes are those who are exposed to a variety of different sporting experiences in their youth. It is thought that this breadth of exposure stimulates not only visual perceptual skills such as anticipatory timing, but also motor development and neuromuscular control in addition to a generalized appreciation for the tactical aspects of ball games and sport in general. There is therefore ample evidence to support the contention that sport specialization should be avoided before 10 years of age in favor of broader sporting experience.

Youth volleyball program design

How, then, does one create a youth program that at once attracts children to the sport while providing opportunities for promising athletes with aptitude to develop their talent? First and foremost, the program should encourage participation. Youth should be encouraged to contact the ball as many times as possible in both skill-enhancing structured drills and during unstructured "play time." Children learn best by playing, and the early emphasis should be on learning the basic skills of the game (Fig. 15.3). Youth also learn a great deal by imitating the skills of more skilled athletes they see on television or in the

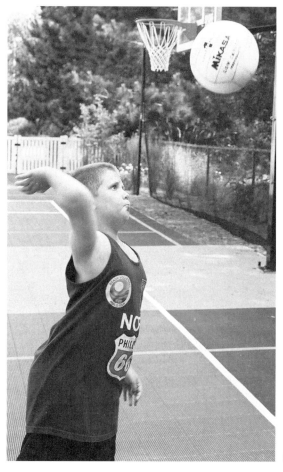

(a)

(b)

Fig. 15.3 Preadolescent athletes should be taught basic volleyball skills using developmentally appropriate equipment and rules. Youth programs should emphasize participation, maximize the number of "touches," and encourage fun and good sportsmanship. (a) Setting, and (b) spiking.

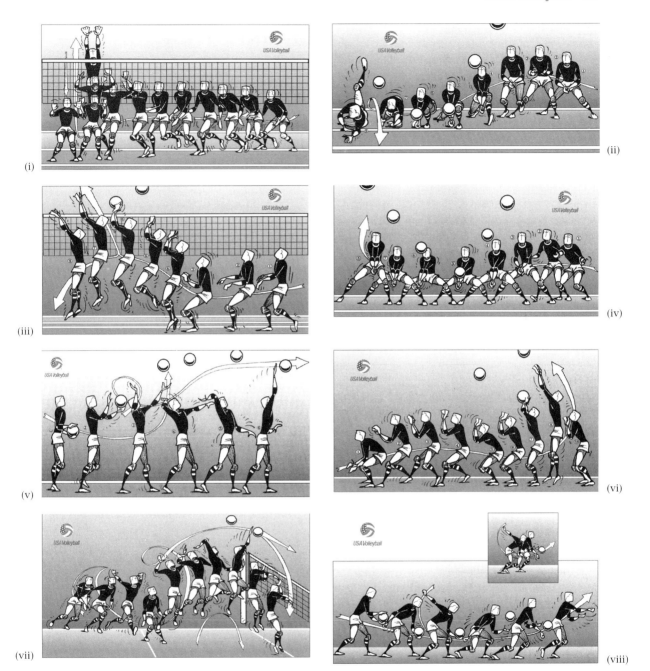

Fig. 15.4 USA Volleyball, the national governing body for the sport in the United States, has developed a series of eight pictograms illustrating the specific movement patterns of the fundamental volleyball skills. These can be used by coaches and players alike to better appreciate the kinematics of the sport. (i) Blocking. (ii) Digging. (iii) Jump-setting. (iv) Passing. (v) Serving. (vi) Setting. (vii) Spiking. (viii) Underhand serving. Used with the permission of USA Volleyball, Colorado Springs.

sporting arena. Coaches should capitalize on this innate mimicry and encourage novice volleyball players to repeat skills such as setting and spiking that have been demonstrated for them. USA Volleyball has developed pictographic instructional guides that provide novice players with a model upon which they can pattern their skill-specific movements and kinematics (Fig. 15.4).

For children aged 9–13 years who demonstrate an interest in the game and wish to play it competitively, a developmentally appropriate version of volleyball has been invented. Called "mini-volleyball," the game is tailored to preadolescent athletes and permits them to learn the essential elements and skills of the sport in a safe environment. Play is co-educational, with three boys and/or girls to a team. Employing a smaller court (9 × 6 m total dimensions), a lower net height (2.1 m), and developmentally appropriate equipment and rules (e.g. larger and lighter weight volleyball), mini-volleyball is not only fast-paced and fun but by design it minimizes the wear and tear on developing skeletal structures that would otherwise occur from playing with adult equipment and rules. Transition to a regulation volleyball court and equipment is recommended only after 14 years of age. As the athlete progresses through the youth and junior stages, appropriate progression is made in technique and strategy, as well as physical training and conditioning.

Conclusion

In conclusion, it is apparent that education is perhaps the most vital ingredient in youth volleyball. Nurturing young volleyball talent requires knowledge of developmental physiology and age-appropriate strengthening and conditioning techniques. Youth coaches should be familiar with developmental sports psychology, and both coaches and parents should have realistic expectations of both the physical and emotional abilities and limitations of young athletes. Sports medicine personnel working with young athletes must remember that they should place the health and well being of the child before the needs of the team or the expectations of coaches or parents. Working together, con-

cerned and knowledgeable adults can create an environment conducive to personal and athletic growth and development that will foster a life-long love of the great sport of volleyball among the world's youth.

References

American Academy of Pediatrics (1997) Adolescents and anabolic steroids: a subject review. *Pediatrics* **99** (6), 904–908.

American Academy of Pediatrics (2000a) Climatic heat stress and the exercising child and adolescent. *Pediatrics* **106** (1), 158–159.

American Academy of Pediatrics (2000b) Intensive training and sports specialization in young athletes. *Pediatrics* **106** (1), 154–157.

American Academy of Pediatrics (2001) Organized sports for children and preadolescents. *Pediatrics* **107** (6), 1459–1462.

American College of Sports Medicine (1998) Current comment: youth strength training. Available on-line at www.acsm.org.

Arendt, E. & Dick, R. (1995) Knee injury patterns among men and women in collegiate basketball and soccer: NCAA data and review of literature. *American Journal of Sports Medicine* **23**, 694–701.

Backx, F.J.G., Erich, W.B.M., Kemper, A.B.A. & Verbeek, A.L.M. (1989) Sports injuries in school-aged children. *American Journal of Sports Medicine* **17** (2), 234–240.

Bijur, P., Trumble, A., Harel, Y., Overpeck, M.D., Jone, D. & Scheidt, P.C. (1995) Sports and recreation injuries in US children and adolescents. *Archives of Pediatric and Adolescent Medicine* **149**, 1009–1016.

Bruns, W. & Maffulli, N. (2000) Lower limb injuries in children in sports. *Clinics in Sports Medicine* **19** (4), 637–662.

De Loës, M. (1995) Epidemiology of sports injuries in the Swiss organization 'Youth and Sports' 1987–89. *International Journal of Sports Medicine* **16**, 134–138.

De Loës, M., Dahlstedt, L.J. & Thomee, R. (2000) A 7-year study on risks and costs of knee injuries in male and female youth participants in 12 sports. *Scandinavian Journal of Medicine and Science in Sports* **10**, 90–97.

Faigenbaum, A.D. (2000) Strength training for children and adolescents. *Clinics in Sports Medicine* **19** (4), 593–619.

FIMS (Federation Internationale de Medecine Sportif) ad hoc Committee on Sports and Children of the FIMS Education Commission (1997) Sports and children. *Olympic Coach* **7** (3), 6–8.

Ferretti, A., Papandrea, P., Conteduca, F. & Mariani, P.P. (1992) Knee ligament injuries in volleyball players. *American Journal of Sports Medicine* **20**, 203–207.

Gualdi-Russo, E. & Zaccagni, L. (2001) Somatotype, role, and performance in elite volleyball players. *Journal of Sports Medicine and Physical Fitness* **41**, 256–262.

Hawkins, D. & Metheny, J. (2001) Overuse injuries in youth sports; biomechanical considerations. *Medicine and Science in Sports and Exercise* **33** (10), 1701–1707.

Jones, S.J., Lyons, R.A., Sibert, J., Evans, R. & Palmer, S.R. *et al.* (2001) Changes in sports injuries to children between 1983 and 1998: comparison of case series. *Journal of Public Health Medicine* **23** (4), 268–271.

Kioumourtzoglou, E., Michalopoulou, M., Tzetzis, G. & Kourtessis, T. *et al.* (2000) Ability profile of the elite volleyball player. *Perceptual and Motor Skills* **90**, 757–770.

Kocher, M.S., Waters, P.M. & Micheli, L.J. (2000) Upper extremity injuries in the paediatric athlete. *Sports Medicine* **30** (2), 117–135.

Maffulli, N., Bundoc, R.C., Chan, K.M. & Cheng, J.C. *et al.* (1996) Paediatric sports injuries in Hong Kong: a seven year survey. *British Journal of Sports Medicine* **30** (3), 218–221.

Metzl, J.D. (2000) The adolescent preparticipation physical examination. *Clinics in Sports Medicine* **19** (4), 577–591.

Micheli, L.J., Glassman, R. & Klein, M. (2000) The prevention of sports injuries in children. *Clinics in Sports Medicine* **19** (4), 821–834.

Thompson, J.L. (1998) Energy balance in young athletes. *International Journal of Sport Nutrition* **8**, 160–174.

Recommended reading

Armstrong, N. & van Mechelen, W. (eds) (2000) *Paediatric Exercise Science and Medicine*. Oxford University Press, Oxford.

Bar-Or, O. (ed.) (1996) *The Child and Adolescent Athlete*. Blackwell Science, Oxford.

Marsh, J.S. & Daigneault, J.P. (1999) The young athlete. *Current Opinion in Paediatrics* **11**, 84–89.

Chapter 16
The female volleyball athlete

David Wang and Elizabeth Arendt

Introduction

Volleyball is one of the most popular participation sports in the world. Although the gender breakdown of participants internationally is not known, in the United States significantly more females participate in organized volleyball than do males. At the secondary school level alone, an estimated 400,000 females participated in volleyball in the United States in 1998. At the collegiate level, female participants far outnumber male participants. According to data provided by USA Volleyball (Colorado Springs, CO, USA), during the 1998–99 season 93% of collegiate volleyball athletes were female. It is therefore important to consider in detail sports medicine issues that pertain specifically to female athletes. Although the majority of injuries and ailments for which the female athlete is at risk are similar to male athletes, there are several issues that apply uniquely to female athletes that are deserving of separate discussion. Table 16.1 lists some of the conditions that are frequently encountered when caring for female athletes and which will be discussed in this chapter.

Disordered nutrition

Nutrition is a critical component of many of the conditions that can affect female athletes. Poor nutrition can contribute to anemia, osteoporosis, and fatigue. Females are at greater risk of disordered

nutrition than are male volleyball athletes. For a number of reasons, the true prevalence of eating disorders among female athletes is difficult to ascertain. Certain individual sports that are judged subjectively (such as gymnastics and ice skating) and which place a premium on leanness and appearance, are thought to foster disordered eating behaviors among their participants to a greater extent than team sports (such as volleyball).

Anorexia nervosa and bulimia nervosa are perhaps the two most publicly recognized eating disorders, and are characterized by typical behaviors and attitudes towards eating and body image (Table 16.2). Note, however, that these two entities do not encompass the entire spectrum of eating disorders. The term EDNOS (eating disorder not otherwise specified) has been used as a diagnosis for those individuals with pathological eating behaviors who do not fulfill the criteria set forth in the *Diagnostic and Statistical Manual of Mental Disorders IV* (American Psychiatric Association 1994). Clinically, it is important to identify and treat any athlete who exhibits pathological eating behavior, rather than focusing only on those who fulfil the formal criteria for a specific diagnosis. In one survey of 182 female collegiate athletes, 14% admitted to self-induced vomiting and 16% indicated that they had used laxatives for weight control. Although volleyball was not found to be a "high-risk" sport, it does rank in the top of the second tier of sports in which eating disorders occur (after such high-risk sports as ballet, figure skating, gymnastics, and diving). Intuitively, female beach volleyball athletes must feel even more pressure to

Table 16.1 Issues of particular importance to female athletes.

Disordered nutrition
anorexia nervosa
bulimia nervosa
disordered eating
Amenorrhea/oligomenorrhea
Anemia
Thyroid disorders
Fatigue
Pregnancy
Musculoskeletal issues
bone health
stress fractures
sports injuries

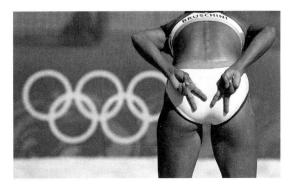

Fig. 16.1 The extent to which the beach volleyball culture encourages skin exposure may place female beach athletes at risk for disordered eating. (© Allsport/Scott Barbour)

Table 16.2 Characteristics of anorexia nervosa and bulimia nervosa.

Anorexia
Refusal to maintain weight at or above 85% of ideal body weight
Intense fear of becoming fat, despite being underweight
Distorted body self-image
Secondary amenorrhea

Bulimia
Recurrent binge eating
Recurrent self-induced vomiting, laxative abuse, or excessive exercise
Overemphasis on body shape and weight

maintain a lean appearance than do their indoor counterparts (Fig. 16.1).

Identification of an individual with an eating disorder usually results from concerns voiced by teammates, coaches, and family members. Less commonly, health questionnaires administered as part of the preseason physical examination successfully detect disordered nutrition. If an eating disorder is suspected, a longer standardized questionnaire such as the EAT-26 or the EDI-2 can be used to screen for disordered eating, although these questionnaires are limited in several respects. The reliability of these instruments is dependent in large measure on the extent to which the athlete's confidentiality is maintained (Garner *et al.* 1998). Furthermore, the "defense mechanism" of denial is common among individuals who suffer from disordered eating. Thus, questionnaires and interviews may not be sufficient to uncover states of disordered nutrition, particularly in the early stages of the condition.

Eating disorders are difficult to treat. Patient denial, underlying depression, and the inherent complexity of the problem may complicate the clinician's ability to effectively treat the female athlete with disordered nutrition. It is recommended that athletes be referred to a clinician experienced in the treatment of athletes with eating disorders, and who is therefore knowledgeable about the demands and stressors placed on athletes by society, their coaches, and by the athletes themselves. The athlete should also be educated regarding the detrimental effects of poor nutrition on sports performance. To help prevent the development of eating disorders it is recommended that coaches be made aware that they have a powerful influence on athletes and that they should not be advising athletes to lose weight without a legitimate reason. One study revealed that 67% of athletes with eating disorders were dieting on the advice of a coach. If weight loss is indicated, it should be undertaken through an appropriately monitored, nutritionally sound program (see Chapter 5).

Amenorrhea

Amenorrhea, defined as the absence of menstruation, can be classified as either primary or secondary

Table 16.3 Potential causes of amenorrhea (after Gidwani 1999).

Hypothalamic	Space-occupying lesions
	Functional disturbances of the hypothalamic-pituitary axis
Pituitary	Hypopituitarism
	Prolactin-secreting tumor
Ovarian	Gonadal dysgenesis
	Tumor
	Polycystic ovaries
	Resistant ovary syndrome
Uterine or vaginal	Absence of uterus
	Complete or partial absence of vagina
	Imperforate hymen resulting in hematocolpos
Other	Pregnancy
	Congenital adrenal hyperplasia
	Hypothyroidism or hyperthyroidism
	Debilitating chronic disease

in aetiology. Primary amenorrhea is the absence of menses in a 16-year-old with normal secondary sex characteristics. Secondary amenorrhea is the absence of three or more consecutive menstrual periods after menarche. There are numerous potential causes of amenorrhea (Table 16.3), of which one is pregnancy. When evaluating primary amenorrhea it is also important to note that menarche is typically delayed in athletes when compared to non-athletes. Secondary amenorrhea can result from reduced energy availability and/or stress. Energy availability is defined as dietary energy intake minus energy expenditure. One can lower the energy availability by decreasing energy intake (as seen with certain eating disorders), or by increasing energy expenditure (e.g. through increased volume or intensity of exercise) without a compensatory increase in caloric intake. It is thought that a deficit in energy availability can lead to amenorrhea by altering the levels of reproductive hormones, including gondadotropin-releasing hormone and luteinizing hormone. The interested reader is referred to one of the suggested readings or to the article by Gidwani (1999) for further information on amenorrhea.

The Committee on Sports Medicine of the American Academy of Paediatrics (AAP) recommends that amennorheic athletes within 3 years of menarche should be counseled on improving their nutritional status and decreasing the intensity of exercise. According to the published AAP recommendations (1989), estrogen supplementation should be considered for hypoestrogenic amenorrheic athletes who are 3 or more years postmenarche. These older athletes should also undergo an analysis of their nutritional status/energy balance. One of the principle reasons to treat amenorrhea with hormone replacement is to maximize bone stock, decreasing the possibility of premature osteoporosis and potential stress fractures.

Anemia

There are multiple factors that can potentially contribute to the development of anemia in female athletes. Inadequate dietary intake of iron is a major causative factor for most anemic female athletes. Vegetarian athletes may be at further risk of developing anemia, since vegetarian diets are typically lower in available iron. Female athletes with recognized eating disorders such as anorexia nervosa will likely not only have a diet deficient in energy, but one which is deficient in iron as well.

Potential causes of iron loss in female athletes include menstruation, gastrointestinal disorders, haemolysis urinary losses, and sweat losses. Menstrual losses account for the majority of iron losses. On average, 34 mL of blood is lost per menstrual period; the average eumenorrheic female athlete must therefore consume an additional 0.55 mg iron · day^{-1} over the course of 1 month to compensate for menstrual losses (Harris 1995). Exercising individuals may also lose small quantities of blood through gastrointestinal, urinary, and sweat losses. Appropriate treatment of anemia is dependent upon a satisfactory understanding of the etiology of the blood loss. In most cases involving female athletes the etiology is nutritional deficiency superimposed upon menstrual losses. Dietary modification and iron supplementation are appropriate therapies for anemia due to nutritional deficiency. Note that simultaneous ingestion of vitamin C on an empty stomach increases gastrointestinal absorption of supplemental iron.

The clinician must also be aware of "pseudoanemia," a condition caused by dilution of the athlete's hemoglobin concentration as a result of the volume expansion induced by endurance training. One can differentiate pseudoanemia from true anemia by evaluating both the athlete's iron stores and a reticulocyte count. Laboratory assessment of the athlete's iron stores and their reticulocyte count should be normal in pseudoanemia, but will be abnormal in true anemia.

Occasionally an athlete may be discovered to have a low ferritin level (reflective of iron stores) but is not anemic. The treatment of the athlete with a low ferritin level but with a normal hemoglobin and hematocrit is controversial. Although most studies suggest that iron supplementation in this situation does not enhance sports performance, some studies suggest that iron supplementation may benefit performance in such cases. Unfortunately, study design and methodology make comparison of the existing investigations difficult. Some of the variability in these studies may come from the duration of treatment with iron, and the type and dosage of iron used (Nielson & Nachtisall 1998). In practice (D. Wang, unpublished observations), fatigued female athletes with ferritin levels below $15\text{--}17\,\mu g\cdot mL^{-1}$ often benefit from iron supplementation whether or not they are overtly anemic. It is possible that many athletes with a normal hemoglobin level and low ferritin level actually have experienced a relative decrease in hemoglobin concentration, but nevertheless remain within the normal hemoglobin reference range. This relative deficiency can be appreciated only after adequate iron supplementation has succeeded in increasing the hemoglobin concentration.

Thyroid disorders

Thyroid disorders are often ignored when addressing conditions of the female athlete. It is well known that thyroid disease affects women more than it affects men. This difference is felt to be secondary to sex steroids and local cytokines (Mulder 1998). Hypothyroidism is the most common thyroid disorder, affecting 0.6–5.9% of women depending on the diagnostic criteria and the population surveyed. Hypothyroidism may be primary (most commonly) or secondary in etiology. Primary thyroid failure can result from autoimmune disease, iodine deficiency, prior radioiodine treatment, or thyroid surgery. Secondary hypothyroidism may derive from pituitary or hypothalamic tumors, cranial radiation, or head trauma. Whatever the cause, the symptoms of hypothyroidism can include fatigue, weakness, weight gain, constipation, cold intolerance, depression, muscle cramps, and menstrual irregularities.

Hyperthyroidism affects 0.54–2.0% of women, and is 10 times more common among females than males. The most common cause of hyperthyroidism is Grave's disease, an autoimmune disorder in which antibodies are produced that bind to the thyrotropin receptor. Symptoms of hyperthyroidism include palpitations, heat intolerance, weight loss, dyspnea, tremor, hyperdefecation, muscle weakness, and menstrual irregularities.

Since thyroid disorders are more common among females, and can produce symptoms such as fatigue, menstrual irregularities, and weight loss, thyroid dysfunction must be considered when evaluating a female athlete with amenorrhea, an eating disorder, and/or fatigue. Generally, hypothyroidism is treated with thyroid hormone replacement and hyperthyroidism is treated with medical management, radioiodine ablation of the overactive thyroid, or surgical resection. Additional information on this topic may be found in one of the suggested readings listed at the end of this chapter.

Fatigue

Fatigue can result from a multitude of causes, including anemia, thyroid dysfunction, sleep disorders, fibromyalgia, jet lag, and the overtraining syndrome, to name but a few. Calorie malnutrition can also precipitate fatigue, especially in the face of excessive energy expenditure as seen in those athletes who are overtraining. Although not gender-specific, overtraining is a significant cause of fatigue among athletes. Overtraining is discussed in more detail in Chapter 14.

Pregnancy

A detailed discussion of the effects of pregnancy on athletic performance is outside the scope of this chapter. However, all health care professionals caring for female athletes must be aware that pregnancy can cause amenorrhea and fatigue and therefore should be included in the differential diagnosis when evaluating these complaints. Although no volleyball-specific studies regarding the pregnant athlete have been published, the Canadian Academy of Sport Medicine has drafted a position statement on exercise and pregnancy which concludes: "The current data suggest that a moderate level of exercise on a regular basis during a low risk pregnancy has minimal risk for the fetus and beneficial metabolic and cardiorespiratory effects for the exercising pregnant woman" (available on-line at www.CASM-ACMS.org).

Musculoskeletal issues

Bone health

Maintenance of bone health through a woman's active, athletic years is critical to maintenance of functional capacity in later life. Factors that contribute to the bone health of the female volleyball athlete include nutritional status and menstrual history, and the volume of ground reactive forces that must be dissipated as the result of repetitive jumping.

Nutrition

Lifelong healthy eating habits, including adequate dietary intake of calcium, helps to maximize bone health. The amount of dairy products consumed during childhood and adolescence is directly related to achieving satisfactory bone density in later life (Chan 1994). Vitamin D intake is also essential to bone health, and results in positive effects on bone tissue, including stimulation of osteoblast activity, increased calcium transport, and decreased parathyroid hormone secretion. In addition to adequate cal-

cium and vitamin D, macronutrients are important in adequate bone health (see Chapter 5). Protein, fat, and carbohydrates are the nutrients from which energy can be metabolically derived. Protein comprises most of the non-mineral composition of bone, and its intake is essential for synthesis of the bone matrix. Indeed, there is a positive correlation between protein intake and bone mass gains in children (Weaver *et al.* 1999).

Menstrual irregularity caused by exercise

The "energy drain" hypothesis suggests that inadequate energy intake relative to energy expenditure results in inadequate hormone synthesis (particularly of estrogen). A negative energy balance has been implicated as the principle mechanism by which training predisposes female athletes to menstrual dysfunction (Loucks *et al.* 1989), which in turn has a detrimental effect on bone health. In addition to the effects of lower estrogen on the menstrual cycle and subsequent bone health, a low body mass index independently correlates with low bone mineral density (Drinkwater *et al.* 1990). Unfortunately, treatment of estrogen deficiency alone may not be enough to re-establish normal bone mineral density. In one study improvement in bone density was found only when estrogen replacement was coupled with weight gain (Bennell *et al.* 1996).

Universally accepted guidelines for the treatment of premature osteoporosis secondary to hypoestrogenic menstrual irregularity have not yet been established. Appropriate interventions would include proper nutrition (including calcium intake), restoring the athlete to a positive energy balance, and encouraging modest weight gain among underweight athletes. There are an inadequate number of well-designed studies investigating the effect of hormone replacement on bone mineral density, but despite this lack of prospective longitudinal data, estrogen replacement is frequently recommended. The use of oral bisphosphates (such as alendronate and risedronate) to treat low bone mass in the premenopausal female remains controversial.

Fortunately, female volleyball athletes appear to maintain higher bone mineral densities of the lumbar spine and bones of the lower limb (femur, tibia, calcaneus) when compared with the general population. Indeed, male volleyball players have also been found to have higher bone mineral densities compared with non-active controls (Calbet *et al.* 1999). One possible explanation for this observation is that regular participation in weight-bearing exercise may cause the principal skeletal structures exposed to the recurrent ground reactive forces to adapt to the imposed demands by laying down new bone in accordance with Wolff's law. Thus, the regular jumping that is part of the sport may help to counterbalance any adverse skeletal effects of hypoestrogenism in the female volleyball athlete.

Delayed menarche

The long-term effects of delayed menarche on developing bone, particularly when coupled with exercise at a young age, is unknown. However, there are a few studies in the literature that implicate osteopenia, stress fractures, and scoliosis as potential complications of delayed menarche.

Stress fractures

Stress fracture represents the ultimate consequence of bone that is exposed to a persistent increased load to which it cannot accommodate through normal repair and remodeling.

The diagnosis of stress fracture in a mature female athlete should alert the clinician to the possibility of concomitant osteoporosis. Although the association of bone mineral density with stress fractures is not well documented, a recent prospective study did demonstrate a relationship between stress fractures and reduced bone mineral density of the lumbar spine, femoral neck, femoral head, and whole body in both male and female collegiate runners. Stress fractures were also associated with low body weight and reduced lean body mass. An association between stress fractures and menstrual irregularity has been observed (Barrows & Saha 1988; Bennell *et al.* 1996). At present there are no accepted recommendations regarding the determination of bone mineral density in young female athletes. However, bone mineral density studies should be considered in those athletes with recurrent stress fractures, and for those with concomitant risk factors for osteoporosis such as amenorrhea and disordered eating.

Clinical studies suggest that female military recruits sustain a disproportionately high number of stress fractures compared with male recruits. This increased risk persists even when training loads are differentially paced, and when incidence rates are controlled for age and race. However, an association between gender and stress fracture incidence among athletes has not been detected to date. A more recent review of collegiate athletes reveals that there is no difference in the incidence of stress fractures in among male and female collegiate runners. However, a recent 10-year retrospective review performed at the University of Minnesota indicates that female athletes may sustain a greater number of stress fractures than male athletes. This retrospective review shows that volleyball athletes have a lower incidence of stress fractures when compared with athletes playing other sports.

Treatment of stress fractures involves identifying and modifying the underlying cause(s) of the stress fracture, including accelerated training programs, suboptimal fitness level, and potential nutritional deficiencies. Menstrual irregularity may be treated with hormonal replacement, if appropriate. In this regard, there are several studies that show an inverse relationship between oral contraceptive use and stress fractures.

Sports injuries

Sports injuries result from a complex interaction of intrinsic and extrinsic risk factors. Early studies assessing injury rates supported the notion that sports injuries sustained by female athletes are no different than those of men (Calvert 1975–76; Haycock & Gillette 1976). Studies of the first female military cadets suggested that many of the observed performance variations between men and women could be attributed to improper conditioning of the young women (Tomasi *et al.* 1977; Lenz 1979; Protzman 1979). Since these variations in performance subsequently proved responsive to improved conditioning of the female cadets, it was therefore concluded that sporting injuries are largely a consequence of the type of sport in which one participates and of the individual's fitness level, but is not influenced by gender.

Gender specificity of injuries in sport has been a much researched topic in recent years. Published studies support the following observations:

• Women report injuries differently than do men.

• Women are capable of equal efficiency and aerobic metabolism compared with men.

• There are gender differences in upper body strength, power, and endurance and lesser (but significant) differences in lower limb fitness parameters.

• A greater number of knee injuries are reported among female athletes than male athletes (Lindenfeld *et al.* 1994; Arendt & Dick 1995). In particular, an increased rate of non-contact anterior cruciate ligament (ACL) injuries has been observed for women compared with men, particularly in sports with skills demanding abrupt deceleration, jumping, and pivoting (Arendt & Dick 1995).

Knee injuries

The knee is at considerable risk of injury in volleyball athletes. The most common volleyball-related knee injuries are overuse injuries involving the extensor (patellofemoral) mechanism. The incidence of acute internal derangement of the knee joint is relatively low among female volleyball players, particularly when compared with such high-risk sports as women's basketball. Data from the NCAA Injury Surveillance System (ISS) best illustrate the magnitude of the disparity between volleyball and other collegiate sports for women. Common clinical and historical features of ACL injury include: (i) ACL injuries occur four times more frequently among females than males; (ii) the most common mechanism of ACL injury in volleyball is the offensive skill of hitting (spiking), with most injuries occurring during the landing phase of a jump; and (iii) most ACL injuries are non-contact in nature.

Sport-injury epidemiological data have conclusively demonstrated a gender-specific difference in the rates of non-contact ACL injury. Reasons for this gender-specific difference have been reviewed in detail elsewhere (Arendt & Dick 1995), and appear to include the female athlete's unique hormonal environment and gender variation in neuromuscular control of lower limb function (Hewett *et al.* 1999; Griffin *et al.* 2000). It has been hypothesized that estrogens or other sex hormones may contribute to in-

creased joint laxity in women, or that ligaments may be intrinsically weaker in females than in males.

Nevertheless, despite a number of studies and significant speculation, there is no consensus on the cause and effect relationship of hormones and gender-specific musculoskeletal injuries. The study of the interrelationship between gender-specific hormone production and sport injuries has revealed that women using oral contraceptives appear to be less susceptible to musculoskeletal injuries compared with non-users. More rigorous studies must be performed before one can accept any relationship between hormone environment and injury as causal, to say nothing of understanding the mechanism of such a relationship.

Currently the most intriguing modifiable risk factor for acute knee injuries in females is the athlete's neuromuscular control of the lower limb, particularly control of the proximal lower limb during jumping and landing maneuvers (Kirkendall & Garrett 2000). Strengthening programs that promote proximal hip control (mediated through gluteus medius and proximal hamstring activation in a closed chain fashion) are thought to be beneficial in injury prevention. A strengthening program consisting in part of plyometrics and skill training, particularly in landing and pivoting maneuvers, should be encouraged.

Shoulder pain

Upper limb overuse injuries occur frequently among volleyball players. Whether there is gender predisposition to upper limb injury in general and shoulder girdle injury in particular is difficult to determine based on the available injury incidence data. The NCAA ISS unfortunately does not include incidence data for male collegiate volleyball. However, there is some minimal evidence to suggest that shoulder injuries may occur more commonly among elite female volleyball athletes than among elite male volleyball athletes. (J. Reeser, personal communication). Factors contributing to the prevalence of shoulder pain syndromes in female athletes include poor upper body strength and repetition of a given upper limb activity or skill without adequate torso strength. Faulty technique in sports skills performed with the upper limbs is also likely to play a role. For example, to perform an overhead volleyball serve or spike, glenohumeral motion needs to be coupled with scapulothoracic motion. Improper body mechanics, including motor function of the torso and pelvis, can lead to overuse of the shoulder girdle musculature. Rehabilitation of shoulder injuries as well as preconditioning for volleyball activity should focus on strengthening the muscles of the rotor cuff and the scapular stabilizers, in addition to evaluation and management of any mechanical issues noted while hitting.

Female athletic diamond

Much has already been written in the literature about the medical care of the female athlete. To draw attention to certain potentially serious conditions affecting female athletes, the term "female athletic triad" was coined. The female athletic triad emphasizes the interrelationship of three predominantly female conditions: amenorrhea, osteoporosis, and eating disorders. The introduction of this term has successfully captured the attention of sports medicine providers as well as the lay press. The increased awareness of the triad by health care providers has likely resulted in improved clinical recognition of its component parts.

However, as we have discussed, more issues confront the female athlete than those described in the triad. Therefore, in an effort to account for more of the conditions that affect female athletes, the concept of the "female athletic diamond" was introduced. The "diamond" serves to summarize the complex interrelationships between the various conditions that can potentially affect female athletes (Fig. 16.2). These female-specific problems are, like a diamond, multifaceted. According to this conceptual grouping, the three central issues in the health of female athletes are exercise, nutrition, and their female gender/physiology. It is from one, or an interaction of two or more, of these central issues that the other conditions are derived, and it is these "secondary conditions" that prompt most female athletes to seek medical attention. It is hoped that the diamond concept will help volleyball medical professionals better understand and recognize some of the conditions that affect the female athlete.

Gender verification

In the post-World War II period, athletic achievement became a source of both national and personal prestige and reward. There were subsequently public

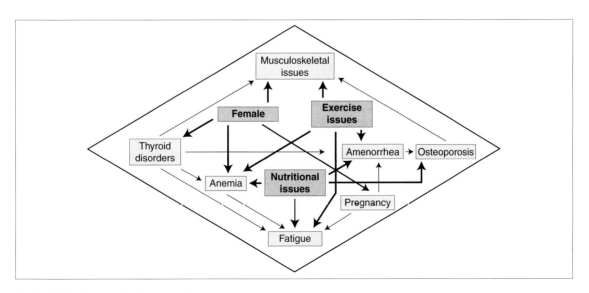

Fig. 16.2 The female athletic diamond.

accounts of "males" impersonating females in sports competitions in order to attain glory by virtue of their superior physical capacities. To deter such apparent fraudulent misrepresentation, the IOC and various international sport federations, such as the IAAF, instituted protocols for "gender verification" of female athletes. In one form or another, such testing was performed before most major international sporting competitions between 1966 and the 2000 Sydney Olympic Games. Significantly, however, gender verification testing was suspended by the IOC prior to the Sydney Olympic Games.

When first instituted, the "sex test" consisted of female athletes parading naked before a panel of female physicians. Through the technology of medical genetics, however, more discreet testing was soon available—at the Mexico City summer Olympiad, female athletes were tested by histological (microscopic) inspection for the presence of a Barr body in cells from the buccal (cheek) mucosa (also commonly referred to as the saliva test). Beginning in 1992 at the Albertville winter Olympics, gender verification has been performed by polymerase chain reaction (PCR) determination of the absence or presence of supposedly unique DNA sequences from the "testes (i.e. male) determining gene" located on the Y chromosome. Unfortunately, at least one report indicates that one of the DNA sequences used in testing athletes during the Barcelona Games was in fact not specific to males, and may have contributed to a significant number of false positive test results (Puffer 1996; Serrat & Garcia de Herreros 1997).

Both of these "advanced" techniques of gender verification test only for the presence of genetic material. Not only are the tests flawed in their execution, resulting in a significant number of false positives and false negatives, the tests also fail to account for the anatomical, physiological, and psychosocial components of gender. There are numerous examples of genetic intersex states that confer no physical advantage on the individual but would result in a "failed" gender verification test. The most common of these is the condition of *androgen insensitivity*. Affecting approximately one in 60,000 "males," these individuals have a 46XY genotype (the typical male chromosomal make up) but fail to develop male sex characteristics since their

cells cannot respond to the circulating male hormone in their bodies. They are phenotypic females (i.e. they appear to have a female body) and are usually raised as females. The presence of the Y chromosome confers no physical advantage on them. According to reports in the scientific literature, at the Atlanta Olympic Games there were eight female athletes who failed gender verification testing (performed by PCR methodology). However, a subsequent physical examination determined that seven of these eight had the condition of androgen insensitivity and were permitted to compete. The eighth athlete was confirmed to have a less common intersex condition and was also allowed to compete in the Games (Elsas *et al.* 1997).

Thus, the present methodology not only frequently fails to identify those individuals whose genetic make up would give them a competitive advantage, but it also unfairly singles out those individuals whose genetic make up—although not "normal"—does not provide them with undue advantage.

It has been argued that gender verification helps to insure a "level playing field" in women's athletics. However, the literature and practical experience both suggest that current testing methods succeed only in identifying rare and practically irrelevant cases of sexual ambiguity. What alternatives exist? One major mechanism for gender verification is already in place: the requirement for direct visualization of the urethra during submission of a doping sample. This requirement, combined with the current uniforms being worn by female athletes (coupled with the scrutiny that international athletes receive from the media), makes it almost inconceivable that a male would be able to successfully impersonate a female in international competition.

Certainly, the need for ongoing gender verification of female athletes has received considerable debate in the international athletic community. Most medical geneticists oppose gender verification testing. Indeed, during the Lillehammer 1994 winter Olympics, the organizing committee was forced to rely on assistance from other countries as no Norwegian geneticist was willing to perform the testing. In many nations gender verification is now illegal. Norway is one of the countries to have passed such legislation, and when the World Championships were held in that country several years ago the International Ski Federation was prohibited from performing gender verification testing. Virtually all organized sports medicine societies have recommended abolishing the process. Perhaps in recognition of the shortcomings of the existing testing methodology, and of the empirical reality that there is no compelling evidence to suggest that males are presently masquerading as females in international sport, the majority of all international sports federations have chosen to abandon routine genetic-based gender verification. The IOC and most international sport federations have, however, also adopted a "failsafe" mechanism reserving the right to investigate special situations in which an athlete's gender comes under question or suspicion. Despite this precedent, the FIVB is one of only four international sport federations that still requires female participants to undergo gender verification. Participants in FIVB-sponsored international competition must therefore present "proof" of their gender in the form of a gender certificate. But while the stated purpose of gender verification testing—to preserve the female athlete's right to fair competition—remains a laudable and worthy goal, in practice the need for such routine measures is suspect.

References

American Psychiatric Association (1994) *Diagnostic and Statistical Manual of Mental Disorders IV*. American Psychiatric Press Incorporated, Washington, DC.

Arendt, E. & Dick, R. (1995) Knee injury patterns among men and women in collegiate basketball and soccer: NCAA data and review of literature. *American Journal of Sports Medicine* **23**, 694–701.

Barrows, G.W. & Saha, S. (1988) Menstrual irregularities and stress fractures in collegiate female distance runners. *American Journal of Sports Medicine* **16**, 209–216.

Bennell, K.L., Malcom, S.A. & Thomas, S.A. (1996) Risk factors for stress factors in track-and-field athletes: a twelve month prospective study. *American Journal of Sports Medicine* **24**, 810–818.

Calbet, J.A.L., Herrera, P.D. & Rodriguez, L.P. (1999) High bone mineral density in male elite professional volleyball players. *Osteoporosis International* **10**, 468–474.

Calvert, R. (1975–76) *Athletic Injuries and Deaths in Secondary School and Colleges 1975–76* National Center for Education Statistics, Department of Health, Education and Welfare, US Government Printing Office, Washington, DC.

Chan, G.M. (1994) Dietary calcium and bone mineral status of children and adolescents. *American Journal of Diseases of Children* **145**, 621–631.

Committee on Sports Medicine of the American Academy of Pediatrics (1989) Amenorrhea in adolescent athletes. *Pediatrics* **84**, 394–395.

Drinkwater, B.L., Bruemmer, B. & Chestnut, C.H. (1990) Menstrual history as a determinant of current bone density in young athletes. *Journal of the American Medical Association* **236**, 545–548.

Elsas, L.J.I.I., Hayes, R.P. & Muralidharan, K. (1997) Gender verification at the Centennial Olympic Games. *Journal of the Medical Association of Georgia* **86**, 50–54.

Garner, D.M., Rosen, L.W. & Barry, D. (1998) Eating disorders among athletes, research and recommendations. *Child and Adolescent Psychiatric Clinics of North America* **7**, 839–857.

Gidwani, G.P. (1999) Amenorrhea in the athlete. *Adolescent Medicine* **10**, 275–290.

Griffin, L.Y., Agel, J., Albohm, M.J. *et al.* (2000) Noncontact anterior cruciate ligament injuries: risk factors and prevention strategies. *Journal of the American Academy of Orthopaedic Surgeons* **8** (3), 141–150.

Harris, S.S. (1995) Helping active women avoid anaemia. *Physician and Sports Medicine* **23**, 35–48.

Haycock, C.E. & Gillette, J.V. (1976) Susceptibility of women athletes to injury, myths vs reality. *Journal of the American Medical Association* **236**, 163–165.

Hewett, T.E., Lindenfeld, T.N., Riccobene, J.V. & Noyes, F.R. (1999) The effect of neuromuscular training on the incidence of knee injury in female athletes: a prospective study. *American Journal of Sports Medicine* **27**, 699–7705.

Kirkendall, D.T. & Garrett, W.E. (2000) The anterior cruciate ligament enigma. *Clinical Orthopaedics and Related Research* **372**, 64–68.

Lenz, H.W. (1979) Women's sports and fitness programs at the US Naval Academy. *Physician and Sportsmedicine* **7**, 41–50.

Lindenfeld, T.N., Schmitt, O.J. & Herdy, M.P. (1994) Incidence of injury in outdoor soccer. *American Journal of Sports Medicine* **22**, 364–371.

Loucks, A.B., Mortola, J.F. & Girton, L. (1989) Alterations in the hypothalamic-pituitary-ovarian and the hypothalamic-pituitary-adrenal axis in the athletic woman. *Journal of Clinical Endocrinology and Metabolism* **68**, 402–411.

Mulder, J.E. (1998) Thyroid disease in women. *Medical Clinics of North America* **82**, 103–125.

Nielson, P. & Nachtisall, D. (1998) Iron supplementation

in athletes: current recommendations. *Sports Medicine* **26**, 207–216.

Protzman, R. (1979) Physiologic performance of women compared to men. *American Journal of Sports Medicine* **7**, 191–194.

Puffer, J.C. (1996) Gender verification: a concept whose time has come and passed? *British Journal of Sports Medicine* **30** (4).

Serrat, A. & Garcia de Herreros, A. (1997) Gender verification in sports by PCR amplification of SRY and SYZ1 Y chromosome specific sequences: presence of DYZ1 repeat in female athletes. *British Journal of Sports Medicine* **30**, 310–312.

Tomasi, L.F., Peterson, J.A. & Pettit, G.P. (1977) Women's response to army training. *Physician and Sportsmedicine* **5**, 32–37.

Weaver, C.M., Peacock, M. & Johnston, C.J. (1999) Adolescent nutrition in the prevention of postmenopausal osteoporosis. *Journal of Clinical Endocrinology and Metabolism* **84**, 1839–1843.

Recommended reading

Drinkwater, B.L. (2000) *Women In Sport*. Blackwell Science, Oxford.

Ganong, W.F. (2001) *Review of Medical Physiology*. McGraw-Hill, New York.

Dickinson, B.D., Genel, M., Robinowitz, C.B., Turner, P.L. & Woods, G.L. (2002) Gender Verification of Female Olympic athletes. *Medicine and Science in Sports and Exercise* **34** (10), 1539–42.

Chapter 17
The disabled volleyball athlete

Jonathan C. Reeser

Introduction

Disabled athletics have become increasingly popular over the last decade, not only in terms of participation but from a public awareness and spectator standpoint as well (Calmels *et al.* 1994). The disabled sporting movement has its roots in post-World War II England, where a physician by the name of Ludwig Guttmann conceived of sport as a means of enhancing the rehabilitation of spinal cord-injured soldiers being treated at the Stoke Mandeville Hospital. Sir Guttmann subsequently organized the first International Wheel Chair Games to coincide with the 1948 London Olympic Games. The first Paralympic Games were held in Rome, 2 weeks after the 1960 Olympics. By 1976, the Paralympic movement had grown to include athletes with disabilities other than paralysis, and by 1996 the Atlanta Paralympics were the second largest sporting event in the world (the Olympics ranking first).

As volleyball has grown and changed over the last half century it has also become more accessible to people with disabilities. Presently, volleyball can be played by individuals with a variety of physical and mental disabilities, including (but not limited to) limb amputation, neuromuscular disorders, hearing impairment, and mental retardation. Moreover, there are a variety of organized competitions for disabled volleyball athletes, ranging from local events and leagues to national and international events such as the Paralympics. For example, volleyball players with a hearing loss of 55 dB or greater in both ears (a standard established by the Comites Internationale des Sports des Sourdes—CISS) are eligible to compete for their national teams in the World Summer Games for the Deaf. Those with mental disability can participate in the volleyball competition of the Special Olympics International World Games. Athletes with cerebral palsy (CP) are eligible to compete in the Paralympics, although there is not at present a CP-specific volleyball competition. The two forms of volleyball that have been contested during the Paralympic Games are sitting volleyball and standing volleyball, although women's sitting volleyball is not yet included (Fig. 17.1). A wheelchair version of the sport may be introduced in the future.

Sitting volleyball

"Sitting" volleyball, considered by some to have evolved from a fusion of volleyball with the German game of "sitzball," was developed in the Netherlands where the first competitive match was played in 1957. Sitting volleyball has subsequently grown into the most popular form of volleyball for individuals with disabilities, particularly in Scandinavia and Northern Europe, where matches are occasionally televised. It has been estimated that at least 40,000 disabled athletes participate in sitting volleyball worldwide. Sitting volleyball varies from the standing version of the sport in three obvious ways: (i) the court is smaller (10×6 m total dimension, compared to 18×9 m for the standing game); (ii) the net is

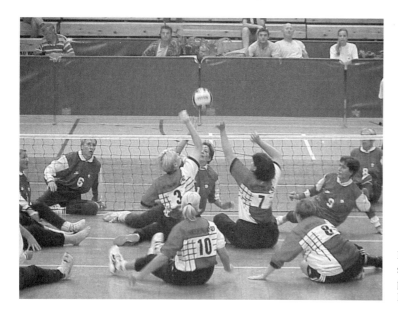

Fig. 17.1 Women's sitting volleyball is scheduled to join the Paralympic program in Athens 2004. (Courtesy of Fritz Klein, WOVD.)

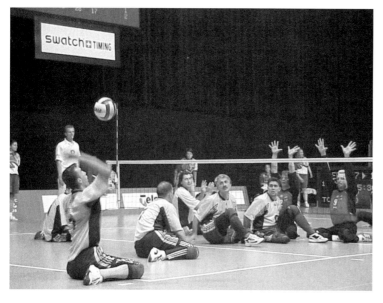

Fig. 17.2 Sitting volleyball is played on a smaller court with a lower net than standing volleyball. Unlike standing volleyball, it is legal to block the serve in sitting volleyball. (Courtesy of Fritz Klein, WOVD.)

lower (1.15 m for men/1.05 m for women vs 2.43 m for men/2.24 m for women in regular volleyball) (Fig. 17.2); and (iii) participants must remain "seated" during competition (the rule stipulates that contact with the floor by a player's buttock or by part of the torso is obligatory) (Fig. 17.3). In order to participate in international competition, the sitting volleyball athlete must meet a "minimum standard of disability" as defined by the World Organization of Volleyball for the Disabled (WOVD), the international governing body for sitting and standing volleyball. Impairments which render athletes eligible for sitting competition include amputation, limb weakness, or disabling joint injuries/conditions. In many countries, however, sitting volleyball is also enjoyed recreationally by able-bodied persons.

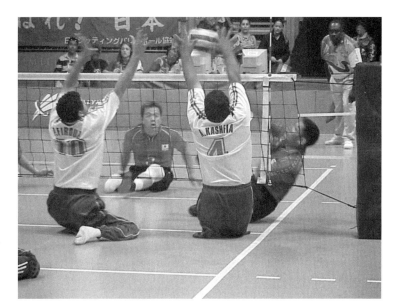

Fig. 17.3 The sitting volleyball athlete must maintain buttock contact with the playing surface at all times while in the front row. In this photograph from the Sydney Paralympics, player no. 10 is at fault for a "lifting" violation. (Courtesy of Fritz Klein, WOVD.)

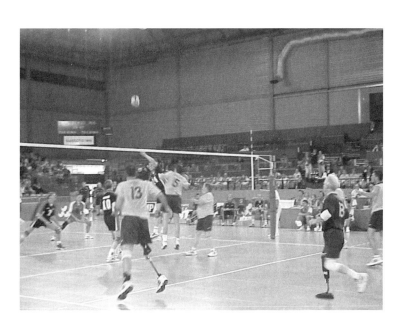

Fig. 17.4 Standing volleyball is favored by limb amputees and is a fast moving sport played on an FIVB regulation size court. (Courtesy of Fritz Klein, WOVD.)

Standing volleyball

A "standing" version of volleyball for athletes with disabilities also has gained considerable popularity (Fig. 17.4). Originally developed in Great Britain, standing volleyball is played by individuals with congenital or acquired limb deficiency ("amputa-tion") or other neuromuscular limb impairment. The rules for disabled standing volleyball are modi-fied only slightly from those of the Fédération Inter-nationale de Volleyball (FIVB). Court size and net height are unchanged, as are the basic rules govern-ing scoring and ball handling. The only significant difference is that each athlete must meet a minimum level of disability as defined by the classification system developed by the WOVD (Table 17.1). This system considers level of amputation, loss of motor function and restricted range of motion, in an effort to group athletes with similar movement potential together. Based on their disability classification, players are assigned to one of three classes: A, B, or C. For example, an individual with a below-knee (transtibial) amputation competing with a prosthetic limb would be classified as class B (4). In general, athletes with greater functional limitations are assigned to class C, while those with lesser disability are assigned to class A. During sanctioned international competitions, each standing team must have no more than one class A player on the court and at least one class C player on the court at all times. The total number of disabled athletes who participate in standing volleyball worldwide is unknown. However, based on data provided by the WOVD (P. Ch. Joon, personal communication) it can be conservatively estimated that there are at least 400 elite disabled standing volleyball players in the world who participate for their respective national teams in international competitions.

Injury patterns

Volleyball—in all its forms—has developed into a sport of explosive, powerful skills. These skills place enormous demands on the musculotendinous units of shoulders, knees, low backs, and ankles and consequently these structures are at increased risk for injury. Since congenital and acquired limb deficiencies, combined with the use of prosthetic limbs, may result in significantly altered biomechanics of sport skill performance, soft tissues may be at even greater risk of overload in this population (Stewart 1983). It would be reasonable to speculate, then, that disabled volleyball athletes are at an increased risk for injury when compared to their able-bodied counterparts. Unfortunately, there is a paucity of published research in this area in the world literature.

Ferrara and Petersen (2000) and Nyland et al. (2000) have investigated the injury trends among disabled athletes, but their studies not focus on disabled volleyball specifically. Although it might be reasonable to infer insight into volleyball injury patterns from research focusing on other forms of disabled athletics, most of the recent literature focuses on wheelchair athletics and on disabled skiing—sports that do not share common movement patterns or physiological demands with volleyball (Shephard 1988; Busconi & Curtis 1995). Ferrara et al. (1991) retrospectively studied injury prevalence among several disabled sports groups and concluded that disabled athletes had injury rates comparable with able-bodied athletes. However, the disabled sport-specific injury patterns differed from those of comparable able-bodied athletes. Other researchers, however, have concluded that disabled athletes are "more vulnerable to stress and fatigue" (Jackson & Fredrickson 1979), and have suggested that "there is a need . . . for better training of disabled athletes" (Calmels et al. 1994). These factors might be hypothesized to present a significant problem for standing volleyball athletes, in view of the fact that most are limb amputees and the use of a prosthesis involves considerable metabolic cost. Studies have demonstrated that an individual with a below-knee amputation expends between 15 and 55% more energy during ambulation than does a non-amputee (Gailey et al. 1997).

Only three studies have been published that investigate the injury history of disabled volleyball athletes. In their survey of injuries occurring among 1992 British paralympians, Reynolds et al. (1994) reported that 90% of the volleyball team members were treated for injuries suffered during training or competition—the highest percentage among any of the 15 British disabled sports teams that participated in the Barcelona Paralympic Games. Unfortunately, the authors did not specify if these were standing or sitting volleyball players, nor did they provide a sport-specific or diagnosis-specific breakdown of the different injuries sustained and treated. The second study investigated the incidence of osteoarthritis in the sound lower limb among male lower limb amputees who play volleyball (Melzer et al. 2001). The authors found that amputees have a higher prevalence of knee joint arthritis in the sound limb than matched healthy controls.

The third study was a self-reported retrospective review of the injury history of disabled standing volleyball athletes participating at the 1996 Atlanta Paralympic Games (Reeser 1999). Based on the ath-

Table 17.1 WOVD standing volleyball classification chart

Class on court	A			B			C	
	1	2	3	4	5	6	7	8
Amputation	Two first fingers of both hands	Chopart one side	Below elbow (A8) long stump	Below elbow (A8) short stump	Chopart both sides	Above elbow (A6)	Exarticulation in hip (A2) with prosthesis	Hemipelvectomy (A2) with prosthesis
	Seven or more fingers (2 hands)	Below knee (A4) through ankle	Lisfranc on 2 feet with prosthesis	Below knee (A4) with prosthesis	Above knee (A2) through knee with prosthesis	Above knee (A2) with prosthesis	Below knee (A4) or above knee (A2) without prosthesis	
	Between MP joint and CM joint *12 one side	Between CM joint and RC joint *12 one side						Below knee 2 sides (A3) above ankle, with prosthesis
	Lisfranc one side							Combination (A9) upper and lower limbs
Shortening upper limb	More than 33%	More than 50%						
Shortening lower limb	7–11.9%	12–15.9%	16–49.9%	50–65.9%		More than 66%		
Loss of muscle points, one upper limb	20–29	30–39	40–49	50–59	60–65	66–70		
Loss of muscle points, both lower limbs	5–10	11–15	16–20	21–25	26–30	31–40	More than 40	
Shoulder, one side	Abduction and flexion not more than 90°			Loss of 20 muscular points with use of arm		Loss of 20 muscular points without use of arm		
Elbow, one side	Stiff in 45° flexion or more	Stiff in 90° flexion or more				Without functional use, one arm		
Wrist, one side	Functional							
Fingers, one hand	Functional							
Hip, one side				Stiff		Loss of 20 muscular points		
Knee, one side			Stiff					
Ankle, one side		Stiff						
CP-ISRA	Class 8	Class 7		Class 6			Class 5	
ISMWSF								

CM, carpometacarpal; MP, metacarpophalangeal; RC, radiocarpal; CP, cerebral palsy; ISRA, International Sports and Recreation Association; ISMWSF, International Stoke Mandeville Wheelchair Sports Federation.

Table 17.2 Summary of injury data for elite disabled standing volleyball players (modified from Reeser 1999).

Rank	Diagnosis	Body part
1	Sprain (32%)	Ankle/foot (21%)
2	Strain (23%)	Shoulder (18%)
3	Tendinopathy (14%)	Wrist/hand (18%)
4	Bursitis (9%)	Knee (14%)

Calculated injury rate: approximately 8.5 per 1,000 athlete exposures.

lete's own estimation of the number of volleyball exposures (practices or competitions) within the preceding year, a time lost injury rate of approximately 8.5 per 1,000 athlete exposures was calculated. The most frequently injured body parts were (in rank order): the ankle/foot, shoulder, wrist/hand, and knee. The most common diagnoses were sprain, strain, tendinitis, and bursitis. Table 17.2 summarizes these data.

The majority of injuries reported by the standing volleyball paralympians who participated in the study were described as new (60%) and occurred during practice or warm-up more often than during competition (64 vs 36%). These percentages are similar to those documented by the Injury Surveillance System for women's collegiate volleyball in the United States by the National Collegiate Athletic Association (NCAA, Indianapolis, IN, USA). As with able-bodied volleyball players, skills involving jumping, such as blocking and spiking, were identified most frequently as the activity leading to injury, and 80% of the ankle/foot injuries reported were caused by contact with another player. The majority of reported injuries involved the lower limb (58%), comparable with the NCAA ISS data (61%). The residual limb or prosthesis was involved in less than half of the lower limb injuries, and in none of the upper limb injuries reported. Fifty-six per cent of the time the athlete returned to participation within 6 days (compared with 73% of the time reported for NCAA women's volleyball during the 1995–96 season by the ISS). However, more time off was taken for injuries occurring earlier in the season than was taken for injuries occurring later in the season. This observation may reflect injury severity or simply indicate that paralympians, like all elite athletes, are

highly motivated to compete—regardless of injury status—for honors in the season-ending major competitions and tournaments.

Comparison between the injured and non-injured groups revealed no significant difference between the length of the volleyball season or the estimated number of exposures per year. Those athletes who reported injuries were more likely to have lower limb impairment as a cause of their disability. However, there was no relationship between the nature of the athlete's impairment and the body part injured, diagnosis, or severity of injury (as gauged by time off from training or competition). Lower limb injuries were associated with a longer time off for healing compared with upper limb injuries. Injured athletes were less likely to participate in strength and conditioning programs during the season than were the uninjured athletes. Finally, players who remained healthy throughout the year were somewhat more likely to have played volleyball prior becoming disabled, or have had a congenital disability, than were players in the injury subgroup (57 vs 43%).

The estimated injury rate for elite disabled volleyball players reported in this study is higher than the injury rates reported in other studies on able-bodied volleyball players (see Chapter 8). Unfortunately, due to differences in study design, meaningful comparison of these data with other existing studies is not possible. The results suggest, however, that disabled standing volleyball players sustain similar kinds of injuries, involving similar etiological factors, as their fellow able-bodied athletes. Disabled volleyball players with lower limb impairment do appear to be at an increased risk of injury when compared to their teammates with upper limb impairment. Adaptive biomechanical alterations or substitutions occurring during performance of volleyball-specific skills involving jumping may contribute to the increased injury incidence in this subgroup (Molnar 1981; Kibler *et al.* 1992), and may also contribute to an increased risk of osteoarthritis in the sound tibiofemoral joint. This suggests that unique, individualized training and conditioning programs should be designed for athletes based on their impairment in order to minimize the risk of injury and to facilitate their rehabilitation from injury. Finally, the observation that players who remained healthy were more likely to have a congenital impairment or learned to play volleyball prior to their disability, while not statistically significant, raises questions regarding motor learning of sport-specific skills following a disabling injury or illness. From a coaching standpoint, it would be prudent for coaches of disabled athletes to pay particularly close attention to form and technique when teaching new volleyball skills in order to minimize the risk of overuse pathology brought on by subclinical biomechanical adaptations or substitutions.

Conclusion

As the Paralympic movement attests, disabled athletics have evolved from therapeutic recreational activities introduced by Sir Guttmann into intensely competitive international sport (McCann 1996). As these elite athletes strive to become stronger, run more swiftly, and jump higher, their risk of injury increases. For reasons yet to be fully elucidated, disabled volleyball athletes may be at increased risk of injury compared with their able-bodied counterparts. As the sport continues to grow, it may be that future volleyball competitions will feature greater integration of disabled and able-bodied athletes. It would therefore behove all volleyball coaching and sports medicine personnel to understand the injury patterns of disabled athletes so that they receive the optimum care they deserve. Clearly, further prospective studies are needed to improve our understanding of the natural history of injuries among disabled volleyball players. In particular, research is needed in the area of sitting volleyball. Because sitting volleyball attracts athletes with different impairments than does standing volleyball, it follows that injury patterns may differ between the two groups (Griffiths 1995).

References

Busconi, B.D. & Curtis, K.A. (1995) Physically challenged athletes. In: Pappas, A.M. (ed.). *Upper Extremity Injuries in the Athlete*, pp. 101–116. Churchill Livingstone, New York.

Calmels, P., Genevrier, M., Braize, C. *et al.* (1994) Medical activity during an international sporting competition for the physically disabled: Saint-Etienne world handicapped sport championships. *Disability and Rehabilitation* 16 (2), 80–84.

Ferrara, M.S., Buckley, W.E., McCann, B.C., Limbird, T.J., Powell, J.W. & Robl, R. (1991) The injury experience of the competitive athlete with a disability: prevention implications. *Medicine and Science in Sports and Exercise* 24 (2), 184–188.

Ferrara, M.S. & Petersen, C.L. (2000) Injuries to athletes with disabilities. *Sports Medicine* 30 (2), 137–143.

Gailey, R.S., Nash, M.S., Atchley, T.A. *et al.* (1997) The effects of prosthetic mass on metabolic cost of ambulation in non-vascular trans-tibial amputees. *Prosthetics and Orthotics International* 21, 9–16.

Griffiths, S. (1995) Physiotherapy in disabled sport — is there a difference? *Physiotherapy in Sport* 18 (3), 10–12.

Jackson, R.W. & Fredrickson, A. (1979) Sports for the physically disabled. *American Journal of Sports Medicine* 7 (5), 293–296.

Kibler, W.B., Chandler, T.J. & Stracener, E.S. (1992) Musculoskeletal adaptations and injuries due to overtraining. *Exercise and Sport Science Reviews* 20, 99–126.

McCann, C. (1996) Sports for the disabled: the evolution from rehabilitation to competitive sport. *British Journal of Sports Medicine* 30 (4), 279–280.

Melzer, I., Yekutiel, M. & Sukenik, S. (2001) Comparative study of osteoarthritis of the contralateral knee joint of male amputees who do and do not play volleyball. *Journal of Rheumatology* 28, 169–172.

Molnar, G. (1981) Rehabilitative benefits of sports for the handicapped. *Connecticut Medicine* 45 (9), 574–577.

Nyland, J., Snouse, S.L., Anderson, M., Kelly, T. & Sterling, J.C. (2000) Soft tissue injuries to the USA Paralympians at the 1996 Summer Games. *Archives of Physical Medicine and Rehabilitation* 81, 368–373.

Reeser, J.C. (1999) Injury patterns among elite disabled standing volleyball players. *International Journal of Volleyball Research* 1, 12–17.

Reynolds, J., Stirk, A., Thomas, A. & Geary, F. (1994) Paralympics — Barcelona 1992. *British Journal of Sports Medicine* 28 (1), 14–17.

Shephard, R.J. (1988) Sports medicine and the wheelchair athlete. *Sports Medicine* 4, 226–247.

Stewart, M.J. (1983) The handicapped in sports. *Clinics in Sports Medicine* 2 (1), 183–190.

Recommended reading

de Haan, J. (1986) *Sitting Volleyball*. Uitgeverij De Vrieseborch, Haarlem, Nethelands.

International Paralympic Committee (1997) *The Triumph of the Human Spirit*. Disability Today Publishing Group, Inc., Oakville, Ontario.

Doll-Tepper, G., Kroner, M. & Sonnenschein, W. (eds) (2000) *New Horizons in Sport for Athletes with a Disability*, Vols 1 and 2. Meyer & Meyer Sport, Aachen, Germany.

Additional information is available at the following internet addresses: www.wovd.com and www.usavolleyball.org/disabled

Chapter 18
The elite volleyball athlete

Steef Bredeweg

Introduction

Competing at the highest level in international volleyball is both physiologically demanding and psychologically stressful. The international indoor volleyball player competes year round. From October to April, elite players are usually active in indoor club/league competition. The national team season starts in May and ends in September. The elite volleyball athlete "lives on the edge," constantly striving for optimal performance, and is therefore vulnerable to physical, mental, and social stress. Consequently, the medical care of the elite volleyball athlete differs in many respects from the care of recreational athletes. While there is a paucity of literature describing accepted practices of care for the elite volleyball athlete, there is a wealth of anecdotal information derived from experience, trial, and error. This chapter, then, will discuss the care of the elite volleyball athlete, drawing upon the experiences of the men's national volleyball team from the Netherlands that won the indoor volleyball gold medal at the 1996 Atlanta Olympic Games.

Winning an Olympic gold medal is for most athletes and coaches the ultimate dream. At the Olympic Games in Atlanta 1996, the men's volleyball team from the Netherlands, known as the "Flying Dutchmen," fulfilled this dream (Fig. 18.1). The start of this "golden period" in Dutch volleyball dates to 1988 when coach Arie Selinger initiated the so-called "Bankras model" for training the national team. The Bankras model refers to the practice of tak- ing all national team members out of club competi- tion so that the national team can train and compete together 12 months per year. The intensive training paid dividends in 1992 at the Barcelona Olympic Games, where the Dutch team won the silver medal in indoor volleyball. After this Olympiad, all of the national team players returned to club competition for the national league season, with many of the best players competing in Italy. In 1993 Joop Alberda was named national team head coach and initiated "the road to Atlanta." By this time the team had gained significant experience and confidence from partici- pating in major tournaments like the World League, the European and World Championships, and the Olympic Games.

The staff

The staff of the Dutch men's volleyball team over this period consisted of the head coach, assistant coach, team manager, physical therapist, and team physician (trained in sports medicine). For impor- tant tournaments, a "scout" was added to assist in analyzing the other teams. Even with the periodic addition of the scout, the Dutch national team staff was small in comparison to those of other national volleyball teams. The major advantage of this small staff was that every member of the staff knew not only their own responsibilities but also the respon- sibilities of the other members. Frequent (often daily) meetings were held at which time the status of

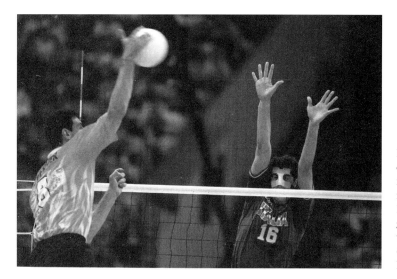

Fig. 18.1 In a match some have described as the greatest volleyball match ever, the "Flying Dutchmen" from the Netherlands defeated the Italian national team 3 to 2 to win the gold medal in indoor volleyball during the 1996 Atlanta Olympic Games. (Photo courtesy of Olympic Museum, Lausanne.)

all the players on the team was discussed. This multidisciplinary approach promoted the exchange of valuable ideas and differing perspectives on each athlete's progress, and allowed optimal individual "fine tuning" to take place.

Preseason physical examination

Each year before the start of the national team season, all players are seen for their preseason medical evaluation. This check-up consists of a standard health questionnaire requesting the athletes to document and describe any illnesses or musculoskeletal injuries and any treatment received for these ailments during the past season. Vital signs and blood pressure are recorded. A thorough examination of the eyes (including vision testing), ears, nose, throat and teeth, heart, lungs, abdomen, and lymph nodes is performed. A screening neurological examination is conducted, and a detailed orthopedic examination carried out on all joints, muscles, and tendons with special emphasis on the shoulders, knees, and ankles.

The athlete's height, weight, and body composition are measured (Table 18.1). For every new player in the national team a resting electrocardiogram (ECG) and baseline pulmonary function tests (PFTs) are obtained. Subsequently, the resting ECG and

Table 18.1 Physical characteristics and experience of the 1996 starting six and bench players of the Netherlands men's volleyball team just before the Olympic Games of 1996.

	Starting six	Bench players
Age (years)	27.5	27.3
Length (cm)	202	201
Weight (kg)	95	90
Body fat (%)	12.8	12.2
$\dot{V}_{O_{2max}}$ (ml·kg^{-1}·min^{-1})	60	56.6
Years played on national team	7	6
Matches played for national team	277	167
Olympic Games*	6	4
World Championships*	8	4
European Championships*	18	8
World Leagues*	33	14

* Sum of tournaments played by the starting six and bench players, respectively.

PFTs are updated every 3 years. Other tests obtained annually include laboratory testing of blood (red blood cell count, white blood cell count, serum glucose, ferritin, and tests of liver and kidney function), and a urinalysis. Cardiovascular fitness ($\dot{V}_{O_{2max}}$) is measured by means of a maximal treadmill test with direct measurement of the oxygen uptake (Table 18.1). Jump testing is performed intermittently. Each athlete's squat jump and countermovement jump with and without the assistance of the arms are analyzed on a jump mat. Block reach and spike reach are measured by a commercially available device (Table 18.2). Perhaps surprisingly, the average jump height for the Dutch men's national team as measured by static jump tests was not all that high. In fact, club-level players participating in the Dutch national volleyball league jumped on average 10% higher than national team members did. However, spike and block reach were both comparable to results from the Canadian national team and universiade volleyball players (Smith *et al.* 1992).

Strength of the major muscle groups acting about the shoulders and the knees are tested isokinetically. These test results were used to monitor an individual's progress and physical development over time. Isokinetic testing provides valuable information on strength, power, and the ratio between external and internal rotation of the shoulder (Hinton 1988), in addition to flexion and extension of the knee. The testing protocol for knee flexion and extension consists of three repetitions at 60° per second, five repetitions at 180° per second, and 20 repetitions at 300° per second while seated (Table 18.3).

Particular attention is given to the measurement of shoulder strength, due to the chronic overload of this joint among volleyball athletes. Elite volleyball players have been estimated to perform from between 30,000 and 40,000 spikes in 1 year. This high demand can lead to an imbalance in the ratio between external and internal rotation, functional instability, and—in time—to shoulder impingement syndrome (Ticker *et al.* 1995). Progressive deterioration of the absolute peak torque of shoulder external rotation can be the first indication of suprascapular nerve entrapment affecting the infraspinatus muscle (Ferretti *et al.* 1987; Holzgraefe *et al.* 1994). Shoulder internal and external rotation are also tested while the athlete sits, with the elbow flexed to 90° and the shoulder abducted to 90°. The shoulder protocol consists of three repetitions at 60° per second, and 20 repetitions each at 180° and 300° per second (Table 18.3). One Dutch athlete was found to have severe infraspinatus atrophy, while two other players had evidence of incomplete infraspinatus

Table 18.2 Performance characteristics for different kinds of jumps performed by the starting six and bench players of the 1996 Netherlands men's volleyball team.

	Starting six	Bench players
Squat jump (cm)	44.6	39.3
CMJ (cm)	47.8	42.2
CMJass (cm)	56.9	50.3
Spike height (cm)	346	342
Block height (cm)	325	323

CMJ, countermovement jump; CMJass, countermovement jump with assistance from both arms.

Table 18.3 Average isokinetic measurements, peak torque (N·m), and ratios, for the knee and the shoulder of the 1996 Netherlands men's volleyball team ($n = 12$).

Degrees per second	Knee			Shoulder		
	Measurement	Peak torque (N·m)	Ratio H/Q	Measurement	Peak torque (N·m)	Ratio ER/IR
60	FR	216	R 65%	ERR	39	R 62%
	FL	235		ERL	43	
	ER	332	L 70%	IRR	63	L 74%
	EL	337		IRL	58	
180	FR	189	R 79%	ERR	34	R 70%
	FL	197		ERL	38	
	ER	239	L 81%	IRR	49	L 81%
	EL	242		IRL	47	
300	FR	177	R 92%	ERR	29	R 69%
	FL	178		ERL	34	
	ER	192	L 90%	IRR	42	L 85%
	EL	198		IRL	40	

EL, extension left knee; ER, extension right knee; ERL, external rotation left shoulder; ERR, external rotation right shoulder; FL, flexion left knee; FR, flexion right knee; IRL, internal rotation left shoulder; IRR, internal rotation right shoulder; ratio ER/IR, ratio external rotation/internal rotation; ratio H/Q, ratio hamstring/quadriceps.

atrophy. As is typical for entrapment of the suprscapular nerve, all of the players were asymptomatic and were treated conservatively.

Supplements

Members of the Dutch national team started using creatine in 1994 in an effort to promote muscle development. Players were initially "loaded" with 5 g orally four times daily for 5 days. After the loading period, 3 g of creatine was taken orally per daily. During the 1996 season, three players did not use creatine because they experienced weight gain and frequent muscle cramps. All of the athletes took a multivitamin and mineral supplement once daily. No other supplement use was authorized.

Immunizations

When traveling internationally, it is important to follow standard preventative medicine precautions, including administration of the appropriate immunizations and vaccinations required in the countries to be visited. All the Dutch athletes receive injections of hepatitis A immunoglobulin annually, because hepatitis A is endemic in countries adjacent to the Mediterranean Sea. Players also receive a typhoid vaccination every 3 years. Tetanus boosters are administered every 10 years, and a toxoid injection is given after a tetanus-prone wound. Other vaccinations, immunizations, or prophylactic medications are given according to the national guidelines for foreign travel.

Injuries and other medical conditions

Because national teams train (and often live) together for months at a time, the medical staff of an elite volleyball team should be prepared to treat non-musculoskeletal conditions, such as upper respiratory infections, other viral illnesses, reactive airways disease (asthma), and environmental allergies. It is important for the team physician to keep the IOC list of prohibited substances in mind when dispensing or prescribing medications. The most common injuries seen in elite volleyball are acute ankle, thumb and finger sprains, and overuse injuries of the shoulder, knee, and lumbar spine (e.g. shoulder impingement, suprascapular nerve entrapment, patellar tendinopathy, and low back pain). This injury pattern does not differ significantly from that observed among non-elite volleyball athletes (Briner & Kacmar 1997; Briner & Benjamin 1999). However, the medical care for an injured elite athlete is typically somewhat different from that a recreational athlete would receive for an equivalent injury. Aggressive diagnostic and treatment strategies are adopted for the injured elite athlete in an effort to minimize time loss and accelerate their return to play. For example, the elite athlete may undergo immediate diagnostic imaging (e.g. magnetic resonance imaging), which may be postponed in the recreational athlete pending a trial of conservative care. Injured national team athletes typically receive frequent treatments from a physiotherapist, often several times a day. Common therapeutic modalities include massage, soft tissue mobilization, ultrasound, iontophoresis, electrostimulation, and ice (or heat if appropriate) applied superficially. Non-steroidal anti-inflammatory drugs (NSAIDs) are used regularly to control pain. Progress is evaluated daily, and the athlete is returned to play as soon as possible. The potential for conflict exists when an important match must be played and the injured athlete's rehabilitation is incomplete. In this situation, the team physician must decide if and to what extent the athlete is capable of playing. The athlete must be fully informed of the risks associated with premature return to play. If, despite medical advice, the athlete insists on playing, the decision must be carefully documented in the presence of witnesses to prevent future liability in the event of serious recurrent injury.

The national team season

The 1997 Dutch national team's season-long itinerary is presented in Table 18.4. In that year, the national team schedule was 132 days long. Of these 132

Table 18.4 The 1997 national team season for The Netherlands men's volleyball team.

Date		Date		Date		Date	
MAY		JUNE		JULY		SEPT	
5	Training	6	Training	24	Rest	1	Rest
6	Training	7	WL Ned.–Russia	25	Training	2	Training
7	Training	8	WL Ned–Russia	26	Training	3	Training
8	Rest	9	Rest	27	Rest	4	Training
9	Training	10	Rest	28	Training	5	Rest
10	Training	11	D South Korea	29	Training	6	
11	Rest	12	A South Korea (+8 h)	30	Rest	7	
12	Training	13	Training	31	D Brazil	8	*European*
13	Training	14	WL Korea—Ned.	AUG		9	*Championships*
14	Rest	15	WL Korea—Ned.	1	A Brazil (–8 h)	10	
15	Training	16	D/A Amsterdam (–8 h)	*2–10 Aug Training/matches in Brazil*		11	
16	Training	17	Rest			12	*6–14 Sept*
17	WL Ned.–Korea	18	D/A Cuba (–8 h)			13	
18	WL Ned.–Korea	19	Training	11	D Amsterdam (+8 h)	14	*First place*
19	Rest	20	WL Cuba–Ned.	12	A Amsterdam		
20	Training	21	WL Cuba–Ned.	13	Rest		*End of*
21	D/A Moscow	22	D Amsterdam	14	Training		*National*
22	Training	23	A Amsterdam (+8 h)	15	Training		*Team*
23	WL Russia–Ned.	24	Rest	16	Training		*Season*
24	WL Russia–Ned.	25	Training	17	Rest		
25	D/A Amsterdam	26	Training	18	Rest		
26	Rest	27	D/A Moscow (+1 h)	19	Training		
27	Training	28	Training	20	Training		
28	Training	29	Training	21	Rest		
29	Training	*30 June–6 July WL Finals*		22	*World*		
		Moscow			*Championships*		
30	Training	JULY		23	*Qualification*		
31	WL Ned.–Cuba	7	D/A Amsterdam (–1 h)	24			
JUNE		*8–20 July Holiday*		25	Rest		
1	WL Ned.–Cuba			26	Training		
2	Rest	21	Training	27	Training		
3	Training	22	Training	28	Training		
4	Training	23	Training	29	Rest		
5	Training			30	Training		
				31	Rest		

D, departure; A, arrival; WL, World League; Ned., The Netherlands.

days, there were 48 training days (36%), 40 rest days (30%), 30 match days (23%), and 14 days of foreign travel (11%). On 6 of the 14 travel days, the team flew across multiple time zones. Two practice sessions lasting 2.5 h each were held on training days. Strength training sessions were held every other day, alternating between morning and afternoon. Players were free to pursue recreational activities of their choice on rest days. All athletes performed stabilizing "preventive" exercises for the shoulder before, during, and after training sessions. Three sets of 10 repetitions of both internal and external rotation were performed, first with the shoulder in a neutral position and the elbow at the side, then with the shoulder abducted to 90°. Team members also performed lumbar stabilization and strengthening exercises before, during, and after training. As can be seen from Table 18.4, the athletes had little time for physiological or psychological recovery during the national team season. Not only is the national team athlete under high physical stress (exacerbated as it is by travel fatigue and jet lag), but in addition he or she can also experience considerable emotional stress during the season, including the pressure of winning matches and medals, superimposed on the inconvenience of being away from home and "on the road."

International travel and jet lag

As mentioned, the international volleyball player must travel all over the world. Unfortunately, long-haul flights (those crossing multiple time zones) produce travel fatigue and jet lag. Not only is traveling inherently inconvenient, but the conditions on board are not generally conducive to rest: airline seats are narrow and cramped, with minimal leg room, and the dry air in the cabin during flight (air humidity approximately 10%) promotes dehydration. During long flights, the athletes are encouraged to drink as much as possible to compensate for insensible fluid losses. Players are also advised to avoid drinking alcohol and coffee because both stimulate urinary water loss. To minimize the hassle of traveling by air it is important to arrange the flights well in advance so that the most convenient travel schedule and the most comfortable seats on the airplane can be reserved. When traveling, the 1997 Dutch national volleyball team tried to arrive at its final destination late in the afternoon or early in the evening (local time). That way, after a flight when everybody was tired, the team could transfer to the hotel and promptly go to sleep.

When rapidly crossing multiple time zones, the endogenous ("body") clock becomes desynchronized with respect to the new local time. This desynchronization is called "jet lag" (Waterhouse *et al.* 1997). The body clock regulates physiological processes according to a circadian (24 h) rhythm (Atkinson & Reilly 1996). Examples of physiological processes that fluctuate according to a circadian rhythm include body temperature, blood pressure, and hormone secretion. Components of sports performance (for example, flexibility, aerobic power,

and strength) appear to have a peak in the evening closely related to the daily maximum in body temperature (Atkinson & Reilly 1996). The adaptation of the body clock to a phase shift in time occurs slowly, taking several days to readjust. So-called "zeitgebers" (time-givers) help to reset the body clock to the new time. "Zeitgebers" include light, darkness, exercise, social cues (e.g. meals), and sleep. For example, when flying from Amsterdam to Tokyo (eastward) there is a phase advance of 8 h (+8 h). Upon arriving in Tokyo, the urge to sleep occurs at 6 a.m. (instead of 10 p.m) and the peak in body temperature (peak in sports performance) occurs around 2 a.m. (instead of 6 p.m). Common symptoms of jet lag include fatigue, sleep disturbance, gastrointestinal disorders (loss of appetite, constipation), loss of concentration, disorientation, loss of vigor, and impaired sports performance. Jet lag tends to be more severe following a long-haul eastbound flight compared with the effects of a long-haul westbound flight. Furthermore, symptoms of jet lag are more severe when more time zones are traversed. Adjustment to the new local time takes approximately 1 day for each hour of time difference.

There are several strategies to help the athlete cope with jet lag. Adjusting the sleep–wake cycle prior to departure is not effective, however, because the "zeitgebers" to which the athlete is most attuned (light, darkness, social contacts) cannot readily be manipulated, so the body clock will not adjust to the destination time prior to departure. After arrival in the new time zone, it is important to focus on the local "zeitgebers" and quickly adopt a (locally) normal schedule for eating, sleeping, and training. During the first several days following arrival in the new time zone, it is not advisable to take naps because naps can "anchor" the body clock in the previous time zone. Exposure to bright light can accelerate adjustment of the body clock (Czeisler *et al.* 1989). The timing of the exposure to bright light is important to achieve the desired result (Table 18.5). For example, when arriving at a westward destination that is 8 h ahead of the previous time zone, exposure to bright light between 14.00 and 20.00 local time may accelerate adaptation. A protein-rich breakfast for stimulating the body and carbohydrate-rich meals in the evening for inducing sleep have been promoted as helpful in combating

Table 18.5 Timing for the use of bright light after time zone travel. See text for discussion.

	Good local times for exposure to bright light
Time zones to the west	
4 h	18.00–24.00
8 h	14.00–20.00
12 h	10.00–16.00
Time zones to the east	
4 h	09.00–15.00
8 h	13.00–19.00
10–12 h	Treat as 12–14 h to the west

jet lag; however, scientific evidence of positive effects is limited. More important than the content of the meal, it seems, is the timing of the meal itself. Sleeping pills (e.g. benzodiazepines) can be used to promote and enhance sleep but some soporifics have a long half-life, which can result in a "hangover" effect the following morning. Therefore, when using a sleeping pill a short-acting benzodiazepine is preferable. Some members of the Dutch national team used midazolam 15 mg at bedtime. The half-life of midazolam is approximately 3 h, so the serum concentration after 8 h of sleep should be approximately one-eighth of its peak. Melatonin has been used more recently to improve the quality of sleep. There is evidence that melatonin is helpful in ameliorating the subjective feeling of jet lag and that it might accelerate adjustment of the body clock to a new time zone (Petrie et al. 1989). The 1997 Dutch national team athletes used melatonin 2.5 mg at 8 p.m. for 3 consecutive days after arrival in a new time zone. Finally, caution must be taken during the initial training sessions following a "jet lag" flight to accommodate the anticipated decreased coordination and alertness of the fatigued athletes (both of which would otherwise serve to increase their risk of injury).

Meals and accommodation in a "foreign" country

Upon arrival in a new city, the first order of business is usually to check into the hotel. The beds in the hotel rooms must be large enough to comfortably accommodate the players, or else sleep will be difficult to come by for reasons other than jet lag. Inadequately cleansed or prepared food and impure water can cause traveler's diarrhea. Practical measures to prevent "tourista" include inspecting the kitchen to insure that foods are appropriately stored, of high quality, and adequately prepared. Avoid consuming raw fruits (if not peeled) and vegetables. Entrees should be thoroughly cooked; try to avoid raw meat or fish. It is not advisable to use ice cubes or to drink unbottled water or other unsealed drinks. Avoid dairy products, such as ice cream, unless they have been carefully prepared and stored.

Longevity of the elite volleyball athlete

The average international volleyball career lasts about 8 years (two Olympic quadrennials). Most elite volleyball players retire due to a combination of "mental" and physical concerns. Because the international volleyball calendar is filled year round, it is difficult for the athlete to remain motivated—especially for the national team season with its attendant stressors of heavy travel and time away from home. As athletes age, the physical challenge seems to be increasingly difficult to tolerate. Perhaps not surprisingly, the incidence of injuries seems to increase with age. Furthermore, older athletes need more time to recover from the demands of training, competition, and from injuries. Well-designed studies are needed to better understand the long-term functional consequences of intensive training and volleyball-related injuries.

The elite female volleyball athlete

The elite female athlete is at risk of developing a syndrome of disordered eating, amenorrhea, and osteoporosis commonly referred to as the female athlete triad (Otis et al. 1997; West 1998). Female athletes who try to lose body weight or body fat may develop a disordered eating pattern, resulting in low caloric intake in the face of increased caloric expenditure. If this pattern persists, the athlete begins to suffer from impaired sports performance and an increased risk of injury. Amenorrhea can result from disordered eating or from emotional or physical stress (Constantini 1994), and can lead to bone loss (osteoporosis) over time. Unfortunately, this bone loss is often irreversible. Therefore it is advisable to screen female athletes for the female athlete triad. Further information on this constellation of conditions, and on other aspects of care of the female athlete, is presented in Chapter 16.

The elite beach volleyball athlete

The elite beach volleyball athlete is somewhat different from their indoor volleyball counterpart. The beach volleyball player needs to be proficient in all of the volleyball technical skills, including the serve, pass, set, spike, block, and defense. The beach game may be more physically demanding than the indoor version, because the beach player must defend a larger area (per player), make more ball contacts per match, and typically cover more distance with each rally on a surface over which it is difficult to move quickly. Beach volleyball athletes also must contend with the environmental stressors of heat and humidity. Lastly, participants on the FIVB Beach Volleyball World Tour travel to a new destination every week during the season, and must therefore constantly adjust to new time zones and cope with the many demands of international travel.

Few studies investigating the injury patterns common to beach volleyball athletes have been published. Aagaard *et al*. (1997) found that beach volleyball players experience more shoulder pain related to overuse when compared with indoor volleyball players. There may be at least three reasons for this observation. First, the beach volleyball player serves and spikes more often than the indoor volleyball athlete. Second, as the result of wind and sand, beach players may have to spike the ball from awkward or unpredictable positions, to which the shoulder is unaccustomed. Finally, outdoor/beach volleyballs are slightly larger in circumference and tend to be a little heavier than indoor volleyballs and

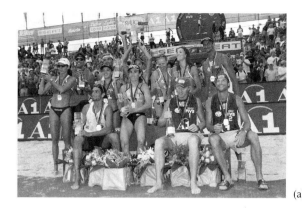

(a)

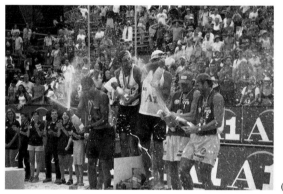

(b)

Fig. 18.2 All athletes aspire to step onto the awards podium at the conclusion of competition. Here, victorious athletes from the 2001 Beach Volleyball World Championships celebrate their triumphs.

thus may produce greater loads at the shoulder with the overhead movements of spiking and serving. Beach volleyball athletes should therefore pay extra attention to shoulder girdle strengthening and coordination training.

Conclusion

The care for the elite volleyball athlete is unique. He or she competes year round and is vulnerable to multiple stressors. It is important to provide the elite athlete with state of the art medical care, including injury prevention, treatment, and rehabilitation. The national team physician may also be responsible for prescribing proper medication, managing doping-related issues, counseling the athlete on nutrition and the use of dietary supplements, and attending to travel-related issues. It is of critical importance to build an experienced support staff around the athlete and team in which all members are open to the suggestions of others and work cooperatively. In doing so, the international volleyball athlete can concentrate fully on the core goal of any elite athlete: *winning*! (Fig. 18.2).

References

Aagaard, H., Scavenius, M. & Jorgensen, U. (1997) An epidemiological analysis of the injury pattern in indoor and in beach volleyball. *International Journal of Sports Medicine* **18**, 217–221.

Atkinson, G. & Reilly, T. (1996) Circadian variations in sports performance. *Sports Medicine* **21** (4), 292–312.

Briner, W. & Benjamin, H. (1999) Volleyball injuries. *Physician and Sportsmedicine* **27** (3), 48–54.

Briner, W. & Kacmar, L. (1997) Common injuries in volleyball. *Sports Medicine* **24** (1), 65–71.

Constantini, N. (1994) Clinical consequences of athletic amenorrhoea. *Sports Medicine* **17** (4), 213–223.

Czeisler, C., Kronauer, R., Allan, J. *et al.* (1989) Bright light induction of strong resetting of the human circadian pacemaker. *Science* **244**, 1328–1333.

Ferretti, A., Cerullo, G. & Russo, G. (1987) Suprascapular neuropathy in volleyballplayers. *Journal of Bone and Joint Surgery* **69A** (2), 260–263.

Hinton, R. (1988) Isokinetic evaluation of shoulder rotational strength in high school base ball pitchers. *American Journal of Sports Medicine* **16**, 274–279.

Holzgraefe, M., Kukowski, B. & Eggert, S. (1994) Prevalence of latent and manifest suprascapular neuropathy in high performance volleyball players. *British Journal of Sports Medicine* **28** (3), 177–179.

Otis, C., Drinkwater, B., Johnson, M., Loucks, A. & Wilmore, J. (1997) American College of Sportsmedicine. Position stand: the female athlete triad. *Medicine and Science in Sports and Exercise* **29** (5), i–ix.

Petrie, K., Conaglen, J. & Thompson, L. (1989) Effect of melatonin on jet lag after long haul flights. *British Medical Journal* **298**, 705–707.

Smith, D., Roberts, D. & Watson, B. (1992) Physical, physiological and performance differences between Canadian national team and universiade volleyball players. *Journal of Sports Science* **10**, 131–138.

Ticker, J., Fealy, S. & Fu, F. (1995) Instability and impingement in the althlete's shoulder. *Sports Medicine* **19** (6), 418–426.

Waterhouse, J., Reilly, T. & Atkinson, G. (1997) Jet-lag. *Lancet* **350**, 1611–1616.

West, R. (1998) The female athlete: the triad of disorded eating, amenorrhoea and osteoporosis. *Sports Medicine* **26** (2), 63–71.

Recommended reading

International Olympic Committee Medical Commission (2000) *Sport Medicine Manual*. International Olympic Committee, Lausanne, Switzerland.

PART 5

PERFORMANCE ENHANCEMENT

Chapter 19
Ergogenic aids

Roald Bahr

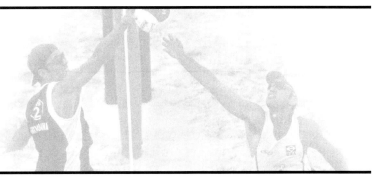

Introduction

Doping may be defined as the illegal use of biochemical substances or methods in an effort to improve or maximize athletic performance. Fortunately, there is very little evidence to suggest that systematic and deliberate doping is common in the sport of volleyball. Very few positive cases have been recorded in international volleyball since doping tests were started. Although systematic doping does not seem to be a problem, it is none the less important for players, coaches, and medical staff to be aware of the antidoping regulations of the Fédération Internationale de Volleyball (FIVB). The team physician must above all avoid inadvertently treating athletes with banned substances, also referred to as "accidental doping." Other important causes of accidental doping include dietary supplements, nutritional ergogenic aids, and self-treatment with herbal medicines.

According to the FIVB medical regulations, doping contravenes the ethics of both sports and medical science, can be harmful to the health of the athlete, and constitutes a clear attempt to cheat in sports competition. The FIVB definition of doping is restricted to the use of certain pharmacological agents as well as other doping methods. The official FIVB doping list is based on the list of banned substances established by the International Olympic Committee (IOC) and the World Anti-Doping Agency (WADA) (2001) (see Table 19.3). These lists are updated regularly, and

represent the standard to which all volleyball players participating in international competition are held accountable. National-level competitions may be governed by doping regulations adopted by the respective national volleyball federation.

This chapter will review the FIVB doping list and discuss the use of nutritional supplements, with particular attention to compliance with the doping rules and avoidance of accidental doping.

To avoid accidental doping it is, of course, essential to confirm that substances legitimately prescribed by the athlete's personal or team physician are not on the doping list. The IOC doping list, which is continuously updated, is available on the internet at www.olympic.org. The FIVB also publishes its own doping list, but it is important to note that the list of banned substances and methods published by the FIVB is not exhaustive in its content. Rather, it contains only selected examples of substances from the different pharmacological classes in order to illustrate which types of agents are banned. Substances belonging to a banned class of pharmaceuticals cannot be used for medical treatment unless used in specific, preapproved situations. This applies to all agents within that drug class, even those not specifically enumerated in the published list. For this reason, the phrase "and related substances" is emphasized throughout the list of banned substances. This term refers to and legally encompasses all drugs that belong in the class by virtue of their pharmacological action(s) and/or chemical structure.

If a banned substance is detected in the doping laboratory, the relevant sports authority (normally the IOC during the Olympic Games, the FIVB in international competitions, or the national federation in national competitions) will act to sanction the athlete. It should be noted that the presence of the drug in the urine constitutes an offence, irrespective of the route of administration. If an athlete is prescribed medication by a physician or uses an over-the-counter preparation, it is ultimately the athlete's responsibility to make sure that the drugs taken do not contain substances on the doping list. In such situations it is important to check with competent medical personnel that the product consumed is safe from a doping standpoint.

In the past, medications used in the treatment of asthma and other common respiratory disorders have caused problems for athletes, since some of the more commonly prescribed drugs for these conditions are powerful stimulants and are therefore banned as doping agents. Cough medications have proven similarly problematic for athletes. Furthermore, because these drugs have many different product names, the status of a particular drug may be confusing. The most prudent approach is the simplest one: never take or prescribe a product for upper respiratory symptoms, common cold symptoms, sore throats, cough, or the flu without first checking with a physician or pharmacist who has special expertise in the area of doping control.

Substances found on the doping list can, according to certain rules, be used to treat illness or, disease. Within certain of the doping classes, for example, special exceptions have been made to allow administration of a particular pharmaceutical if an athlete's health condition necessitates its use.

Nutritional supplements

A vast array of nutritional supplements is available to athletes. These products all claim to improve physical performance, often in unique ways. However, there is little to no scientific evidence to support the majority of these claims. Nevertheless, there are specific situations when athletes may benefit from the use of certain nutritional supplements. Generally, athletes cite three principle reasons to justify their supplement use: (i) to compensate for less than adequate diets or lifestyles; (ii) to meet unusual nutrient demands induced by heavy exercise; and (iii) to produce a performance-enhancing (i.e. ergogenic) effect. In the following discussion nutritional supplements (also referred to as "nutriceuticals") will be classified either as dietary supplements or nutritional ergogenic aids (Burke *et al.* 2000).

Dietary supplements

According to one proposed definition (Burke & Read 1993; Burke *et al.* 2000), a dietary supplement should:
• Contain nutrients in amounts generally similar to the recommended dietary intakes and similar to the amounts found in food.
• Provide a convenient or practical means of ingesting these nutrients, particularly in the athletic setting.
• Permit or facilitate the attainment of known physiological or nutritional requirements in athletes.
• Contain nutrients in large amounts for use in treating a known nutrient deficiency.
• Have been shown to meet a specific physiological or nutritional need that improves sports performance.
• Be generally acknowledged as a valuable product by sports medicine and science experts.

Supplements that meet the definition of dietary supplements are summarized in Table 19.1. However, it is important to appreciate that dietary supplements do not improve sports performance *per se*. Rather, the use of a dietary supplement may help the athlete achieve a specific sports nutrition goal that in turn creates an environment that permits optimal performance. In most cases, the use of a supplement should be part of a larger plan of optimal sports nutrition or the clinical management of a nutritional problem. This means that education is important to highlight the general importance of optimal nutrition for athletes, and to insure that dietary supplements are only used when they are beneficial to the player.

Table 19.1 Supplements that meet the definition of dietary supplements (Burke *et al.* 2000).

Sports drink
Sports gel
High-carbohydrate supplement
Liquid meal preparation
Sports bar
Vitamin/mineral supplement
Iron supplement
Calcium supplement

Table 19.2 Nutritional ergogenic aids classified according to the scientific evidence for their efficacy in sports (Burke *et al.* 2000).

With scientific support
Creatine
Caffeine
Bicarbonate

With mixed scientific support
Antioxidant supplements
Protein and amino acids
Glycerol

Lacking substantial scientific support
Ginseng and related herbal products
Carnitine
Coenzyme Q10
Inosine
Chromium picolinate
Medium-chain triglycerides

Nutritional ergogenic aids

The second category of supplements, nutritional ergogenic aids, are described by the following characteristics (Burke & Read 1993; Burke *et al.* 2000):
• They contain nutrients or other food components in amounts greater than the recommended daily allowances, or the amounts typically provided by food.
• They claim to have a direct ergogenic (work-enhancing) effect on sports performance, often through a pharmacological rather than a physiological effect.
• They often rely on anecdotal support rather than on documented support from scientific trials.
• They are generally not supported by sports nutrition experts, except where scientific trials have documented a significant ergogenic effect.

Well-conducted scientific trials have produced evidence that some ergogenic aids can enhance sports performance. The documentation available for some ergogenic aids has been summarized in Table 19.2. However, it should be noted that each ergogenic aid works in a specific and narrow set of exercise situations, and thus may not have any effect on (or could conceivably prove to be detrimental to) the volleyball athlete's performance.

There are three nutritional ergogenic aids for which there is some scientific support—creatine, caffeine, and bicarbonate. Creatine is a high-energy muscle fuel. Stored primarily in skeletal muscle, there is some evidence to show that the oral intake of large doses can increase muscle stores of phosphocreatine. Since creatine provides a rapidly available, but transient, source of cellular energy, it appears to increase performance during repeated maximal

efforts of 5–10 s duration in laboratory tests. In other words, volleyball players may experience a performance-enhancing effect from creatine loading. However, it is important to note that about 30% of individuals appear to be non-responders. Creatine loading consistently leads to a weight increase of 1–3 kg, probably the result of water retention within muscle. Such an increase in body weight is clearly detrimental to the jumping athlete. Furthermore, those studies that have been published have not been conducted with elite athletes, nor are the protocols and performance outcome measures directly relevant to volleyball. Reports have also suggested that creatine use can precipitate compartment syndrome of the lower limbs. For these and other reasons, including the lack of large-scale studies, a cautious approach to creatine use seems warranted.

Caffeine stimulates the central nervous system as well as cardiac muscle, and promotes both diuresis and epinephrine release and activity. There is no clear mechanism to explain the "beneficial" effects of caffeine supplementation. Whereas caffeine has been shown to increase performance during steady-state endurance exercise (such as running and swimming), studies examining caffeine's effect on sports like volleyball, which require intermittent maximal performance, are lacking. The few studies available on short-term maximal exercise generally show no effect of caffeine supplementation. Moreover, since caffeine is a restricted substance according to the doping rules, care must be taken not to exceed a urinary concentration of $12 \mu g \cdot mL$. This level can be reached with a caffeine intake above $6–10 mg \cdot kg$, or $500 mg$ for a $70 kg$ person. A cup of coffee typically provides $100 mg$, but some sports drinks contain much higher levels per serving.

Bicarbonate increases the buffering capacity of muscle, and there is some evidence that bicarbonate supplementation may increase an athlete's anaerobic capacity. A positive effect on performance might therefore be expected in athletes who participate in events of medium duration that demand maximal effort, such as the 800 m race in track and field (or other predominantly anaerobic sporting events). There is therefore no reason to expect that bicarbonate loading would be physiologically beneficial to the volleyball athlete. Furthermore, many athletes suffer from gastrointestinal distress and nausea after sodium bicarbonate loading.

In conclusion, with a possible exception for creatine, there is no evidence to support the use of nutritional ergogenic aids among volleyball players.

Accidental doping through nutritional supplements

As stated earlier, it is vitally important for athletes, coaches, and sports medicine personnel to understand that nutritional supplements and herbal medicines may contain banned substances. These nutritional supplements are generally produced by a (poorly) self-regulated industry of food manufacturers and marketers in which product labeling and advertising is often purposely incomplete or misleading. Consequently, sports nutritional supplements may contain banned substances and inaccurate labeling information (Catlin *et al.* 2000). There are several documented cases of athletes testing positive after consuming nutritional supplements or herbal medication that, unbeknown to the athlete, contained a banned substance that had not been identified on the list of ingredients.

Moreover, since supplements purchased via international mail order, through internet sales, or by personal marketing schemes are not subject to any

scrutiny in the country of destination, it is important to have a global understanding of the regulation of supplements. In many countries, there is minimal regulation of production and marketing. When considering the enthusiasm and emotive nature of the advertising claims made, it is important to realize that such advertising is not regulated. This is especially the case with products that target the bodybuilding or resistance training industry, where testimonials and multilevel marketing "rackets" abound.

Consequently, the use of nutritional supplements or herbal medication in connection with sports is strongly discouraged without careful consideration, including one-on-one nutritional counseling with a sports nutritionist. If, after thoughtful deliberation, the athlete and their support personnel decide to proceed with supplement use, it is advisable to select products from large companies that also manufacture conventional dietary supplements such as vitamins and minerals. It is reasonable to expect that companies involved in the preparation of "mainstream" pharmaceutical products are likely to demand and achieve better quality control than should be expected from less invested companies.

The doping list

The doping list is based on classes of banned substances and methods (Table 19.3). As mentioned, in addition to the substances that are mentioned in the FIVB and IOC doping lists, "related substances" are also banned.

Class IA: stimulants

Stimulants comprise various types of drugs that increase alertness, reduce fatigue, and may increase competitiveness and aggressiveness. Their use can also produce loss of judgement, which may lead to accidents in some sports. Amphetamines and related compounds have the most notorious reputation for producing problems in sport. Some athletes have died while taking "normal" doses of these agents under conditions of maximum physical activity.

Comparable effects, although less pronounced,

Table 19.3 The doping list (World Anti-doping Agency/International Olympic Committee 2001).

I: *Doping classes*
A Stimulants
B Narcotic analgesics
C Anabolic agents
D Diuretics
E Peptide and glycoprotein hormones and analogues

II: *Doping methods*
A Blood doping
B Pharmacological, chemical, and physical manipulation

III: *Classes of drugs subject to certain restrictions*
A Alcohol
B Marijuana
C Local anesthetics
D Corticosteroids
E Beta-blockers

---

exist for a group of sympathomimetic amines. These are stimulants that are used in lower doses in medication for colds and as asthma and allergy medication, of which ephedrine is an example. In high doses, this type of compound produces mental stimulation and increased blood flow. Adverse effects include elevated blood pressure and headache, increased and irregular heart beats, anxiety, and tremor. In lower doses, they are often present in cold and hay fever preparations, which can be purchased in pharmacies and sometimes from other retail outlets without the need for a medical prescription.

Another group of stimulants is the beta-2 agonists. These drugs are unusual because they are classified as both stimulants and anabolic agents. When taken by mouth or by injection they exert powerful stimulatory and anabolic effects. However, when taken as an aerosol, they do not have an anabolic effect. Of the beta-2 agonists, only salbutamol and terbutaline are permitted, and only by inhalation.

There is an upper limit to the allowable urinary concentration of caffeine, above which the athlete is considered in violation of the doping code. Fortunately, the upper limit cannot be exceeded by moderate consumption of most caffeine-containing beverages including coffee, tea, and colas. Note, however, that some sports drinks contain very high levels of caffeine, which could result in a positive doping test if consumed in large quantities.

Class IB: narcotic analgesics

Drugs belonging to this class, which are represented by chemical and pharmacological analogues of morphine, act fairly specifically as analgesics for the management of moderate to severe pain. In addition, they have a pronounced cough-inhibiting effect, and can therefore be found in cough medication. Most of the active substances in this class have considerable side effects, including dose-related respiratory depression, and carry a high risk of physical and psychological dependence. These drugs are banned because there is evidence indicating that narcotic analgesics have been and are abused in sports. This ban is also justified by international restrictions affecting the movement of these compounds, and is in keeping with the recommendations of the World Health Organization regarding narcotics.

Exceptions have been made for some compounds in this class, such that medical use as a pain reliever or a cough medication may be permitted. In these cases the athlete must be able to document the diagnosis and need for treatment by supplying written documentation from his or her physician.

Class IC: anabolic agents

The anabolic androgenic steroids include testosterone and substances that are related in structure and activity to it. Anabolic steroids have been misused in sport to increase muscle strength and bulk, and to promote aggressiveness. Also, beta-2 agonists, usually administered by metered dose inhaler for the treatment of asthma, may have an anabolic effect on muscle if used in tablet or injectable form. This use of beta-2 agonists is therefore banned, as are anabolic steroids and testosterone.

The use of anabolic androgenic steroids is associated with potentially serious adverse effects, particularly when used over prolonged periods. The adverse effects most commonly reported are boils, gynecomastia, water retention or edema, stretch marks, and testicular atrophy. In women these substances lead to menstrual disorders, clitoris growth, and masculine traits (such as a deepening of the voice, increased body hair, male-pattern baldness), and more pronounced muscle bulk and skin vessels. It is important to realize that the use of anabolic androgenic steroids in children or teenagers may lead to premature closure of the epiphyseal plates, which may stunt growth. Adverse psychological effects are also commonly reported, including sleep disturbances, aggressiveness, loss of temper, mood swings, depression, and personality changes. There is evidence to suggest that psychological changes are the most problematic side effect for long-term steroid users.

Most of the side effects connected with the transient use of anabolic steroids are "reversible" and normalize to a certain degree—even after continuous use over several years. However, some adverse effects, such as a deepening of the voice and increased clitoris size in women and growth arrest in children and adolescents, are permanent. In addition, there is evidence to suggest that long-term use of anabolic steroids may lead to an increased risk of cardiovascular disease, increasing the athlete's risk of premature myocardial infarction.

Class ID: diuretics

Athletes abuse diuretics for two main reasons: to reduce weight rapidly, and to mask other drug use. In sports where athletes are categorized by weight, diuretics are often used to reduce weight quickly. This is unlikely to occur among volleyball players. Diuretics are also used to reduce the concentration of other drugs in the urine by increasing the rate of urine production. This is a familiar strategy used to dilute the concentration of drug metabolites in the urine, thereby making their detection more difficult or lowering the drug concentration below an acceptable threshold. Diuretic use is therefore unacceptable on ethical grounds, and, moreover, diuretic misuse carries with it the risk of potentially serious side effects that may compromise the athlete's health and well being.

Class IE: peptide and glycoprotein hormones and analogues

This class consists of a number of hormones that help regulate various life-sustaining functions, including growth hormone, erythropoietin, insulin, and insulin-like growth factor. Insulin administration is, however, permitted if used in the treatment of insulin-dependent diabetes. The athlete must in

such cases be able to document the diagnosis and need of treatment by a written declaration from his or her physician.

Class IIA: blood doping

Blood doping refers to the intravenous administration of red blood cells, related blood products, or artificial oxygen transporters for reasons other than necessary medical treatment. The usual indication for therapeutic intravenous administration of blood in medicine is acute blood loss. In sport, however, the goal of blood doping is to improve endurance by increasing the athlete's oxygen-carrying capacity. Blood doping can be accomplished by transfusing blood products obtained from the athlete him/herself, or from a different person. In addition, the non-medicinal use of erythropoietin, a naturally occurring hormone that stimulates the production of red blood cells, also constitutes doping.

Blood doping contravenes the ethics of medicine and sport. There are significant risks involved in the transfusion of blood and related blood products, including, but not limited to, allergic transfusion reaction, transmission of infectious diseases, circulatory overload, and metabolic shock. Sadly, a number of deaths of young endurance athletes have been connected to use of erythropoietin.

Class IIB: pharmacological, chemical, and physical manipulation

All methods and substances used to alter the integrity and validity of urine samples used in doping control are banned. Examples of banned methods include bladder catheterization, urine substitution and/or tampering, inhibition of renal excretion, and epitestosterone administration. Any attempt at sample manipulation is considered a violation of the doping rules, whether the attempt is completed or not.

Class IIIA and IIIB: alcohol and marijuana

Alcohol and marijuana are not viewed as doping substances, but breath and/or blood alcohol levels may be tested if requested by the responsible authority. Similarly, urine may be tested for cannabinoids.

Class IIIC: local anesthetics

Injectable local anesthetics are permitted provided they are used as part of medical treatment or dental treatment. However, only certain local anesthetics are permitted and only local or intra-articular injections may be administered. In connection with the Olympic Games or other international championships, it may be required to report the use of local anesthetics to the responsible authority.

Class IIID: glucocorticosteroids

Because of their anti-inflammatory properties, the naturally occurring and synthetic corticosteroids are widely used in medicine to treat many conditions, including, but not limited to, the inflammatory arthropathies. Glucocorticosteroid use is prohibited, with the exception of topical or inhalational administration, and intra-articular or local injection. However, in connection with the Olympic Games or other international competition there may be a requirement to report the use of corticosteroids to the responsible authority, regardless of the route of administration.

Class IIIE: beta-blockers

Beta-blocker use is permitted for the treatment of high blood pressure or cardiac arrhythmia. The athlete must in such cases be able to document the diagnosis and need of treatment by a written declaration from his or her physician.

Doping tests

The National Olympic Committees, FIVB, IOC, and WADA all conduct doping tests on a regular basis. Urine tests are normally sent for analysis to IOC-accredited laboratories around the world. According to FIVB procedures for doping control, competent personnel should conduct the control in accordance with written guidelines. Notification for doping control can occur either in writing or orally.

Sampling procedures

The urine sample is submitted under the supervision of one or more doping control officers. After the sample has been given, the urine is sealed in two containers, one labeled container A and the other container B. The doping control officer uses the rest of the urine to measure specific gravity and pH. The volume, specific gravity, and pH of the urine have to meet certain requirements for the sample to be accepted as a valid sample.

Information about the athlete and sample are carefully noted on a doping control form. The doping control form is the only document connecting the athlete's identity to the code number of the sample. After the doping control has been completed, the doping test is sent to the doping control laboratory, while the doping control form is sealed and sent to the sports governing body requesting the sample. In this way nobody can connect the result of the analysis and the identity of the athlete until the analysis of sample A has been conducted, and the sports authority has received a report from the laboratory.

Laboratory analysis

After the samples have arrived in the laboratory, detailed written procedures are followed for the handling and analysis of all urine samples. This is done to insure that samples are not exchanged by mistake or that anything should happen to the sample (which in a worst-case scenario might lead to reversing the result of the analysis).

If the first analysis is suspicious for banned substances, a repeat follow-up test is performed. A confirmatory analysis is also performed on sample A. If the suspicion is confirmed, and the substance can be identified by means of mass spectrometry, the laboratory reports which substances have been detected to the sports authority. The requirements for identification of substances in a sample are strict, and all doubt regarding the identity of the substance will be in favor of the athlete. These strict standards mean that, in some cases, documentation is inadequate to permit reporting a positive finding after the confirmation analysis.

After the sports authority has received information on a positive doping test, the athlete will normally be informed. The athlete will be asked to give a statement and is at the same time informed about the possibility of analyzing sample B. If sample B is negative, the case is closed without sanction of the athlete. If sample B is positive, the sports authority considers the case and a decision will then be made as to the consequences for the athlete.

Penalties for doping offences

The punishment for a first-time violation of the doping regulations is usually a 2-year ban on sporting participation (including both competition and organized training). For repeat offences the athlete is normally banned from the sport for life. In addition to disqualification and loss of the right to participate in competition and training, the athlete may also lose medals, prize money, or records from competitions in which the accused athlete may have participated under the performance-enhancing effects of doping.

Doping-free volleyball

Although that there is little evidence to suggest that doping is a widespread problem in volleyball, there is certainly reason to be "on guard." Athletes must guard against accidental doping, e.g. unknowingly taking banned substances when ill or as a nutritional supplement. Common sense dictates that athletes should check all medications taken and supplements used against the FIVB doping list, and should avail themselves of expert advice if uncertain as to the status of these products.

Conscious, deliberate doping typically involves the use of anabolic steroids. Unfortunately, the abuse of steroids seems to be widespread in certain youth training environments, in which consumption appears to be driven as much by a desire for improved physical appearance as by a desire for improved sports performance (Buckley *et al.* 1988; Perry *et al.* 1992; Kersey 1993; Yesalis *et al.* 1993; Fields *et al.* 1994; Elliot & Goldberg 1996; Korkia 1996; Melia *et al.* 1996; Korkia & Stimson 1997; Laure 1997). It is therefore very important that the coaching staff and the medical staff remain sensitive to this phenomenon, so that proper guidance can be given to athletes at risk.

References

Buckley, W.E., Yesalis, C.E., Friedl, K.E., Anderson, W.A., Streit, A.L. & Wright, J.E. (1988) Estimated prevalence of anabolic steroid use among high school seniors. *Journal of the American Medical Association* 260, 3441–3445.

Burke, L., Desbrow, B. & Minehan, M. (2000) Dietary supplements and nutritional ergogenic aids in sport. In: Burke, L. & Deakin, V. (eds). *Clinical Sports Nutrition*, pp. 455–553. McGraw-Hill, New York.

Burke, L.M. & Read, R.S.D. (1993) Dietary supplements in sports. *Sports Medicine* 15, 43–56.

Catlin, D.H., Leder, B.Z., Ahrens, B. *et al.* (2000) Trace contamination of over-the-counter androstenedione and positive urine test results for a nandrolone metabolite. *Journal of the American Medical Association* 284, 2618–2621.

Elliot, D. & Goldberg, L. (1996) Intervention and prevention of steroid use in adolescents. *American Journal of Sports Medicine* 24, 46–58.

Fields, L., Lange, W.R., Kreiter, N.A. & Fudala, P.J. (1994) A national survey of drug testing policies for college athletes. *Medicine and Science in Sports and Exercise* 26, 682–686.

Kersey, R.D. (1993) Anabolic-androgenic steroid use by private health club/gym athletes. *Journal of Strength and Conditioning Research* 7, 118–126.

Korkia, P. (1996) Anabolic steroid use in adolescents. *Sports Exercise and Injury* 2, 136–140.

Korkia, P. & Stimson, G.V. (1997) Indications of prevalence, practice and effects of anabolic steroid use in Great Britain. *International Journal of Sports Medicine* 18, 557–562.

Laure, P. (1997) Epidemiologic approach of doping in sport. *Journal of Sports Medicine and Physical Fitness* 37, 218–224.

Melia, P., Pipe, A. & Greenberg, L. (1996) The use of anabolic-androgenic steroids by Canadian students. *Clinical Journal of Sport Medicine* 6, 9–14.

Perry, H.M., Wright, D. & Littlepage, B.N.C. (1992) Dying to be big: a review of anabolic steroid use. *British Journal of Sports Medicine* 26, 259–261.

World Anti-doping Agency/International Olympic Committee (2001) *List of Prohibited Substances and Methods. Olympic Movement Anti-doping Code.* IOC/WADA, Lausanne, Switzerland.

Yesalis, C.E., Kennedy, N.J., Kopstein, A.N. & Bahrke, M.S. (1993) Anabolic-androgenic steroid use in the United States. *Journal of the American Medical Association* 270, 1217–1221.

Chapter 20
Visual perception and decision making in volleyball

Darlene A. Kluka

Introduction

Visual perception and decision-making skills play indispensable roles in volleyball performance. Fundamentally, the eyes serve to gather information from and transmit details about an individual's environment. The retina of the eye encodes the visual world, transforming optical images into nerve impulses that are conducted by the optic nerve to the brain. These electrical messages are translated into "sight" by the vision center, located in the occipital lobe of the cerebral cortex. Visual perception and decision making depend upon the athlete's ability to discern shapes and colors, and to coordinate visual input with voluntary, purposeful movement of the musculoskeletal system so that efficient and effective action can occur. The ability to appropriately interpret what is perceived is a learned skill, just as spiking, blocking, and serving are learned.

Research suggests that there are at least three vision-related components to the successful acquisition of volleyball skills: (i) the visual information gathered by the athlete; (ii) perceptual decision-making strategies mediated by connections between the visual system and the frontal lobes of the brain; and (iii) efficient production of volleyball-specific actions, resulting from integrated connections between the visual system, the brain, and the body (Kluka 1997). It has also been theorized that there are at least nine factors that contribute to an individual's relative inability to successfully learn volleyball skills (Ahrabi-Fard & Huddleston 1991). Of these, four involve the visual/perceptual system and decision making: (i) lack of recognition (reading); (ii) late reading; (iii) lack of inner focus for accuracy; and (iv) poor selection of inner options that can result in inappropriate motor program execution. These components and factors, on which volleyball success depends (in large measure), are themselves related to a core set of visual and perceptual skills which include static and dynamic visual acuity, convergence and divergence, central and peripheral awareness, glare recovery, contrast sensitivity function, fusion, color perception, and total reaction time. These skills, when integrated with quick action plans (decision making), enable volleyball athletes to anticipate impending events so that their actions and reactions are timed appropriately.

Visual perceptual skill enhancement

Because the volleyball environment is quite dynamic, it is important that each athlete has sharp static visual acuity. Once relative motion begins, both visual clarity and image contrast rapidly deteriorate. The sharper the static focus, the slower the erosion of clarity and contrast while tracking an object in motion. The athlete should therefore undergo a detailed examination by a sports vision/eye care professional (optometrist or ophthalmologist) at least once every 2 years, or when environmental clarity is suspect. If the athlete's vision requires a correction, spectacles (sport frames with polycarbonate lenses) or contact lenses (soft or rigid, gas permeable) are available at low cost. Because the body generates heat during play, spectacles may fog. Spectacle frames may also impair peripheral vision. Contact lenses are, as a rule, cleaner and clearer than spectacles. Contact lenses, particularly disposable soft lenses, are therefore generally more appropriate than spectacles for use during athletic contests, and are typically well tolerated by the athlete. The athlete should be carefully fitted by a sports vision/eye care professional to insure that the contact lenses do not move away from the center of the pupil during extreme or rapid eye movements. The athlete should have at least two extra pairs of lenses in case a lens is lost, torn, or otherwise not wearable. Once the athlete's static visual system is at its sharpest, the athlete and coach may attend to other visual/perceptual skills (Kluka & Planer 1998).

Although attempts to correlate enhanced visual skills with enhanced motor performance have in the past proven inconclusive, there is increasing evidence that several of the core visual/perceptual skills previously mentioned can be enhanced through training. For example, it has been shown that convergence and divergence, central and peripheral awareness, contrast sensitivity function, fusion, and speed of recognition can be enhanced in volleyball athletes after 6 weeks of volleyball-specific training combined with general sports vision training. Training sessions should be conducted three times per week during regular practice times on a regulation volleyball court so that the drills and procedures are contextually based. Stations and activities might include: (i) overhead passing while on a minitrampoline illuminated by a strobe light; (ii) training central/peripheral awareness via a random light display (an AcuVision instrument may be helpful); (iii) measuring speed of recognition (with a tachistoscope); (iv) training object acquisition and tracking by having the athlete pass a volleyball served from behind a barrier; or (v) tracking and detecting a volleyball after a full body turn (Kluka *et al.* 1996; Adolphe *et al.* 1997; Vickers & Adolphe 1997). Additional drills that can easily be incorporated into practice sessions are described in detail in Box 20.1.

Decision making

Research has demonstrated that when vision affects performance and decision making, there are at least three visual perceptual skills that form the foundation of the athlete's capacity for such decision making: visual search, selective attention, and anticipation (Kluka 1999). In this context, it is important to briefly discuss the four types of eye movements that athletes use to survey their volleyball environment: vergence (the ability to maintain focus on an object traveling towards or away from you), smooth pursuit (tracking an object with smooth eye motions), saccadic (the rapid movements the eyes make as they track an object from side to side), and vestibulo-ocular (eye movements influenced by the body's balance organ in the inner ear) (Wilkinson 1992). When combined with the focal and peripheral visual systems, these eye movements facilitate information gathering. When playing defense, for example, the middle back follows the served volleyball as it travels across the net to the opponent's first pass (vergence and smooth pursuit), then tracks the ball toward the opposing setter's hands (smooth pursuit), quickly scans the net for potential attackers (saccadic), and then finally locks in on the ball just before the attack, all the while maintaining dynamic balance (vestibulo-ocular). There are, however, limits to the capacity of this system: at contact, a spiked volleyball can approach speeds of $160 km \cdot h$, producing visual angular velocities in excess of $500° \cdot s$ (Kluka & Dunn 2000). Based on these figures, it can be calculated that the last time the middle back defender actually "sees" the volleyball before making a play on it is at the moment of the opponent's attack. Volleyball athletes must therefore learn to anticipate events in these (and other) situations, based on a probability analysis of the environment and conditions in comparison to past experiences under similar circumstances. Those athletes who can correctly extrapolate to the end result of a play based upon the preliminary conditions are more likely to quickly formulate an appropriate action plan. For example, defenders will distinguish themselves if they are able to quickly process the visual information presented to them and, based on those data, correctly anticipate the location of

Box 20.1

The following drills (Kluka & Love 1988) can also easily be incorporated into practice sessions.

1 *Equipment*: A 75 × 125 mm file card. Place four volleyball terms (e.g. spike, pass, block, serve) on the card so that one is located near the center on each side of the card. Place the card on the floor in the line of vision when in a push up position.
Drill: While focusing upon one of the words on the card, perform a push up. Keep the word on the card in focus as long as possible.
Goal: Complete 40 push ups, focusing upon each word on the card ten times.
Variations: Focus upon each word, going in a clockwise direction; focus in the form of a cross (up/down, left/right); place the card on a wall at eye level. Perform wall push ups; perform one-arm push ups; perform triangular push ups; perform push ups with a clap.

2 *Equipment*: None.
Drill: Jog at a leisurely pace around the court.
Goal: Focus for 5 s on your shoestrings. Focus for 5 s on something you see in the distance on the right. Focus on your right hand for 5 s. Focus on something you see in the distance on the left for 5 s.
Variations: Increase your speed. Decrease the time of your focus to 3 s; without moving your head, focus upon something which is diagonally to your left on the floor, then diagonally to your right, then near the ceiling.

3 *Equipment*: A balance board, a volleyball, and a partner.
Drill: While maintaining your balance on the board, a partner gently tosses the ball to you. Focus upon the ball as it comes to your hands in an overhead pass. Pass it in balance back to your partner.
Goal: Successfully pass ten consecutive tosses in balance.
Variations: Use two balance boards, one for each foot. Repeat the above drill.

4 *Equipment*: A wall, a 75 × 125 mm file card with a 25 mm darkened dot in the center, a volleyball, masking tape, and a partner.
Drill: Place the file card on the wall with masking tape so that the card is at eye level. Stand 4.5 m (15 feet) from the wall. While focusing on the dot, serve the ball into the wall. As the ball rebounds off the wall, continue to focus on the dot and pass the ball to a partner who is positioned as a setter.
Goal: Repeat for 2 min or ten successful sequences while focusing on the dot.
Variations: Change the position of the card on the wall to simulate blocking level.

5 *Equipment*: A partner and a volleyball net.
Drill: With your partner, face each other so that you are about 90 cm (3 feet) apart, with the net between the two of you. Focus on each other's eyes. Move your right hand slowly. Your partner should mirror the movement by moving the left hand, without moving the eyes. If the right hand is moved forward, your partner's left hand should move backward. Move various body parts slowly and have your partner mirror the movements without moving the eyes.
Goal: Be the leader in the drill for 1 min; change roles for another minute.
Variations: Make the movements progressively more rapid; make the movements more complex, resembling spiking and blocking.

6 *Equipment*: VCR, television or monitor, videotape of a match, and a pencil with an eraser.
Drill: Place the videotape into the VCR. Stand directly in line with the television screen 3 m (10 feet) away. While the videotape is playing, hold the pencil vertically with one hand at arm's length in front of the body and focus upon the eraser. Verbally describe what is occurring on the videotape.
Goal: Focus on the eraser for two 30 s intervals, allowing 1 min rest by closing the eyes.
Variations: Turn to the left so that you are standing at a 30° angle to the television. Repeat the drill.

7 *Equipment*: Three sets of volleyballs, one colored primarily white, another red, another green—designate what color will be used for a particular response (for example: white, off speed shot; blue, hit line; red, hit crosscourt)—partner, and volleyball passing machine.
Drill: Using the passing machine, execute the appropriate attack pattern according to ball color.
Goal: Successfully complete nine color-coded responses.
Variations: Increase the number of balls available (e.g. 12 balls—4 red, 4 blue, 4 white).

the volleyball so as to be in position to make the defensive play.

Some researchers (Allard & Starkes 1980; Ahrabi-Fard & Huddleston 1991; Starkes *et al.* 1995) have suggested that appropriate visual search strategies assist athletes in making good decisions by helping to focus their attention. Attention has been catego-

rized (Nideffer 1976) into four styles: broad internal, broad external, narrow internal, and narrow external. Volleyball athletes typically use a broad external focus to read and recognize information. They learn to "zoom out" externally (a blocker reading or scanning the opposition to identify potential attackers, for example) (Fig. 20.1), then "zoom in" externally

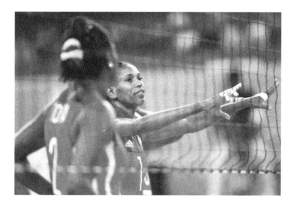

Fig. 20.1 Blockers tend to use a broad external focus of attention to read and recognize information, such as identifying the opponent's potential attackers before the service. (Photo courtesy of Olympic Museum, Lausanne.)

to intensely read or focus on a specific attacker (narrow external focus of attention). The blocker then identifies potential scoring opportunities (a broad internal focus permits selection of the appropriate motor program based on the possibilities within each player's ability), and finally produces a controlled contact by executing the motor program selected (positioning the hands correctly while blocking requires a narrow internal focus of attention) (Ahrabi-Fard & Huddleston 1991).

Recently, other researchers (Williams *et al.* 1999; Ford *et al.* 2000) have theorized that visual focus may be refocused without making eye movements. Task-specific knowledge structures that control visual search strategies seem to be stored in memory. These structures may result from previous game experience. If true, this perspective suggests that states of peak volleyball performance may be consciously triggered by visual perception. Indeed, there is increasing anecdotal evidence that players who are in a "peak performance state" use their eyes in a dramatically different way than the traditional "keep your eye on the ball" pattern. It has also been theorized (Ford *et al.* 2000) that the volleyball athlete is capable of performing in several operating modes simultaneously. In this model, the athlete in a normal performance state is operating in a *serial* mode, while the athlete in a peak performance state (said to be in "the flow" or in "the zone") is operating in a *parallel* mode.

The human visual system is capable of configuring visual information to the brain using different strategies: variable depth of focus (VDF) strategy (asymmetry), fixed depth of focus (FDF) strategy (symmetry), or a combination of VDF and FDF strategies. The visual strategy used by the athlete in every contact sequence (a discrete occurrence, having a beginning, middle, and end) determines the efficiency as well as the accuracy of the available information being formulated in the brain. More importantly, it also determines the temporal dimension in which the athlete performs actions within the space and time of every contact sequence. A VDF strategy engages the athlete in the past temporal dimension during the action, while a FDF strategy engages the athlete in the present temporal dimension during the action. The end result for the athlete is action in the "past" (normal performance state) versus action in the "present" (peak performance state).

From a performance perspective, the fundamental building block of volleyball is the contact sequence. Each individual contact sequence begins with the movement of the ball ("ball"), followed by the athlete's movement to intercept the ball ("athlete"), and ends with contact ("contact"), the event that occurs when ball movement and athlete movement come together at a single point in space and time— the "contact point." This construct has originally been referred to as *coincidence anticipation timing* in the motor learning literature.

Every contact sequence is a discrete occurrence, meaning spatial and temporal relationships can be established between the athlete as a system of movement and the other elements of the contact sequence—ball movement and contact. In temporal relativity, the contact sequence resembles this in time:

$$\text{Ball} \rightarrow \text{Athlete} \rightarrow \text{Contact}$$
$$1 \qquad 2 \qquad 3$$
$$\text{Past} \quad \text{Present} \quad \text{Future}$$

In spatial relativity, the contact sequence resembles this in space:

$$\text{Ball} \rightarrow \text{Contact} \rightarrow \text{Athlete}$$
$$1 \qquad 3 \qquad 2$$
$$\text{Past} \quad \text{Future} \quad \text{Present}$$

When athletes focus on the ball (VDF input), visual countermovements are used to input temporal information about "ball" movement only. This means that visual countermovements are used to input temporal information to the brain about the past only. The unequal distribution of the temporal elements of the contact sequence around the common temporal axis of the athlete can be referred to as temporal asymmetry or "contacting in the past."

In contrast, a FDF input configuration sets up a completely different distribution of temporal information in every contact sequence. When an athlete fixes focus on the contact zone and locates the contact point along a predefined depth of focus, temporal information is distributed equally on both sides of the temporal axis of countermovement. By simultaneously inputting equal temporal information about the "ball's" movement and the depth of "contact," the athlete effectively inpatterns equal temporal information about past and future simultaneously. The athlete's brain receives equal distributions of the past and the future simultaneously, creating a third dimension, the dimension of the present. This equal distribution of the temporal elements of the contact sequence around the common temporal axis of the athlete is temporal symmetry, or "contacting in the present."

Jump serve reception serves to illustrate this process. In traditional visual tracking, the athlete uses smooth pursuit eye movements and vergence to focus on the ball throughout its trajectory from the moment of contact with the server's hand to the point of contact with their forearms. However, when the volleyball travels faster than $70° \cdot s$ (as is often the case when the ball is spiked or jump served), the athlete is unable to continuously track it. Consequently, most athletes use a VDF strategy to track the ball from the moment of contact with the server's hand to the moment of contact with the passer's forearms. As a result of this strategy, however, at the moment of contact the receiving athlete's last working visual image of the ball's position is obsolete. In other words, by the time the athlete processes the last visual image of the approaching volleyball, the ball has moved out of that position—forcing the athlete to rely on anticipatory skills described earlier.

Utilizing a FDF strategy requires the athlete to initially focus on a "window" which is approximately an arm's distance away from and in front of the body. In this strategy, the volleyball athlete relies on his or her peripheral vision to determine the direction and speed of the oncoming ball to calculate the window's location, and is then free to contact the ball at the point where the ball hits the window in time and space. The athlete is therefore able to play the ball in the "visual present" rather than in the "visual past." Although anecdotally effective and of sound theoretical basis, well-designed studies are needed to prove that this fixed depth of focus visual strategy improves volleyball performance.

Systematic observational skills for the coach

A discussion of the importance of visual perception and decision making in volleyball must also include a consideration of the coach's need to observe and critique the athlete's performance of volleyball skills. Coaches who possess the ability to evaluate critical environmental and technical cues affecting an athlete's performance have more opportunities to provide that athlete with meaningful feedback and instruction. The observant volleyball coach can also help minimize overuse injuries by being attentive to subtle alterations in technique that may herald subclinical adaptations to chronic tissue overload. Knowing how to look, when to look, where to look, and what to look for are some of the keys to successful observation. In short, the coach seeks to answer the following questions: What should the athlete keep doing? What should the athlete stop doing? What should the athlete begin doing?

A framework has been devised that facilitates systematic observation and analysis of volleyball skills (Barrett 1979; Kluka 1999). The methodology consists of a logical six-step process employing visual perception and decision-making strategies that coaches can employ to develop efficient and effective observational and descriptive skills:

1 Classify each volleyball skill.
2 Understand the biomechanics associated with each of the skills, and how the skills are used in the context of the rally, game, and match.

3 Divide each skill into phases.
4 Focus on key body areas when observing skill performance.
5 Interpret meaningful information collected during the performance.
6 Provide effective and efficient feedback to the athlete.

Most volleyball skills can be classified as either "closed" or "open." A closed skill may in this context be considered to be one that depends predominantly on internal timing. It involves the appropriate sequencing of movement that is manifested as a coordinated independent performance. Performing a floater serve can be classified as a closed skill, as its execution is entirely dependent on the athlete's ability. An open skill adds the element of external timing. Blocking is an example of an open skill, in which successful execution is dependent upon the tempo of the attacker, the spiked volleyball, and the blocker's jumping and timing ability so that the blocking action coincides with the arrival of the ball. An understanding of timing is therefore beneficial to both open and closed skill analysis.

Coaches can establish a basis for performance cue acquisition through careful study and practice. By analyzing the technique of efficient and elite-level athletes (either in person, on film, or through computer simulation or mental imagery and visualization), coaches can begin to apply the principles of biomechanics to skill performance. For example, each volleyball skill can be divided or codified into five temporally sequential phases. These include: (i) the ready position; (ii) preparation for action; (iii) the action or contact; (iv) follow-through; and (v) preparation for the next movement. Thus, when analyzing an outside block the coach should:
• Focus on the torso at the ready position to identify the body's initial balance.
• Visually release from the initial starting (ready) position and visually search up the body to the shoulders, arms, and elbows as the blocker prepares for action.
• Focus on the hands at the moment of contact with the ball.
• Visually release from the ball at contact, shifting focus to the athlete's head, shoulders, and navel; view the body's dynamic balance upon landing (follow-through).

• Focus on torso movement during the preparatory phase for subsequent actions.

Because only 3° of visual angle are in focus at a given instant (an area roughly the size of a thumbnail), the coach uses the ambient (peripheral) visual system to detect much of the overall movement. It is therefore important for the coach to observe from sufficient distance to be able to view the athlete's entire movement sequence in relationship to other concurrent events in the environment. Furthermore, when focusing on the core of the body, the visual search should be in a straight line from navel to nose up the body, or nose to navel down the body. The following questions may benefit the coach who is learning to utilize visual perception to identify and interpret performance-related cues (Barrett 1979; Kluka 1999):
• Where is the head/torso aligned in relation to the goal of the skill?
• What is the position of the head through the action sequence?
• What impact does head positioning have on performance?
• Where are the athlete's eyes focused (e.g. on the ball, on the target, in between, or unfocused)?
• Where is the body's center of gravity during performance of the skill?
• How is body weight distributed during each of the phases of skill performance?
• Is the base of support sufficient to provide stability?
• Is there dynamic stability in relation to up/down, side/side, front/front, front/back?
• Is force produced by a logical series of progressive movements through connected body segments (the "kinetic chain")?
• What is the range of motion within each joint that contributes to force production?
• What is the role of the legs and/or arms in this skill?
• Is hip movement important? If so, how much and in what direction(s)?
• Where are the shoulders in relation to the hips and feet?
• Where are the hands in relation to the desired outcome before, during, and after contact with the ball?
• What is the extent of follow-through?
• What is the outcome of the movement in relationship to the goal?

One way in which coaches (and athletes) can enhance their decision-making capacity and their ability to interpret performance cues is through videotape analysis. It is recommended that before any feedback or analysis is provided to the athlete, the coach should observe their movements/performance a minimum of three times—once from the rear, once from the side (perpendicularly), and once from the front. By videotaping the action from these three sides, more complete information can be collected through repetitive viewing. For some skills, such as blocking and attacking, videotaping from directly above can also provide beneficial information (e.g. overhead viewing permits assessment of rotation around the vertical axis). Viewing actions in slow motion can also help the coach "break down" and analyze the athlete's technique. Pausing the video during the preparation and action phases permits the coach to make predictions about the result(s) of each action.

The ultimate goal of this undertaking is, of course, to provide efficient and effective feedback to the athlete that will enable him or her to improve his/her performance and on-the-court decision-making capacity. To this end, the coach and the athlete should agree on a set of succinct verbal and visual instructional cues that provide meaningful information to the athlete. Short, descriptive action, emotional, or spatial area words or phrases (e.g. crush, reach, explode, roof, smash, 11 o'clock, flat platform) can facilitate rapid communication between the coach and athlete during both training sessions and matches. These types of words should be used at least 3 s prior to the desired initiation of movement so that the athlete can process the cue and translate its message into the intended action.

Developing observational skills therefore enables the volleyball coach to select appropriate information for detailed processing and performance analysis. Such skills enhance the coach's visual perceptual and decision-making capacity and thereby facilitate skill and tactical instruction essential to developing talented volleyball athletes. As athletes attain consistently higher levels of performance, coaches should create even more challenging practice environments that include misleading motor cues—making it increasingly difficult for actions to be anticipated. For example, setters should be encouraged to eliminate advanced cue information as they prepare to contact the ball for a variety of sets, thereby making it more difficult for opposing blockers to read the direction of the attack. Attackers should be encouraged to deceptively vary their spiking motion just prior to contact to create uncertainty among the defenders, thereby reducing the defender's ability to correctly anticipate the play and maximizing the probability of scoring a point. Finally, coaches are encouraged to re-examine the volleyball-specific drills used during practices, with the goal of reconstructing each drill "from the eyes down." By using drills that prioritize visual perception and decision making, the coach can foster peak performance by facilitating the volleyball athlete's ability to formulate quick, accurate action plans.

References

Adolphe, R.M., Vickers, J.N. & Laplante, G. (1997) The effects of training visual attention on gaze behaviour and accuracy: a pilot study. *International Journal of Sports Vision* **4** (1), 28–33.

Ahrabi-Fard, I. & Huddleston, S. (1991) The attentional demands of volleyball. *Coaching Volleyball Journal* **6**, 12–14.

Allard, F. & Starkes, J.L. (1980) Perception in sport: volleyball. *Journal of Sport Psychology* **2**, 22–33.

Barrett, K. (1979) Observations for learning and coaching. *Journal of Physical Education, Recreation and Dance* **50** (1), 23–25.

Ford, S., Hines, W. & Kluka, D. (2000) Volleyball and four-dimensional visual/cognitive/motor symmetry: a model for performance enhancement. *International Journal of Volleyball Research* **3**, 12–16.

Kluka, D. (1997) Observational skills: qualitative analysis for competitive excellence. *The Coach* **3**, 24–27.

Kluka, D. (1999) *Motor Behavior: from Learning to Performance*. Morton Publishing Co., Englewood, CO.

Kluka, D. & Dunn, P. (2000) *Volleyball*, 4th edn. McGraw-Hill, Boston.

Kluka, D. & Love, P. (1988) *Visual Skills Enhancement Exercise Cards*. EyeSport, Inc., Ruston, LA.

Kluka, D., Love, P., Kuhlman, J., Hammack, G. & Wesson, M. (1996) The effects of a visual skills training program on selected intercollegiate volleyball athletes. *International Journal of Sports Vision* **3** (1), 23–34.

Kluka, D.A. & Planer, P.A. (1998) Improving volleyball decision making through visual/perceptual skills training. *Performance Conditioning for Volleyball* **6** (2), 7–8.

Nideffer, R.M. (1976) *The Inner Athlete*. Thomas Crowell, New York.

Starkes, J.L., Edwards, P., Dissanayake, P. & Dunn, T. (1995) A new technology and field test of advance cue usage in volleyball. *Research Quarterly in Exercise and Sport* **66** (2), 162–167.

Vickers, J.N. & Adolphe, R.M. (1997) Gaze behaviour during a ball tracking and aiming skill. *International Journal of Sports Vision* **4** (1), 18–27.

Wilkinson, S. (1992) A training program for improving undergraduates' analytic skill in volleyball. *Journal of Teaching Physical Education* **11**, 177–194.

Williams, A.M., Davids, K. & Williams, J.G. (1999) *Visual Perception and Action in Sport*. E. & F.N. Spon, London.

Chapter 21
Applications of sports psychology to volleyball

Heiner Langenkamp and Michael Gasse

Introduction

If I look in three stages to coaching, the thing I do first is I know the process of reaching a goal. Second I know the route towards the goal. The third thing is, players whom I select I have to trust! (Joop Alberda, coach of the Dutch Men's National Team, 1996 Olympic Gold Medallists)

I like to . . . make my practice environment and the structure of the drill shape the behaviour. If I want my position 4 attacker to learn how to hit the ball at an angle cross-court, I put her in the situation where I demand for her to hit angle cross-court against the block. I have to put her in that environment in the same situation in a stress orientation, where she must receive a serve, has to dig, then go hit—just like in a game. And then I add to that a goal: "You must do this to get seven out of 10." (Taras Liskevych, coach of the USA Women's National Team, 1992 Olympic Bronze Medallists, 1995 International Coach of the Year)

So the preparation of the match is to reflect, to focus on those things which are most important— but not everything! When we give too much information, it is worse than if we would give no information. We make our players confused, because the player thinks "Oh, I cannot use all this information, so I am not a good player!" (Julio Velasco, coach of the Italian Men's National Team, 1990 and 1994 World Champions)

For the coach you have to know your players really well. The coach needs to give their players a lot of confidence! During the game for me the coach has to be really calm. For instance the player, the one who gets nervous, watches the coach. She will get more and more nervous, if she sees the coach in the same condition. So it is very important to be a role model for your players. (Lang Ping, coach of the Chinese Women's National Team, 1996 Olympic Silver Medallists)

These four quotes from experienced and highly successful volleyball coaches illustrate how knowledge of sports psychology may help to optimize the work of the coach and the team. Sports psychology can influence all aspects of the game, from the role and demeanour of the coach (Alberda, Lang Ping), to the structure of drills and training exercises (Liskevych), to match preparation (Velasco). The discipline of sports psychology provides an essential theoretical basis for understanding both individual and team athletic performance, and it offers practical and effective methods for team building and sharpening individual athlete and team focus. Knowledge of sports psychology will help a coach find solutions to problems encountered by the athlete, the team, and the coaching staff during training and competition.

The principle objective of sports psychology is to optimize a team's effectiveness. To the individual untrained in sports psychology, it may appear that its utility is limited to identifying and correcting individual or collective psychological weaknesses and deficits. On the other hand, we also intuitively understand that sports psychological advice and care aims to support and enhance individual athletic performance so that the team realizes its potential and attains its goal of success. A volleyball match between two competitive, equally talented teams can produce significant mental stress for athletes and coaches alike if both teams compete to their full physical potential. In such situations, successful teams often rely on learned sports psychology concepts and strategies to optimize their collective psychophysical will to succeed.

Psychological activities should be integrated routinely into volleyball-specific training and team drills. Only rarely, or at specified intervals, should "sports psychology" stand alone as a separate component of the team's training program. In the preseason or precompetition phase of training, sports psychology concepts can assist the coach, athletes, and team as a whole define their level of individual and collective commitment and their respective goals for the season. During the season, the training program should—through specific exercises—intermittently focus on psychological parameters such as perception, decision making, mental flexibility and adaptability, and stress management. Furthermore, it is important for both the athlete and coach to gain experience and self-confidence through game simulation. Having prepared for such situations, when confronted with a similar problem in a match the coach and/or athlete will be able to quickly identify an efficient solution because they: (i) know the relevant volleyball-specific techniques and tactics very well; and (ii) were trained how to employ them under match conditions. Note that the athlete and coach alike should be prepared for adverse "match conditions" that may be extremely demanding both psychologically and physiologically (e.g. raucous, noisy competition venues, poor lighting, short rest intervals, created disharmonies or conflict between teams, teammates, player and referee, etc.) (Fig. 21.1).

Sports psychological achievement control: training problem solving

Psychological factors influencing achievement may be considered "soft" control parameters, partic-

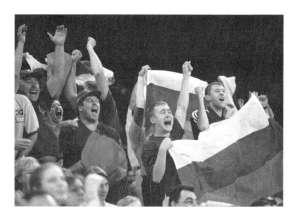

Fig. 21.1 Elite volleyball athletes must be able to focus on the match situation despite raucous, cheering spectators. (Photo courtesy of Olympic Museum, Lausanne.)

ularly when contrasted with "hard" biomechanic, physiological, or medical factors that affect performance. Nevertheless, sports psychology is not without a basic scientific structure and methodological underpinnings. The coach's task (or that of the team sports psychologist, often in collaboration with the coach) is to adapt and apply the fundamental knowledge and methods of the discipline to each player individually through an integrated program of instruction and practice/implementation.

The coach should expect athletes to quickly assimilate and understand the "outer conditions" of a game situation. This skill depends in large part on the athlete's visual perceptual ability (see Chapter 20), and includes an assessment of the competitive environment: the court space, colors of the opponent's uniforms, the movements of the opposing players, the referees and spectators. Furthermore, each player should monitor his or her own immediate "inner" psychological and "outer" physical condition depending on the game situation. Each player must focus on their next action (block the opposing outside attacker, set the middle) within the context of team goals and strategy. Each athlete's action on the court is therefore contingent upon continuous information processing and problem solving.

A problem, in psychological terms, consists of a (mostly unsatisfying) starting point, against which is set an aim or a goal. The plan of action selected by the athlete or coach should seek to overcome, eliminate, or avoid the obstacles to achieving that goal. It is important to convey to the players that encountering a problem in a volleyball match is not psychologically "problematic." Indeed, it should be anticipated since such situations are inherent to sporting competition. The challenge, of course, is to solve the problem(s) effectively and efficiently.

Effective skill execution can become a problem, if a "tactical–technical" difficulty arises as the result of an insufficient assessment of the game situation. For example, one player's performance may suffer as a consequence of a teammate hitting into the block more often than the rest of the team. The player might become distracted by the difficulty his or her teammate is experiencing hitting past the block. This creates an obstacle to that player's own success, negatively affecting his or her performance.

This example of problem solving within a volleyball match emphasizes the need for training situational game competencies. Other situations and questions encountered by coaches for which knowledge of sports psychology is useful include:

1 *Team dynamics*. How is it possible to bring together 12 individuals with different expectations and needs to form a united team?

2 *Motivation*. What is motivation, and how can coaches responsibly manipulate it?

3 *Action control*. How do motivation, will, and personal development influence action control?

4 *Stress management*. What is stress? How does one identify the "keys" to stressful situations?

Team dynamics

In volleyball, as in any team sport, tasks are assigned to specific players at certain times based on the athlete's known abilities and performance history, and by the tactical demands of the match. The coach's decisions in such instances influence team dynamics, which are typically built and actively developed through daily training and shared competitive experience. In general, team dynamics tend to reflect the personality and values of the coach and the players on the team. It is the coach's responsibility to create a dynamic that propels the team forward, enabling it to develop and (ultimately) win. In this regard, a conceptual understanding of leadership behavior frequently used in the business world may

prove useful to coaches as they seek to maximize team success (Blake & Mouton 1990) (Fig. 21.2).

Ideally, a coach should first establish a trusting working relationship with members of the team. Once a solid working relationship is established, the coach and players can together identify both individual and team goals and devise ways to meet those shared goals. It is imperative that all members of the team believe in the goals and the strategy devised to attain those goals. Thus, when critical situations and problems arise, all those involved can return to the solid foundation of the team "rules" that were agreed upon. The more all members of the team internalize the team's goals as their own, and acknowledge the methods of training as a practical means of reaching those goals, the more clearly the coach can emphasize *task orientation* during the season, thereby keeping the team focused on its goals. If all players on the team agree to do what is necessary to reach their goals, then no player should feel offended if the coach pushes them occasionally in order to stoke their competitive fire and maintain their motivation. Although this form of training may seen by some as "authoritarian," the player knows that the coach will do what is necessary to bring the team within reach of its goals, and that the method(s) employed may change depending on the mood and psychological state of the team. Such "rules" improve team cohesion and reduce the experience of stress for each player of the team, since they can rest assured that any disciplinary action or pressure to perform will not be based on an external, imposed standard but rather on the basis of a commonly agreed upon team-coaching "contract" (Fig. 21.3).

One benefit of team coaching can be appreciated in the ongoing assessment of team performance. A team's actual performance varies from what is theoretically achievable according to the following formula developed by Scherm (1998):

Actual game performance (i.e. productivity) = Potential game performance – loss of process

"Actual game performance" represents the on court performance of the team. "Potential game performance" is a product of the team's available physical and cognitive abilities (e.g. level of drive and energy, physical conditioning, tactical knowledge,

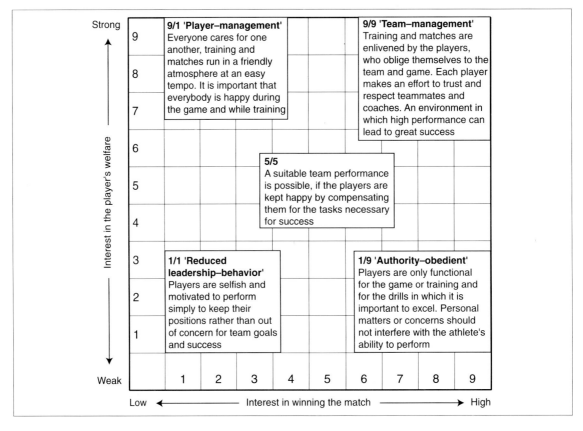

Fig. 21.2 The management grid (modified from Blake & Mouton 1990).

problem-solving abilities, etc.), adjusted for the impact of other resources available to the team (e.g. match preparation, equipment, etc.). "Loss of process" refers to the extent to which performance is limited by various individual and team factors, including lack of motivation, injury, and/or communication breakdowns between teammates or between the coach and players. Although it is virtually impossible to totally eliminate "loss of process," respected team leadership and cohesive team dynamics help to minimize its effect on actual game performance.

As a game of strategy, team success in volleyball demands that each player understand and follow the tactics and action concepts mutually agreed upon by the coach and team. This submission of the individual to the team is especially hard for a "star" athlete who enjoys talent and has skills surpassing

those of his teammates, and who receives special public attention as a result of spectacular individual performances (Fig. 21.4) Team coaching would appear to be a sensible solution to the problem, since it encourages common decision making and an understanding of team goals by all the players. Thus, everyone on the team should appreciate that strategic decisions are made, not based on personal preferences, but rather on *game functional* considerations. Team building is a critical component to the success of team coaching. One method that has proven itself effective is to create a phrase that triggers in each player the vision of the collective goals shared by the team. Excellent examples of such devices are the acronym adopted by the Dutch national team: "TEAM = Together Everyone Achieves More" and the former exhortation of the US Olympic team: "Go for the Gold!"

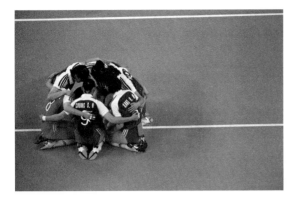

Fig. 21.3 Success often depends on creating a team dynamic of unity and perseverance in the face of adversity. (Photo courtesy of Olympic Museum, Lausanne.)

Motivation: how can it be influenced?

Motivation can be defined simply as the need or desire that causes an individual to act. Motivating others typically involves identifying a goal towards which people feel compelled to work. Ideally, a goal should be of such importance that the desire to reach it is sufficient to stimulate action. Motives are adopted or learned in the course of one's life so that they become embodied in one's character. Motives are also transferable, however. To be able to motivate or stimulate someone to act in pursuit of a specific goal, that individual must have a fitting basic motive for that action, e.g. achievement, power, success, etc. For example, "having fun" is a nearly universal motive among young people today. Table 21.1 lists commonly identified motives for sports participation.

The end result of motive is action, which in turn almost always gives rise to a consequence. In sports, the possible consequences include success (winning) and failure (losing). The individual's hope for success or fear of failure can be defined as the tendency of a particular motive. Although most of the time tendencies do not consciously control the decision to act, people may nevertheless be labeled as either *success optimistic* or *failure scared*. Success-optimistic people tend to have experienced predominantly positive results from their previous

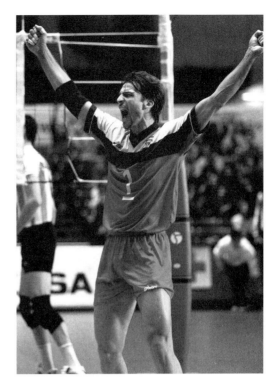

Fig. 21.4 Team coaching encourages goal setting by consensus and thus helps to minimize potential distractions from "star" athletes. (Photo courtesy of Mauro De Sanctis, FIVB.)

Table 21.1 Basic motives for sports (action-stimulating values) (modified from Rieder 1996).

• Enjoyment of movement
• Achievement (technique, comparison, challenge, conquest, self-control)
• Communication ("connection motivation," sociability)
• Stress relief (care-free romping about)
• Regeneration (mental or physical recovery)
• Health maintenance
• Body experience (self-control, body awareness, self-experience)
• Appearance (fitness, shape)
• Self-confidence (consciousness of one's own skills, experiencing a feeling of certainty)
• Social prestige (recognition, image—particularly among youth participants)

actions. This creates task-specific confidence, and typically results in a generalized self-confidence and faith in one's own ability. Because of this self-confidence, success-optimistic individuals tend to undertake difficult tasks. They risk making mistakes or failing because they are looking for a challenge. Sports teams generally profit from the self-confidence of these success-oriented athletes.

For example, if a player thinks he is in a complicated situation during a match, and feels that a hard deep hit down the line will demoralize the opposing team and turn the match in favor of his team, the player's motivation in this situation could be described as success oriented and achievement motivated. If however, the player risks the attack simply to provoke other people's reactions, the action would be primarily "connection motivated."

Conversely, failure-scared people tend to have experienced negative outcomes as the result of prior action or commitment. Failure-scared individuals usually lack self-confidence, doubt themselves, and generally avoid taking risks. Rather, they accept tasks they can confidently handle (i.e. tasks that are much too easy for them), or they may take on tasks from which no one could accurately judge their true skill level since the undertaking was destined for failure anyway. After a while the failure-scared person misjudges their own limitations and repeatedly chooses tasks that are beyond their capability. Unfortunately, neither of these tasks (too easy or too difficult) generates results that raise the individual's low self-confidence.

Motivation and will

Motivation is the actual willingness to act by an individual or a team. The *intent to act* is by itself not sufficient—a concrete plan of action and the will to carry out the plan must be present. This process of motivation is crucial for the action of the game/match and training. Figure 21.5 presents in schematic form the process of motivation. A player can be simultaneously motivated to perform a spike to diffuse anger directed toward a less-involved teammate, to quiet the noisy crowd of spectators, and so on. These goals compete with each other for the athlete's attention, and the athlete will choose an intended course of action based on their relative importance (value) and appeal. The more confidence the athlete has in their ability to reach the goal through their own talents and physical and mental capacity, the higher the priority they will assign to working toward the goal (decision to act), and the higher the probability of success.

The more willingly an athlete puts the plan into action, the more obviously the action becomes separated from other *motivated action possibilities*. Upon completion of the action, the athlete assesses its outcome. If the goal has been accomplished and the intent of the action realized, the entire process of the motivated action is "closed," and the athlete is able to turn their attention to other aims and goals. If on the other hand the intended goal was not achieved, a period of analysis follows during which time the plan of action is re-examined, and the appropriateness of the goal is reassessed. If after each failure an athlete becomes preoccupied with the analysis, and overinterprets the significance of each unmet goal, the athlete may experience a psychological block and further action or subsequent action (performance) could be adversely affected. The individual who reacts to failure in this manner will remain

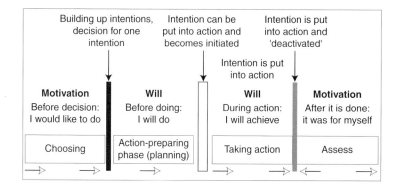

Fig. 21.5 Schematic representation of the process of motivation (modified from Heckhausen 1989).

cognitively stuck on the mistake or failure, and thus become unable to correct the situation through further action (Fig. 21.6). For example, a promising young player makes a series of mistakes while being scouted by the national team coach. The athlete's irritation and preoccupation with their mistakes, coupled with the distraction of knowing that the national team coach is present, might negatively affect their performance and prevent their selection to the squad.

Action control

The extent to and way in which a player is able to control their actions is a function of their personality and the way in which they process information. This ability develops in concert with an individual's personality, and remains malleable and adaptable even into adulthood. Control of one's actions depends to a great extent on the interaction between two basic constructs of information processing that coexist in varying proportions in most people: *action (or goal) orientation* and *state orientation*. The manner in which we look for and work with information to solve problems may be described as predominantly action oriented or state oriented.

This theory, presented in tabular and oversimplified form in Fig. 21.7, has been thoroughly studied and its applicability to sports and problem solving during competition has been validated (Beckmann & Kazén 1994). For competitive sports like volleyball, high-level players and coaches should be proficient at both types of information processing, and should be able to switch easily between both modes. For example, when involved in *goal planning* it is beneficial to be open to receiving information (state orientation), and then based upon that information be willing to take action in pursuit of the desired outcome or goal (action orientation). Upon making the decision to act, the action-oriented athlete approaches the action with a positive attitude, and will remain focused on the action.

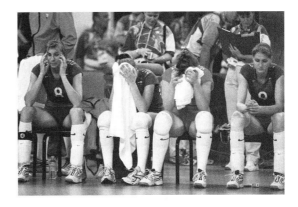

Fig. 21.6 To achieve success, athletes and teams must be able to learn from their mistakes and losses and must then move forward to focus on the next goal.

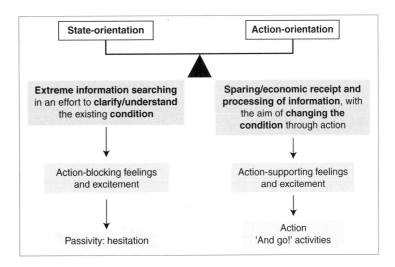

Fig. 21.7 Styles of action control: (extreme) state orientation and (extreme) action orientation.

According to Heckhausen (1989), seven factors influence the athlete's ability to translate intention into action. These factors are discussed below.

1 *Selective attention.* The athlete's attention remains focused exclusively on information that pertains to the immediate situation and relevant action plan. *Action-deviating* thoughts and emotions are ignored or actively suppressed.

Example: An attacker intentionally ignores the temptation to glance at the scoreboard, on which the obvious situation of the match is visible, and instead watches the setter for instruction on the next offensive play.

2 *Deepened insight into the relevance and importance of information.* Information relevant to the immediate goal(s) will be analyzed more carefully and in greater detail, so that it is immediately available for consideration in relation to subsequent information collected.

Example: During warm-up two attackers on the opposing team repeatedly alternate their position next to the principle passer, who plays the ball to the coach at the sideline. The focused athlete attempts to remember the positional relationships and passing tendencies, although the significance of the observation may not be immediately apparent.

3 *Emotional control.* An athlete's emotional state influences their performance and their ability to efficiently execute action plans. The focused athlete knows their optimal emotional state and attempts to recreate it to improve the likelihood of success.

Example: Many athletes participate in individualized rituals prior to competition to put them in an optimal emotional state. Similarly, following a bad play or match, the focused athlete does not withdraw and dwell on the negative but rather concentrates on the next action.

4 *Control of motivation.* An athlete who understands their goals and appreciates what actions are necessary to attain those goals will be better able to manage the occasional conflict between competing goals and incentives, and is capable of prioritizing her actions accordingly.

Example: An athlete whose goal is to make the national team understands that during a special training camp led by the national team coach his energies will be better spent (i.e. bring him closer to his goal) working hard in practice than by carousing at night with his friends.

5 *Control of the environment.* If distractions exist in an athlete's environment that negatively influence their motivation, the environment should be reorganized in a manner consistent with their stated intentions and goals. In so doing, others learn of the athlete's priorities and in turn the athlete becomes rededicated to fulfilling his action plan and meeting his goals.

Example: By encouraging fans to attend their matches, a team not only increases attendance but also improves the atmosphere during the competitions. As a result of the increased fan support and cheering, team performance improves.

6 *Economical information processing.* Information processing can be regarded as economical if data collection is both reliable and reproducible, and results in information that is useful toward attaining a reasonable (reachable) goal. Beyond these criteria, no further details or clarification would improve the likelihood of success.

Example: The blockers have consistently "read" the opponent's attack correctly and implemented the tactically appropriate defence in every instance. Therefore, in the decisive situation there is no reason for the blockers to alter the blocking scheme.

7 *Coping with failure.* If the athlete's goal is not met or if they have failed at an assigned task, then after an appropriate analysis of the relationship between the requested task and their own competencies the athlete should no longer dwell on the failure (particularly if other tasks lie ahead). The same can be said for team goals that are not attained. Instead, the athlete (or team) should focus on the next goal, and the actions needed to meet that goal (accurately passing the next serve, hitting past the block on the next set, etc.).

Example: Players are prone to "second guessing" themselves (or perhaps their coach) after meeting with failure. Rather than succumb to the frustration, anger, and doubt that detract from the ability to concentrate on the play at hand, the focused athlete dismisses the negative thoughts and instead tries to make a positive contribution with their next action.

Beckmann and Strang (1991) have researched the effect of behavior orientation among athletes from

Table 21.2 Action control and characterization of behaviour.

The inner reference of processing orientation towards:	Rough characterization of behavior with more or less strong development of:	
	State orientation	Action orientation
Failure, mistakes	Gets "caught" by mistake	Thinks mistake is "stupid" and is obviously annoyed, but pushes on for repetition or new action plan
Planning and decision making	Includes more and more new information, but does not come to a decision	Briefly plans, then pushes for decision. Realizes the plan could fail, but takes a chance
Follow-through	Is easily attracted to new, "spur of the moment" possibilities; easily changes activities if they are not routine	Pushes activities through ("under any circumstances"); is not easily distracted by alternatives that were already there or that just suddenly appear

different sporting disciplines, and conclude that performance is most influenced by the athlete's ability to control action in three areas (summarized in Table 21.2):
- Dealing with failure and mistakes.
- Coping with conditions requiring *planning and decision making.*
- Carrying out agreed-upon tasks, i.e. *follow-through.*

Stress management

A player who wants to block the ball is confronted with a task that demands technical skill, the ability to process multiple pieces of information concurrently, and a convenient condition of motivation and arousal. In a competitive situation, such a task would be considered by most players to be demanding, and possibly stressful given the proper context. Preparing the athlete for these types of situations, it could be argued, is the principle goal of practice and training. The axiom "athletes play like they practice" implies that there should be a psychological component to training, to ready them for the demands of competition. With trained competencies, the player can experience similar situations during a match without becoming overly excited to the point of "stress." Coaches can prepare the team for the demands of competition through careful analysis of the mental and physical demands of volleyball tasks, and by then developing appropriate drills, exercises, and training plans (Voigt & Richter 1991).

To achieve this, it is essential that the athlete experience a degree of inner psychological tension or anxiety, which could also be termed arousal or excitement. The nature of this state varies from person to person within the same task. This has been graphically depicted by an upside down "U" as shown in Fig. 21.8. The implication of the graph is clear: there exists for every athlete a unique, optimal level of arousal. Above and below this optimum, performance suffers. For example, an athlete would probably have difficulty serving accurately immediately after waking from sleep.

Management of tasks and problem solving becomes easier if one is physically and psychologically prepared for the specific functional demands of the situation or task at hand. The psychological components of performance (such as attention, concentration, knowledge, and perception) are accompanied by correspondingly intense moods, feelings, and thoughts that reflect the athlete's valuation of, and motivation for, the action plan. Certainly, positive as well as negative emotions influence the management of tasks. The more a player permits negative thoughts to influence their emotional state before or during an action, the more complex and difficult—indeed stressful—the task becomes. It is also stressful for an athlete to attend to two or more tasks simultaneously, and if the athlete is expected to excel at both tasks the situation quickly becomes overtaxing.

Everyone experiences stress, but the definition of what constitutes stress is unique to each individual. In general, however, it can be said that stress results when one perceives a disadvantageous relationship

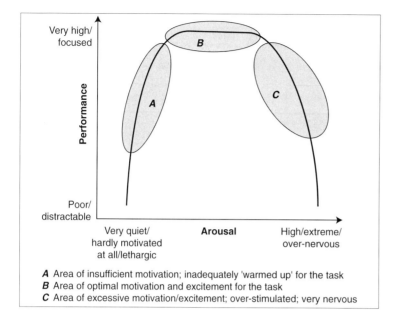

A Area of insufficient motivation; inadequately 'warmed up' for the task
B Area of optimal motivation and excitement for the task
C Area of excessive motivation/excitement; over-stimulated; very nervous

Fig. 21.8. Levels of arousal and performance.

between their own capacities and the demands of a situation (demand (D): capacity (C) relationship). If the demands of a situation exceed the individual's ability to effectively act or respond, the individual may feel their image or reputation threatened by the possibility of an unfavorable outcome. This sense of insecurity creates what has been termed "negative" stress. Alternatively, some individuals may view an unfavorable D:C relationship as a challenge. Achieving the desired goal under such circumstances would undoubtedly cause a certain amount of stress, but for this optimistic and self-confident individual the challenge of the undertaking could be termed "positive" stress. The emotional and physiological consequences of positive and negative stress are quite different.

Stress, then, is based on an assessment of the demands of a situation or task and the individual's ability to fulfil the task. One authoritative, current psychological model describes stress as originating from a three-step process:
• A *primary appraisal* of the D:C relationship of the immediate situation.
• A *secondary appraisal* of the individual's anticipatory reaction to the situation.
• A continuous *reappraisal* of the success of one's efforts and the evolving D:C relationship as the task unfolds (Lazarus & Launier 1978; Lazarus 1991).

How a person initially reacts in a defined situation is dependent on their primary appraisal of the circumstances. This initial assessment requires accurate knowledge about the situation as well as an understanding of their own abilities. This latter perception may be biased based on the individual's degree of self-confidence. In the secondary appraisal the individual analyzes and judges: (i) the possibilities for action and their own competency for coping with the given task; (ii) their expectations of how the demands of the task will change over time; and (iii) the extent and nature of any new responsibilities that may derive from the outcome of the action plan. The interaction of the first two steps leads to a third level of ongoing assessment termed *reappraisal*, which may also be characterized as the "task–person relationship." This relationship determines in what way and to what extent the individual is successful in coping with the stress created by the situation as it unfolds. Depending on the effect of the reappraisal, the level of stress the individual experiences could be very high or quite minimal (Fig. 21.9). In sports, athletes often use a similar process termed "mental imagery" to project and plan or rehearse their response(s) and coping strategies to a set of imagined or possible circumstances.

Physiological and psychological responses to stress include:

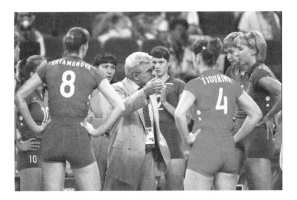

Fig. 21.9 Coaches can help minimize player stress during competition by remaining calm and focusing on problem solving. (Photo courtesy of Olympic Museum, Lausanne.)

• A heightened level of arousal, characterized by a resting tachycardia, pallor, clammy extremities, increased perspiration, tachypnea, and tremor.
• A stressful experience often triggers negative emotions like anger, fear, helplessness, frustration, and depression. The outward behavior of the individual may appear unusual or disjointed, and cognitively the individual may have difficulty concentrating or focusing. Performance tempo often accelerates out of anxiety, or may become excessively deliberate and slow. Changes of orientation towards other persons (or teammates) may become noticeable. A naturally aggressive, confident athlete may suddenly become passive and insecure, looking around for help from the coach or their teammates.
• The athlete may experience a shift away from task-orientated thinking (focusing on the immediate task at hand, visualizing a successful outcome) to task-irrelevant thinking (losing concentration, questioning strategy, thinking too far ahead). Such extraneous thoughts clearly do not help the athlete find a solution to the problem confronting them, and often prove fatal to focused, task-specific thinking. Performance may therefore suffer, and in turn stress may lead to a loss of confidence — further deteriorating the athlete's capabilities and shifting the balance in the existing D : C relationship.

Measures for coping with stress

On a practical basis it is useful to distinguish between strategies that help the athlete cope with

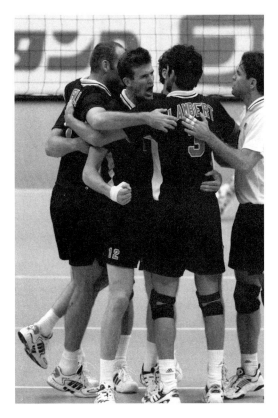

Fig. 21.10 Successful teams also develop strategies to avoid overexcitement, which can impair decision making and problem solving during competition. (Photo courtesy of Mauro De Sanctis, FIVB.)

acute stress and long-term plans for preparing the athlete for the psychological demands of competition-related stressors. The principles, however, are similar. Obviously, stress in sports cannot be entirely prevented, but competition-related stress can be minimized thorough preparation and practice. Training in four areas of action control and planning can assist the athlete in better managing their response to stressful situations:
• Measures for regulating *excitement*. Unbridled excitement and arousal hampers problem solving and decision making during competition, as does apathy (recall the inverted "U") (Fig. 21.10). Positive, task-specific action plans and goal-directed thinking help the athlete stay focused and even tempered. Practice and drills, including mental rehearsal, should prepare the athlete for different situations and provide them with potential solutions to problems which may occur. Athletes should be encouraged to ap-

proach obstacles constructively and with a positive attitude, and negative "automatic" thoughts should be discouraged.

• Measures for influencing a *situation*. Situational planning facilitates making tactical decisions and adjustments that could keep stress to a minimum by permitting both the coach and player to feel confident and flexible in their secondary appraisal.

• Measures for influencing a *person/people*. If a player becomes overconfident to the point of cockiness or carelessness, it is important that the coach and team members have a strategy for bringing the player back to goal-orientated action and minimizing task-irrelevant thinking.

• Measures to regulate *interaction* (compare Laux & Weber 1993). Taunting an opponent and "trash talking" can often detract from the performance of the athlete engaged in such behavior. Team rules should govern athlete conduct, and strategies should be in place to minimize these regrettable incidents.

Stress inoculation training

"Stress inoculation training" was developed by Meichenbaum and has since been adapted for application to sports. After a period of instruction and training, the athlete tries to manage stressful situations in which they immediately feel overtaxed. In this confrontation phase of training, the athlete works to develop the skills identified in the following steps:

Step 1: Identify and consciously acknowledge the stress: *"There 'it' is!"*

Step 2: Ask yourself: *"What was it that I wanted to do now?"*

Step 3: Provide a concrete task directed at the goal identified in step 2: *"I just wanted to do 'this' . . . "*

Step 4: Carry out *"this"* action.

Step 5: Assess the outcome of the action in relation to the action itself but not, for the moment, in relation to the final goal (if indeed they differ).

Step 6: Constructively dialogue with yourself, offering praise whenever possible: *"Well done! That was*

what I wanted to do, and that's what I have accomplished!" If the outcome has fallen short of the intent, repeat step 2.

Thus, the *inner dialogue* becomes a tool in the constructive search for solutions to problems. Through this structured approach, the athlete learns to break down a problem into component parts to which solutions are more easily identified and designed. In time, such stress management training should help the athlete perform better in critical situations, ultimately elevating their own capacity and, as a direct result, that of their team.

References

Beckmann, J. & Kazén, M. (1994) Action and state orientation and the performance of top athletes. In: Kuhl, J. & Beckmann, J. (eds). *Volition and Personality: Action versus State Orientation*, pp. 439–451. Seattle.

Beckmann, J. & Strang. H. (1991) Handlungskontrolle im Sport. *Sportpsychologie* 1, 5–10.

Blake, R.R. & Mouton, J.S. (1990) In: Eunson, B. (ed.). *Betriebspsychologie*, p. 395. McGraw-Hill, Hamburg. (Originally published as *Behaving. Managing Yourself and Others*, 1987. McGraw-Hill, Australia.)

Heckhausen, H. (1989) *Motivation und Handeln*. Springer Verlag, Berlin.

Laux, L. & Weber, H. (1993) *Emotionsbewältigung und Selbstrarstellung*. Kohlharnmer.

Lazarus, R.S. (1991) *Emotions and Adaptation*. Oxford University Press, New York.

Lazarus, R.S. & Launier, R. (1978) Stress-related transactions between person and enviroment. In: Pervin. L.A. & Lewis, M. (eds). *Perspectives in Interactional Psychology*, pp. 287–327. Plenum Press, New York.

Rieder, H. (ed) (1996) *Sport mit Sondergruppen. Ein Handbuch*. Hofmann (Schorndorf).

Scherm, M. (1998) Synergie in Gruppen mehr als eine Metapher? In: Ardelt-Gattinger, E., Lechner, H. & Schlögl, W. (eds). *Gruppendynamik*, pp. 62–70. Göttingen, Seattle.

Voight, H.F. & Richter, E. (1991) *Betreuen, Fördern, Fordern: Volleyballtraining im Kindes und Jugendalter*. Philippka.

Index

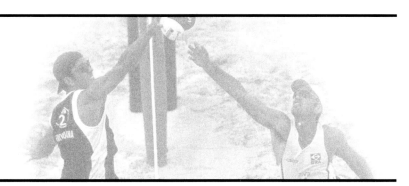